The Ecology of Health

This book is dedicated to my son, Linden, and to the memory of Helen Nearing, who spent her life living simply that others might simply live.

The Ecology of Health

Identifying Issues and Alternatives

Jennifer Chesworth
Editor

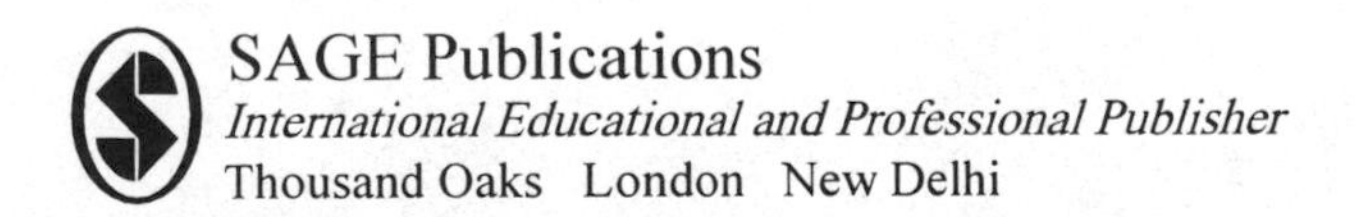

For information address:

SAGE Publications, Inc.
2455 Teller Road
Thousand Oaks, California 91320
E-mail: order@sagepub.com

SAGE Publications Ltd.
6 Bonhill Street
London EC2A 4PU
United Kingdom

SAGE Publications India Pvt. Ltd.
M-32 Market
Greater Kailash I
New Delhi 110 048 India

Printed in the United States of America

Library of Congress Cataloging-in-Publication Data

Main entry under title:

The ecology of health: identifying issues and alternatives / editor, Jennifer Chesworth.
p. cm.
Includes bibliographical references and index.
ISBN 0-8039-7302-0 (cloth: acid-free). — ISBN 0-8039-7303-9 (pbk.: acid-free)
1. Environmental health. 2. Health—Philosophy. 3. Nature, Healing power of. 4. Medical policy. I. Chesworth, Jennifer.
RA566.E26 1996
610—dc20 95-32538

96 97 98 99 10 9 8 7 6 5 4 3 2 1

This book is printed on acid-free paper.

Sage Production Editor: Diana E. Axelsen
Sage Typesetter: Danielle Dillahunt
Sage Cover Designer: Candice Harman

Contents

II: Policy Issues in Health and Health Ecology

III: New Paths: Toward an Ecology of Health

As if our birth had at first sundered things, and we had been thrust up through and into nature like a wedge, and not until the wound heals and the scar disappears, do we begin to discover where we are, and that nature is one and continues everywhere.

—Henry David Thoreau,
A Week on the Concord and Merimack Rivers (1849)

Acknowledgments

The authors who contributed to this volume did so out of simple love of profession and commitment to public education. I extend my sincere gratitude to each. Special thanks are accorded to Carl Mitcham, an excellent and dedicated teacher, whose advice, and editorial skills helped me in innumerable ways throughout the evolution of this book; Janice Morse, for her kind assistance and guidance; Dr. Wayne B. Jonas, for pointing me in new directions; Bruce and Marcia Bonta, for encouraging me to persevere; Christine Smedley for "going to bat" for me; to Mary Paliotta, for creating the index; and to Diana Axelsen, Jacqueline Tasch, and Jennifer Morgan at Sage Publications, for their undying patience and editorial support. I wish also to extend thanks to my parents for a lifetime of loving guidance.

The production of this book was dependent on considerable use of technology—word processors, fax machines, printing services, and so on. In a book that calls for a rethinking of the role of technology in our society, I cannot help but hope that in the future, we will find new methods of production that more closely complement an ecology of health.

Introduction

When Ivan Illich was consulted in the early stages of the development of Clinton's health care reform plan, he refused an invitation to meet at the White House. There is little point in discussing health care reform when, he said, "no matter what would come out, people would be hooked more on the pursuit of health than they already are. The pursuit of health is the most important pathogen in the United States today."[1]

But why would one make such a claim?

As Illich points out in Chapter 2 of this volume, health is a plastic word. It means something different to each and every one of us, and its meaning changes over time within a broader, cultural context. The arena in which "health care" is practiced also changes from person to person, culture to culture, and era to era. However, as more synthetic drugs and more complicated, specialized, technological controls of "health" are developed and used, requiring more and increasingly specialized doctors to orchestrate health care, people lose the wisdom, judgment, and skills they need to achieve good health. If this is the result of our current methods of defining health and practicing health care, the pursuit of such a goal is, indeed, a pathogen.

Meanwhile, the cost of drugs and technological fixes, along with the cost of insurance against every conceivable misfortune or misuse, dominates public debate on health care. Convinced that the bottom line can always be expressed in dollars, we fret over the best way to afford "total access" and "universal coverage." But the real costs of technological fixes are not fully realized even in the gross dollar estimates of the bottom line. For this reason, the topics of dollar values and insurance are only peripherally addressed here. Instead, this volume attempts to add new interdisciplinary perspectives on health and environmental issues, to counterbalance the overwhelming presence and empowerment of brokers, lawyers, and the people who hire them.

Part One, Philosophical Reflections on Health and Ecology, explores health, ecology, and human nature from a variety of perspectives. Beginning with Carl Mitcham's critique of biomedicine and the ethics of rejecting nature, essays in this section address the place of humans in the world with regard to our concepts of self, health, and nature. How we perceive ourselves in relation to our bodies and to our environment, as well as our own beliefs about what is healthy, determine how we act in and on the world and in society. Furthermore, our attitudes toward other species, explored in this section by Strachan Donnelley (Chapter 5) and Michael W. Fox (Chapter 4), help reorient our individual and collective actions. The moral and ethical principles that inform our science, our politics, and our personal beliefs require reexamination and reform in a world troubled by dis-ease and an unfolding ecological crisis. As Frank B. Golley (Chapter 3) suggests, "a much deeper, different, even radical approach seems to be required" (p. 30)

To address this need, both Ivan Illich (Chapter 2) and B. K. S. Iyengar (Chapter 10) call for *renunciation,* although the two men define it in slightly different terms. Illich revives the Greek word *askesis* to describe a "courageous, disciplined, self-critical renunciation accomplished in community" (p. 26). Iyengar's definition, rooted in the yogic sutras of Patanjali (Iyengar, 1993), is simply "knowledge with devotion to God" (p. 121). Renunciation, for both, empowers the individual and provides an alternative to the hopelessness and helplessness prevalent in contemporary technological society.

In addition to exploring concepts of self, health, and nature, chapters in this section address the relationship between the patient and the healer. Medical anthropologists Robbie E. Davis-Floyd (Chapter 7) and Janice Morse (Chapter 8) expose the incongruities of medical practice in the context of the hospital setting, from the points of view of patients and hospital staff. Davis-Floyd, in her analysis of birth in the technocracy, holds the patient particularly accountable for choices made, whereas Morse and her colleagues, Helen Whitaker and Maritza Cerdas Tasón, explore the role of doctors, nurses, family, and society at large. An interesting contrast arises between Morse's assertion that society *silences* suffering and Hunter "Patch" Adams's observation (Chapter 24) that "suffering permeates popular culture" (p. 261). These two viewpoints are not necessarily incompatible. Morse describes the silencing of patients' personal suffering and the shared suffering of the caregiver, whereas Adams alludes to our modern fascination with violence and misfortune, which promotes "negative emotions such as suspicion, envy, and unhappiness" (p. 261).

The cultural context of healing adds new dimensions to health and to the patient/healer relationship. Anthropologist David E. Young (Chapter 9) suggests that "many individuals are turning to traditional cultures for a more holistic set of values" (p. 112), and David Hufford and Mariana Chilton (Chapter 6) conclude, "the environmental and spiritual dimensions of alternative health traditions are genuine insights that serve all aspects of health" (p. 59). Finally, B. K. S. Iyengar (Chapter 10) offers a dynamic view of health and self as seen through practice and mastery of the ancient Eastern art and science of Yoga.

Part Two, Policy Issues in Health and Health Ecology, discusses the public concerns and challenges inherent in linking health and environmental quality. Policy expert William D. Ruckleshaus (Chapter 11), a former director of the U.S. Environmental Protection Agency, opens this section with an overview of the political interplay between science, the public, and the democratic system. Historian Robert N. Proctor (Chapter 12) explores "the social construction of ignorance" in matters of environmental and occupational cancer, followed by a detailed analysis of the problem of ionizing radiation in the biosphere by Judith H. Johnsrud (Chapter 13), a dedicated champion of public and ecosystem health. David Morris's molecular basis for development (Chapter 14) addresses the need for public policy to guide us toward a safer, saner, and more self-reliant society now and into the future.

Public health and environmental issues are illuminated in a new light through the interdisciplinary chapters included in this section. Medical ethicist Janice Raymond (Chapter 15) discusses reproductive technologies and their effects on women's lives and on public health policy. The Primary Health Care goals of the World Health Organization are delineated and critiqued by Marilyn Mardiros (Chapter 16), with an emphasis on social justice, cultural diversity, and community empowerment. Ethnoveterinary scientist Constance M. McCorkle (Chapter 17) and ethnobotanist Michael J. Balick (Chapter 18) describe approaches to public health that integrate concerns for traditional cultures, nonhuman species, environmental conservation, and equitable health care delivery. Economic botanist James Duke (Chapter 19) explores the herbal alternative to drug therapy and public policies that help and hinder freedom of choice. Internationally renowned agricultural economist and rural sociologist, the late Robert Rodale (Chapter 20), describes the relationships between farming, diet, and health, advising us to "get together with people from all over and start to work on new ideas" (p. 219).

The final section, New Paths: Toward an Ecology of Health, presents innovative approaches and refreshing alternatives in health and ecology. Psychologist Phil Nuernberger (Chapter 21) discusses personal empowerment through self-mastery, offering the principles of yoga science as a means for developing the knowledge and skills necessary to live a healthy and disciplined life. The importance of community in this process is stressed. Jim Johnson's discussion of the Twelve-Step recovery fellowships (Chapter 22) asserts that the success of these programs is primarily due to their partial re-creation of the original human social organization, the tribe. Philip Blackford and Stephen Couchman (Chapter 23) emphasize group effort and community environment in their presentation of the Canadian Outward Bound Wilderness School. Hunter "Patch" Adams (Chapter 24) and Edna McHutchion (Chapter 25) describe innovative contexts for healing that integrate community, companionship, and cultivation of the aesthetic qualities of life.

The body's natural healing abilities are also explored in this section. Breakthroughs made in environmental allergy research are presented by William Rea (Chapter 26), using an approach that views the human body as an ecosystem that responds to pollution in much the same way as the earth's systems. Wayne B. Jonas (Chapter 27), director of the Office of Alternative Medicine at the U.S. National Institutes of Health, compares and contrasts the conceptual basis of homeopathic and conventional drug treatment. These approaches to health and healing challenge the tenets of modern biomedicine and suggest new avenues of exploration.

Particular attention is paid in this book to the relationships between health and agriculture. As Wendell Berry (1976) has pointed out elsewhere, the farmer who cares little for human health is as absurd as the doctor who ignores the patient's diet, environment, and lifestyle. In this volume, Dorothy Blair (Chapter 28) discusses the ethical and practical considerations of eating locally produced foods within the context of ecocentric principles. Bill Mollison (Chapter 29) combines traditional wisdom and modern perspectives to describe *Permaculture*, a philosophy and design system for ecologically sound and sustainable "living in-place." Finally, a compilation of excerpts from Helen and Scott Nearing's *Living the Good Life* (1970) tells of their "personal search for a simple, satisfying life on the land" (p. 312).

Globally, the ecological perspective on health is gaining voice and weight. At a time when both health care and the environment are at the forefront of public debate, a comprehensive discussion of the ethics, issues, and choices emerging at the end of this century in health and ecology is desperately required. It is my hope that this volume will bring us closer to reaching informed consensus in our search for an ecology of health. When we achieve this, we will, as Ruckleshaus (Chapter 11) concludes, be preparing ourselves "to cope as citizens of a free, democratic society moving into a future that will be dominated by barely imaginable technologies and fraught with unfamiliar risks" (p. 133).

REFERENCES

Berry, W. (1976). *The unsettling of America: Culture and agriculture.* San Francisco: Sierra Club Books.

Iyengar, B. K. S. (1993). *Light on the yoga sutras of Patanjali.* San Francisco: HarperCollins.

NOTE

1. Personal communication, January 31, 1995.

PART I

Philosophical Reflections on Health and Ecology

1 Biomedical Technologies and the Environment

Rejecting the Ethics of Rejecting Nature

CARL MITCHAM

> Therefore it appears to me that every physician must be skilled in and strive to know nature.
>
> —Hippocrates (1962, p. 20)

> Do you think it possible . . . to understand the nature of the soul apart from the nature of the whole?
>
> —Plato (*Phaedrus*, p. 270)

Despite the initial conception of bioethics as an environmental ethics (Potter, 1971) and progressive attempts by the *Encyclopedia of Bioethics* (Reich, 1978, 1995) to include environmental ethics, the fields of biomedical ethics and environmental ethics have developed along quite different lines. These divergent paths raise questions about the relation between human health and ecology—and challenge what can be termed the ethics of a rejection of nature in contemporary biomedicine.

BIOMEDICAL ETHICS: ITS HISTORY AND PRINCIPLES

The primary concern in biomedical ethics is the physician-patient relationship—and especially the health and rights of the individual patient.

As Edmund Pellegrino (1993) has pointed out, a fundamental metamorphosis of medical ethics into bioethics and biomedical ethics took place during the 1970s. Until this time, medical ethics existed within the 2,500-year-old Hippocratic tradition, more or less independent and isolated from philosophy. On the basis of an oath to help the sick without causing harm, not to cause abortions, to lead a pure life, not to undertake surgery or have sexual relations with patients, and to preserve patient confidences, medical ethics provided guidelines for the maintenance of a relatively autonomous community of practice. Although the Hippocratic tradition of medical ethics focused on physician responsibilities in the physician-patient relationship, it did so in the context of a larger humility before nature and with the aim of cultivating a human-nature relationship. For Hippocrates, the aim of medicine is "preserving nature, not altering it" (*Precepts,* 1962, p. 19), and the physician must "refuse to treat those overwhelmed by disease, since in such cases medicine is powerless" (*On the Art*, p. 3).

This idea of working with nature to preserve and perfect what already exists is articulated in Aristotle's distinction between cultivation and construction. For Aristotle the *technai* of agriculture, education, and medicine help nature to produce more perfectly or abundantly things that are already produced by nature. Such technai are contrasted to those skills, such as carpentry, which impose on nature forms that cannot be found in nature alone.

Beginning in the 1960s, the Hippocratic tradition of medicine as cultivation came under fundamental attack from two quarters: changes in society and changes in science and technology. In the United States, societal changes included a more critically educated public, one more willing to question authority and to assert individual values in the face of a declining sense of community. The autonomy of physician decision making was stigmatized as paternalistic and elitist. At the same time, advances in medical science (now transformed by psychology, molecular biology, and other life sciences) and in medical technology (transformed by bio- and related forms of engineering) overwhelmed the last vestiges of cultivation in the name of a systematic construction and control of nature. At the same time, stimulated in part by their own failures in other areas, academic philosophers undertook the ethical colonization of now renamed *biomedicine* (Toulmin, 1982).

This professional-ethical colonization of biomedicine was itself part of a broad attempt to apply the principles of modern philosophical ethics to assessing the unique challenges of scientific technology—its new capacities and its expanded knowledge. Although scientific technologies had, since the Industrial Revolution, been subjecting society to radical transformation, the first half of the twentieth century witnessed the rapid acceleration of this process across an expanding field of human activities with deepening impact and power. Examples include the invention and industrial exploitation of the airplane, radio, television, antibiotics, the atomic bomb, artificial contraceptives, dialysis machines, computers, organ transplants, prenatal diagnosis, artificial respirators, in vitro fertilization, genetic engineering, and more. Within this context, *applied ethics* undertook to project modern ethical principles into the techno-lifeworld in order to assist the human appropriation of science and technology.

But the typically modern principles of ethics are cut off from any substantive respect for nature. Neither the Kantian categorical imperative (Treat all human beings as ends in themselves) nor the utilitarian calculus (Maximize the good of the greatest number of human beings) contains any reference to the nonhuman world. The effect of their extended application is thus to enhance the artificiality of the world of artifice, to destroy any semblance of art as an imitation of nature. This enhancement of artifice is especially apparent in biomedical practice. Patients are now placed in hospitals no longer designed to promote contact with the curative powers of nature (as was the case, for instance, with traditional sanitoriums). They are diagnosed by means of techniques that increasingly diminish direct physician-patient contact—from the thermometer and stethoscope through X-ray machines to electromagnetic resonance tomography and expert computer diagnostic systems (Reiser, 1978). And then they are treated with injection, drug, radiation, and surgical therapies as abstract and disembodied in their own way as algebra and electricity. In such a context, that conceptual artifice known as principlism appears increasingly acceptable—and as acceptable, required.

The fundamental principles of biomedical ethics (as advanced in the single most influential bioethics textbook, by Tom Beauchamp and James Childress, 1st ed., 1979, to 4th ed., 1994) are those of respect for autonomy, nonmaleficence, beneficence, and justice. This four-principle approach, also known as the Georgetown School of bioethics, has been taught to hundreds of health care professionals over more than twenty years. In that period of time, in a culture dedicated to change and modulated by fashion, there have, of course, been criticisms. But the two primary criticisms have done little to alter its pervasive influence. The first simply argues that the four principles are an eclectic mix calling for unification in some one principle or in a systematically related set of principles; this is simply principlism intensified. A second points out that principles cannot be exercised without certain enabling character traits, that is, virtues. But by and large, the importance of virtue has simply been accommodated to principlism, as pointing up the kind of moral character necessary to exercise principles correctly. Nature is left out in the cold.

ENVIRONMENTAL ETHICS: ITS HISTORY AND PRINCIPLES

The distinguishing concern in environmental ethics is precisely the opposite of that in biomedical ethics. It is the nonhuman world—nature. (And yet the fact that this nature is renamed *environment,* or that which surrounds the human, reveals the continuing dominance of what would otherwise be challenged.)

Prior to the modern period, nature served as a fundamental touchstone for ethics. From Aristotle through Cicero to Thomas Aquinas, natural law ethics—although fractured by the Christian theological enclosure of nature within divine creation—presented the ultimate human good as harmony with the nonhuman whole, of which the human is no more than a part. Similar ideas of a natural or transhuman order as the ultimate ground of all human good can be found in Chinese theories of the Tao and in both Hindu and Buddhist teachings about the Dharma. But nature is conspicuous by its absence in modern ethical theory.

As Roderick Nash (1989) has argued, however, a fundamental movement in moral understanding (if not philosophical ethics), from the Magna Carta of 1215 to the Endangered Species Act of 1973, has been to enlarge the realm of the morally considerable. And although for the first five hundred years of this movement, the expansion remained within the strictly human realm—from kings to nobles to white male property owners to former slaves and to women—the last century has witnessed provisional extensions beyond the anthropological. For instance, although from a philosophical perspective Darwinian evolution leads to the reduction of natural rights to human rights—because there are no rights in nature—a less technically sophisticated ecological awareness reaffirms the interrelationship of humans with the natural world and readily opens the way toward the postulation of rights for animals, plants, life, mountains, ecosystems, and the planet. In his epilogue, Nash makes explicit comparison between the nineteenth-century abolitionists and the contemporary altruistic anarchist ecowarriors of Earth First!, who wage guerilla warfare to liberate the rest of nature.

There are, however, two basic approaches to the theoretical defense of nature: the anthropocentric and the nonanthropocentric. The founding book of the contemporary environmental movement, Rachel Carson's (1962) *Silent Spring,* was profoundly ambiguous in this respect. Although she called attention to the unwitting destruction of the environment by DDT and related petrochemicals, Carson as humanist pointed up the harmful effects these could have on people and, as naturalist, described the harm they impose on nature itself. Even when human beings are freed from disease and prosper unrestrained by the rhythms of the seasons, birds no longer burst into song as the days lengthen after the winter solstice.

The anthropocentric approach argues that moral analysis must be expanded to include nature—because of the value nature has for human beings. Nature must be respected, but only as a means to human ends. This approach is fully compatible with the Kantian imperative and with utilitarian calculations. Indeed, it is usually justified because of them. In the absence of any vision of another way, the only solution to the problems of modern technology is thought to be simply more, and more modern, technology. But whether or not this is really the case ultimately remains a contested issue.

By contrast, the nonanthropocentric approach—which comes in many versions, from animal liberation and ecofeminism to deep ecology, biocentrism, and ecocentrism—in one way or another argues that nature in itself, independent of any human utility function, has value and requires moral consideration. Human beings have a moral obligation to recognize that they are only part of a larger reality and that at least on occasion they must sacrifice their individual interests to those of the whole. Often based on a new perception of nature as ecology, this in effect points toward a reformulation or recovery of premodern natural law theory, which under the influence first of Christianity and then of modernity, had been severely anthropomorphized. To say the same thing in a different way: What is called for is de-anthropomorphization of ethics under the auspices of moral reflections on nature.

FROM BIOMEDICAL VERSIONS OF ENVIRONMENTAL ETHICS TO ENVIRONMENTAL VERSIONS OF BIOMEDICAL ETHICS

One attempt to construct a bridge between biomedical and environmental ethics has been creation of that discipline known as *environmental health.* But despite what environmental health might be thought to imply—that one is concerned not just about human health but the health of that larger whole of which humans are only a part—in fact this discipline is no more than an expanded and updated version of what was once called *public health.*

Public health is again a discipline that can be traced back to Hippocrates—to his treatise "On Airs, Waters, Places," which reflected on the ways in which climate and geography affect human life. For more than two thousand years, until the coming of bacteriology and immunology, public health practices remained essentially unchanged. Build away from swamps. Bring fresh water into and take sewage out of the home. Keep public spaces open. Then in the mid-1800s, Edwin Chadwick in England, as founder of the sanitary reform movement, turned public health into the sanitary engineering of industrial cities. His efforts were followed closely by the work of Louis Pasteur in France and Robert Koch in Germany, who established medical laboratories to research and develop vaccines for mass public inoculation against smallpox, diphtheria, whooping cough, cholera, yellow fever, polio, measles, and so on.

But quantum increases in the human population and in the production and consumption of goods; shifts in the substance out of which these goods are produced, from natural materials to synthetic chemicals, many of which are toxic; and the export of expanded technological capacities from the developed to the developing countries led to the pollution of even the nonindustrialized world, created unprecedented health hazards, and resulted in the need for medical action beyond a local urban or even national level. As standard environmental health textbooks, such as that by Dade Moeller (1992), define it, "environmental health is the subfield of public health concerned with assessing and controlling the impacts of people on their environment . . . and the impacts of the environment on them" (p. 1).

Although one may appeal to the American Medical Association (1989), which calls for "a protective and nurturing philosophy toward the environment at both the personal and societal levels" (p. 2) in a policy statement on *Stewardship of the Environment,* the very idea that humans might nurture the environment as a whole (rather than gardens therein) highlights modern technological attitudes. Moreover, the environment so construed includes the industrial workplace, urban artifice, and technological means of transportation. Environmental health is as concerned to mitigate worker accidents, automobile injuries, and airplane crashes as it is hazardous pollution. And from the first, textbooks in the field have stressed the human survival value of environmental health research and action. As another popular text says, "Controlling man-made, as well as naturally occurring environmental conditions by environmental health practice provides *people's first line of defense against disease*" (Morgan, 1993, p. 24, italics in the original). Clearly, environmental health remains fundamentally anthropological in its central orientations.

As if in contrast to prevailing impulses in environmental health, the first edition of the *Encyclopedia of Bioethics* (Reich, 1978) contained an article on "Environmental Health and Disease," subsumed under the general heading "Environmental Ethics." In the revised edition (Reich, 1995), however, a similar article is given a status independent of the greatly expanded four-part entry on environmental ethics, and it is complemented by a second one on "Hazardous Wastes and Toxic Substances." Both articles express the anthropological and activist agendas implicit in the major textbooks. For instance, the primary ethical problems in both entries concern equity issues. In the first, it is the problem of *environmental racism.* In the second, it is geographical and intergenerational equity. But in neither case is there any discussion of equity with regard to animals, plants, or mountains and rivers. What about the impact of a biomedically enhanced human population on the natural environment? Why is it that no article considers the effect on nature of hazardous wastes and toxic substances from the pharmaceutical industry and mass diagnostic processes and therapies of continuous-flow hospitals?

Biomedical versions of environmental ethics thus fail to integrate the distinctive insights of environmental ethics. A more promising tack grows out of the attempt by Leon Kass (1985) "to search for a yet newer and richer biology that will do justice to matters of human significance" (p. 9). As Kass notes, modern "natural science is, quite deliberately, most *un*natural, not only in what it enables us to do to one another, but even more in what it teaches us to think about who and what we are" (p. xi). This is because "nature, as seen by our physicists, proceeds deterministically, without purpose or direction, utterly silent on matters of better and worse, and without a hint of guidance as to how we are to live." For that biological science modeled on physics, likewise, "nature is indifferent even as between health and disease; since both healthy and diseased processes obey equally and necessarily the same laws of physics and chemistry, biologists conclude that disease is just as natural as health" (pp. 5-6). However,

> despite the tremendous achievements of our nonteleological and mechanistic natural and human sciences, there is ample reason to believe that the fundamental questions about the nature of nature and the being of man are far from closed. For example, should not the remarkable powers of self-healing, present in all living things, make us suspect that dumb nature in fact inclines purposively toward wholeness and is not simply neutral between health and disease? (p. 8)

Yet the approach of Kass remains, like that of Carson, deeply ambiguous in its commitment to the issue of human significance. On the one hand, his reconception of biology draws on environmental, ecological, and evolutionary insights to challenge any narrowly focused or individualist and human-centered ethics. On the other, Kass (1985) builds his case for such a reconceived, ecological biology on the distinctly humanistic and individualist problems of biomedicine. Although he espouses the heretical view that "the natural, rightly understood, might . . . provide some guidance for how we are to live" (p. 346), his moral conclusions remain disappointingly thin. Although he claims his philosophical biology "would show us the folly of seeking to prolong life indefinitely and the wisdom of reaffirming procreation, regeneration, and self-sacrifice against the narcissistic prejudices connected with a strictly survivalist principle of life," the most it seems able to do with regard to such concrete issues as organ transplants is "to oppose the practice of buying and selling of human organs" (p. 348). The practice of transplanting organs remains untouched—as does the buying and selling of animal organs for human use and, indeed, all propaganda for the charitable donation of human organs.

The qualified effectiveness of interactions between biomedical and environmental ethics is further argued by Ruth McNally and Peter Wheale (1994) in an analysis of the late modern contest over the exercise of biomedical powers. Within biomedical ethics a host of arguments "for the protection of workers, consumers, the environment and animal welfare, the safeguarding of civil liberties, freedom from the threat of biological weaponry, equitable distribution of the world's genetic resources, and sustainable development" (p. 221) tend to limit the exercise of biomedical science and technology. But this points to nothing more than the inherent slowing down of a complex techno-scientific social system, not toward any reappreciation of nature as it is in itself.

TOWARD AN ETHICS OF THE RETURN TO NATURE

Biomedical ethics, as it has emerged in the last quarter century, remains essentially an ethics of the rejection of nature in order to promote individual human physical welfare. As such it is fundamentally opposed to almost three millennia of medical tradition. At the same time, its rejection is not simply a contingent feature of twentieth-century medicine, but the progressive construction of more than five hundred years of intellectual and cultural history. In one sense, of course, modern science and technology are based on an acceptance and understanding of nature. But nature as grasped by modern science is so methodologically attenuated and remote, disembedded from the lifeworld and its immediate experience, that it can provide no substantive guidance for human action. This nature is essentially artificial: made up of forces interacting across subatomic particles, the buildup of complex molecular structures, and blindly competing DNA systems. The only thing to do with such a reality is to control and manipulate it on the basis of strictly human interests—while keeping a wary eye on the New Age metaphysicians who find comfort in scientific cosmological speculations. Biomedical ethics is simply the latest and most developed response to such a worldview.

As such, there can be no easy return to that nature which lies behind and beyond the modern worldview. In the first place, nature is no longer the unquestioned presence it was before nuclear weapons, before the ozone hole, before global climate change. The image of Earth photographed from space—which does celebrity guest appearances in environmental propaganda—technologically circumscribes nature just as subtly as once did the Christian theology of creation. As Bill McKibben (1989) and before him, even more profoundly, Hans Jonas (1979) have argued, nature has become thoroughly contaminated with, if not dependent on, the human. The ultimate implication and occasionally explicit claim is that nature itself has become artifact, not just conceptually but physically. The perfection of such an attitude will be its systematic global management—monitored by metatechnical sensors and satellites, attended by cyborgs and robots.

But just as nature cultivated is still nature, so nature as contaminated by the human or as existing in a pure state only with human consent is still not an artifact—that is, an intentionally designed human construct. Indeed, the repeated discovery of the unknown and unknowable even in the midst of the most intensive human construction belies the modern epistemology of conquest, *verum factum*, "to make is to know" (Giambattista Vico). In unanticipated side effects, in technological disasters and catastrophes, nature reasserts herself as fundamentally beyond human grasp. Even more is this the case in those mutations of disease which, both within and without the biomedical realm, continually escape medical control (see, e.g., Preston, 1994).

Onto this stage of medical impotency stride a number of nonscientific medical techniques, from acupuncture, Tai Chi, massage, and homeopathy to macrobiotics, biofeedback, crystal therapy, and ethnopharmacology. The claims for this divergent constellation of medical techniques outside the bounds of accepted Western frameworks are that they are "complementary" or "alternative" medicines. In the first instance, such techniques are presented as subordinate and destined to be subsumed within the dominant biomedical system. In the second, there remains a question. Are alternative medicines simply striving to do more effectively what Western biomedicine does? To help human beings exist against and independently of the natural world? Or is it possible that they are true alternatives, struggling to help people discover and live in some kind of harmony with nature? The first interpretation is a rationalist superstition, the second a perhaps fragile hope.

The fundamental thrust of any hopeful interpretation is an attempt to recover the Hippocratic tradition by folding biomedical ethics back into a medical or environmental ethics—or, more boldly stated, a natural law ethics. At the foundation of a *truly natural* natural law, ethics must be a renewed humility before and respect for nature. To respect nature will entail a recovery of instruments and therapies that fit within, of uses and treatments that adjust to, and of practices that ultimately allow nature to balance herself in association with that part of nature which is the human. This in turn will entail a renewed recognition of the primacy, not of individuals, but of communities if not species and landscapes. In the words of Wendell Berry (1995), "it may be that *community* in the fullest sense—a place and all its creatures—is the smallest unit of health, and that to speak of the health of an isolated individual is a contradiction in terms" (p. 18).

From this perspective, biomedicine is itself the less real part of a larger reality and is simply not adequately evaluated solely on its contributions to individual human welfare. Biomedical technologies, although beneficial to individuals, must be recognized as harmful to the environment in their origins, in their uses, and in their results. In their origins, biomedical technologies are part and parcel of an industrial production system that, even in its environmentally regulated forms, progressively exploits and contaminates the natural world. In their uses, they single out and separate human beings from nature, just as they themselves are singled out and separated from it. And in their results, they preserve human life at the expense of all other forms of life, as well as the natural in its many nonliving forms. To quote Berry (1995) again, although surely "rest and food and ecological health [should be] the basic principles of our art and science of healing . . . industrial medicine is as little interested in ecological health as is industrial agriculture" (p. 23).

The eclipse of nature is a function of technology, so that its recovery will depend on a countereclipse of that uniquely modern artifice—including its manifestations across the spectrum of techno-scientific biomedical practices. What is needed is thus not so much a new ethics as a new ascetics, a self-disciplined austerity in the face of the biotechnical onslaught. Human beings must wean themselves from an excessive dependence on high-science diagnosis and high-tech therapy, to replace demands for techno-medical cures to cancer and AIDS with simple practices such as healthful eating and chaste sexual behavior. And ultimately they must learn once again to suffer pain rather than trying to kill it, to accept death rather than prolonging it. For assistance in the practice of this new ascetics, some may also legitimately turn to alternative medical traditions.

Guidance and encouragement can be found as well in at least two other traditions. One of these is represented by Robinson Jeffers's (1948) struggle for "a certain philosophical attitude, which might be called Inhumanism, a shifting of emphasis and significance from man to not-man: the rejection of human solipsism and recognition of the transhuman magnificence" (1948, p. vi). In "The Eye," a poetic meditation in the midst of World War II, he looks West from the California coast and sees our ships and planes as no more than minor perturbances on the Pacific Ocean,

> this dome, this half-globe, this bulging
> Eyeball of water, arched over to Asia,

> Australia and white Antarctica: those are the eyelids that never close; this is the staring unsleeping
> Eye of the earth; and what it watches is not our wars. (p. 126)

For *wars* one might well substitute *technologies* and *biotechnologies.*

Complementing Jeffers's tradition of the poetic appreciation of trans-human magnificence is a apophantic religious tradition, of which Simone Weil (1957) and her equally if not even more profound critique of personalism can be taken as representative. For Weil, "far from it being his person, what is sacred in a human being is the impersonal in him" (p. 16).

> Science, art, literature, and philosophy, which are only the flowering forms of the person, constitute a domain of glittering and glorious achievements. . . . But above this domain, far above, separated from it by an abyss, is another domain where there are things of the first order. These things are essentially anonymous. (pp. 16-17)

Such "passage into the impersonal does not come about except through an extraordinary kind of attention, which itself is not possible except in solitude" (p. 17)—a solitude that surely excludes biomedical technologies, but is open to the presence of nature. For as Weil also observes, although the Christian tradition often speaks of God as a person, when

> Christ proposes God himself as a model of perfection for human beings . . . , he enjoins not only the image of a person but also that of an impersonal order: "so that you may be sons of your Father who is in heaven; for he makes his sun rise on the evil and on the good, and sends rain on the just and on the unjust" [Matthew 5:45]. (p. 43)

Against the background of such traditions of poetic and religious affirmation of the moral significance of nature, one may not only wonder about but strive for disciplined restrictions on the decision-making analytics and calculating behavior of contemporary biomedical ethics. As two observers of the contemporary scene have proclaimed, "We consider bio-ethics irrelevant to the aliveness with which we intend to face pain and anguish, renunciation and death" (Illich & Mendelsohn, 1992, p. 233).

For one professional philosopher, medicine is thought to have "saved the life" of analytic ethics (Toulmin, 1982). For another, bioethics has enabled an escape from Puritan moralism and the attainment of a higher plane of probabilistic reasoning (Jonsen, 1991). The more comprehensive interpretation, however, is to see contemporary responses to the ethical challenges of biomedicine as undermining the last vestiges of a tradition of moral thought and praxis once embedded in culture and attuned to nature, thereby cutting the techno-lifeworld ever more freely adrift in its own virtual reality. For those who find virtual glamour less sustaining than the substantive splendor of the natural, this final interpretation provides still further warrant for piecemeal ascetic efforts to reject the ethics of rejecting nature.

REFERENCES

American Medical Association, Council of Scientific Affairs. (1989). *Stewardship of the environment*. Chicago: Author.

Beauchamp, T., & Childress, J. (1994). *Principles of biomedical ethics* (4th ed.). New York: Oxford University Press. (1st ed., 1979; 2nd ed., 1983; 3rd ed., 1989, 4th ed., 1994)

Berry, W. (1995). Health is membership. *Plain Magazine*, No. 7, pp. 17-27.

Carson, R. (1962). *Silent spring*. Boston: Houghton Mifflin.

Hippocrates. (1962). *Hippocrates* (Loeb Classical Library, Vols. 1 and 2; W. H. S. Jones, Trans.). Cambridge, MA: Harvard University Press.

Illich, I., & Mendelsohn, R. (1992). Medical ethics: A call to de-bunk bio-ethics. In I. Illich, *In the mirror of the past: Lectures and addresses, 1978-1990*. New York: Marion Boyars.

Jeffers, R. (1948). *The double axe and other poems*. New York: Random House.

Jonas, H. (1979). *Das prinzip verantwortung: Versuch einer ethik für die technologische zivilization* Frankfurt am Main: Shurkamp. English translation: Jonas, H. & Herr, D. (1984). *The imperative of responsibility: In search of an ethics for the technological age*. Chicago: University of Chicago Press.

Jonsen, A. R. (1991). American moralism and the origin of bioethics in the United States. *Journal of Medicine and Philosophy*, *16*(2), 113-130.

Kass, L. (1985). *Toward a more natural science: Biology and human affairs*. New York: Free Press.

McKibben, B. (1989). *The end of nature*. New York: Random House.

McNally, R., & Wheale, P. (1994). Environmental and medical bioethics in late modernity: Anthony Giddens, genetic engineering, and the post-modern state. In R. Attfield & A. Belsey (Eds.), *Philosophy and the natural environment* (pp. 211-225). Cambridge, UK: Cambridge University Press.

Moeller, D. W. (1992). *Environmental health*. Cambridge, MA: Harvard University Press.

Morgan, M. T. (1993). *Environmental health*. Madison, WI: Brown & Benchmark.

Nash, R. (1989). *The rights of nature: A history of environmental ethics*. Madison: University of Wisconsin Press.

Pellegrino, E. D. (1993). The metamorphosis of medical ethics: A 30-year retrospective. *Journal of the American Medical Association*, *269*(9), 1158-1162.

Potter, V. R. (1971). *Bioethics: Bridge to the future*. Englewood Cliffs, NJ: Prentice Hall.

Preston, R. (1994). *The hot zone*. New York: Random House.

Reich, W. (Ed.). (1978). *Encyclopedia of bioethics* (4 vols). New York: Free Press/Macmillan.

Reich, W. (Ed.) (1995). *Encyclopedia of bioethics* (rev. ed., 5 vols.). New York: Simon & Schuster.

Reiser, S. J. (1978). *Medicine and the reign of technology.* Cambridge: Cambridge University Press.

Toulmin, S. (1982). How medicine saved the life of ethics. *Perspectives in Biology and Medicine,* 25(4), 736-750.

Weil, S. (1957). La personne et le sacré: Collectivité, personne, impersonnel, droit, justice [The person and the sacred: Collectivity, person, impersonal, right, justice]. In *Écrits de Londres et dernières lettres* (pp. 11-44). Paris: Gallimard.

2 Brave New Biocracy

A Critique of Health Care From Womb to Tomb

IVAN ILLICH

Physicians in the Hippocratic-Galenic tradition were pledged to restore the balance or "health" of their patients' constitutions but forbidden to use their skills to deal with death. They had to accept nature's power to dissolve the healing contract between patients and physicians. When the Hippocratic signs indicated that the patient had entered into agony, the "atrium between life and death," the physician had to withdraw from what was now a deathbed. Both *quickening*—coming alive in the womb—and *agony*—the personal struggle to die—defined the boundaries between which a subject of medical care could be treated.

In our world, these boundaries have been obliterated. By the early twentieth century, the physician came to be perceived as society's appointed tutor of those who, having been placed in a patient role, lost their own competence. Physicians are taught today to consider themselves responsible for life from the moment the egg is fertilized through the time of organ harvest. They have become the socially responsible professional manager not of a patient, but of a *life* from sperm to worm.

Physicians have become the bureaucrats of the brave new biocracy that rules from womb to tomb.

In societies confused by the technological prowess that enables us to transgress all traditional boundaries of coming to life and dying, the new discipline of *bioethics* has emerged to mediate between pop science and law. It has sought to create the semblance of a moral discourse that roots personhood in the scientific ability of bioethicists to determine who is a person and who is not through qualitative evaluation of the new fetish of "a life."

What I fear is that the abstract, secular notion of a life—his life, her life—will be sacralized, thereby making it possible that this spectral entity will progressively replace the notion of person in which the humanism of Western individualism is anchored. A life is amenable to management, to improvement, and to evaluation in a way that is unthinkable when we speak of a person. The transmogrification of the person into a life is a lethal operation, as dangerous as reaching out for the tree of life in the time of Adam and Eve.

The churches—one of the most important agencies for defining moral issues in public affairs—bear a particular responsibility as a lost civilization turns to them for guidance on such issues as abortion, euthanasia, organ transplant, embryo cloning, and eugenics. Life is the most powerful idol the church has had to face in the course of its history. More than the ideology of empire or feudal order, more than nationalism and progress, more than gnosticism or Enlightenment, the acceptance of life as a God-given reality lends itself to a new corruption of the Christian faith.

The Christian West has given birth to a radically other kind of human condition unlike anything before it. Only within the matrix that Jacques Ellul (1977) calls the *technological system* has this type of human condition come to full fruition. A new role opens for myth making, moralizing, legitimating institutions, a role that cannot quite be understood in terms of old religions, but that some churches rush in to fill. The new technological society is singularly incapable of generating myths to which people can form deep and rich attachments. Yet, for its rudimentary maintenance, it needs agencies that create and legitimate fetishes to which epistemic sentimentality can attach itself. Life has become this fetish; it has come to constitute an essential referent in current ecological, medical, legal, political, and ethical discourse. Consistently, those who use it forget that the notion has a history. It is a Western notion, ultimately the result of a perversion of the Christian message.

When the Lord announced to Martha, "I am Life," he did not say "I am *a* Life." He says, "I am Life" *tout court.* This Life has its historical roots in the revelation that one human person, Jesus, is also God. This one life is the substance of Martha's faith. In the Christian tradition, we hope to receive his Life as a gift; and we hope to share it. We know that this Life was given to us on the Cross, and we cannot seek it except on the *via crucis.* This Life is gratuitous, beyond and above having been born and living. But, as Augustine and Luther constantly stress, it is a gift without which being alive would be dust.

Life in the Christian tradition is personal to the point of *being* one person, both revealed and promised in John 19. It is something profoundly other than the life that appears as substantive in all the headlines about abortion or euthanasia in Western newspapers. At first sight, the two have nothing in common. On the one side, the Bible says: Emmanuel, God-man, Incarnation. On the other, the term is used to impute substance to a process for which the physician assumes responsibility, which technologies prolong and atomic armaments protect; a substance that has standing in court, can be wrongfully given, and about whose destruction without due process or beyond the needs of national defense or industrial growth the so-called pro-life organizations are incensed.

However, at closer inspection, life as a property, as a value, a national resource, a right, is a Western notion that shares its Christian ancestry with other key verities defining secular society. The notion of a human life as a distinct entity that can be professionally and legally protected has been torturously constructed through a legal-medical-religious-scientific discourse whose roots go far back into theology. The emotional and conceptual connotations of life in Hindu, Buddhist, or Islamic traditions are utterly distinct from those evident in the current debate on this subject in Western democracies.

In the United States, the politicized pro-life movements are sponsored mainly by Christian denominations. It is for this reason that it is mainly up to the churches to demystify life. The Christian churches now face an ugly temptation: to cooperate in the social creation of a fetish that, in a theological perspective, is the perversion of revealed Life into an idol.

A HISTORY OF THE IDEA OF LIFE

Biblical scholars are well aware of the limited correspondence between the Hebrew words for blood, *dam,* and for breath, *ruah,* and the

Greek term we would render as soul, namely, *psyche*. Neither comes anywhere near the meaning of the substantive, life. The concept of life does not exist in Greco-Roman antiquity; *bios* means the course of a destiny and *zoe* something close to the brilliance of aliveness. In Hebrew, the concept is utterly theocentric, an implication of God's breath.

Life as a substantive notion appears two thousand years later, along with the science that purports to study it. The term *biology* was coined early in the nineteenth century by Jean-Baptiste Lamarck. He was reacting to the baroque progress in botany and zoology, which tended to reduce these two disciplines to the status of mere classification. By inventing a new term, he also named a new field of study, the science of life.

Lamarck's genius confronted the tradition of distinct vegetable and animal ensoulment, along with the consequent division of nature into three kingdoms: mineral, vegetable, and animal. He postulated the existence of life that distinguishes living beings from inorganic matter not by visible structure but by organization. Since Lamarck, biology searches for what is sometimes called the *stimulating cause of organization* and its localization in tissue cells, protoplasm, the genetic code, or morphogenetic fields.

What is life? is, therefore, not a perennial question, but the pop-science counterfoil to scientific research reports on a mixed bag of phenomena such as reproduction, physiology, heredity, organization, evolution, and, more recently, feedback and morphogenesis.

Life appears during the Napoleonic wars as a postulate that is meant to lead the new biologists beyond the competing descriptive studies of mechanists, vitalists, and materialists. Then, as morphological, physiological, and genetic studies became more precise toward the middle of the nineteenth century, life and its evolution become the hazy and unintended by-products reflecting in ordinary discourse an increasingly abstract and formal kind of scientific terminology.

A thread that runs back to Anaxagoras (500-428 B.C.E.) links a number of otherwise profoundly distinct philosophical systems: the theme of nature's aliveness. This idea of nature's sensitive responsiveness found its constant expression well into the sixteenth century in animistic, idealistic, gnostic, and hylomorphic versions. In these variations, nature is experienced as the matrix from which all things are born. In the long period between Augustine and Scotus, this birthing power of nature was rooted in the world's being *contingent* on the incessant creative will of God.

By the thirteenth century, and especially in the Franciscan school of theology, the world's being comes to be seen as contingent not merely on God's creativity, but also on the graceful sharing of his own being, his life. Whatever is brought from possibility (*de potentia*) into the necessity of its own existence thrives by its miraculous sharing of God's own intimacy—for which there are no better words than His "life."

With the scientific revolution, contingency-rooted thought fades, and a mechanistic model comes to dominate perception. Caroline Merchant (1990) argues that the resulting "death of nature" has been *the* most far-reaching event in changing human vision and perception of the universe. But it also raised the nagging question: How to explain the existence of living forms in a dead cosmos? The notion of substantive life thus appears not as a direct answer to this question but as a kind of mindless shibboleth to fill a void.

The ideology of possessive individualism progressively affected the way life could be talked about as property. Since the nineteenth century, the legal construction of society increasingly reflects a new philosophical radicalism in the perception of the self. The result is a break with the ethics that had informed Western history since Greek antiquity, clearly expressed by the shift of concern from the good to values.

Society is now organized on the utilitarian assumption that humans are born needy and that needed values are by definition scarce. It becomes axiomatic that the possession of life is then interpreted as the supreme value. *Homo economicus* becomes the referent for ethical reflection. Living is equated with a struggle for survival or, more radically, with a competition for life. For more than a century, it has become customary to speak about the "preservation of life" as the ultimate motive for human action and social organization.

During this same period, *homo economicus* was surreptitiously taken as the emblem and analogue for all living beings. A mechanistic anthropomorphism has gained currency. Bacteria are imagined to mimic economic behavior and to engage in internecine competition for the scarce oxygen available in their environment. A cosmic struggle among ever more complex forms of life has become the anthropic foundational myth of the scientific age.

Ecology, the new framework for this struggle, can mean the study of correlations between living forms and their habitat. The term is also and increasingly used for a philosophical way of correlating all knowable phenomena. It then signifies thinking in terms of a cybernetic system that, in real time, is both model and reality: a process that observes and defines, regulates and sustains itself. Within this style of thinking, life comes to be equated with the system; it is the abstract fetish that both overshadows and simultaneously constitutes it.

Epistemic sentimentality has its roots in this conceptual collapse of the borderline between cosmic process and substance and the mythical embodiment of both in the fetish of life. Being conceived as a system, the cosmos is imagined in analogy to an entity that can be rationally analyzed and managed.

Simultaneously, this very same abstract mechanism is romantically identified with life and spoken about in hushed tones as something mysterious, polymorphic, weak, demanding tender protection. In a new kind of reading, Genesis now tells how Adam and Eve were entrusted with life and the further improvement of its quality. This new Adam is potter and nurse of the Golem, his artificial creation.

In the sickening manufactured environment we have made for ourselves, health in the Hippocratic tradition has become an impossibility; balance has become hope-less. The hope once symbolized in the mystery of the unborn has been corrupted; now there is only the legal entity of the fetus monitored on the sonogram. Agony, too, has been corrupted by the medicalization of death. Dignity will not be found in the universal health care or socialized medicine now demanded, but in hygienic autonomy and in a newly recovered art of suffering and dying. In modern sickness, I see the occasion for this discovery.

A HISTORY OF THE IDEA OF HEALTH

The concept of health in European modernity represents a break with the Hippocratic-Galenic tradition familiar to the historian. For Greek philosophers, health was an idea of harmonious mingling, balanced order, a rational interplay of the basic elements. People were healthy when they were integrated into the harmony of the totality of their world according to time and place.

For Plato and Aristotle, health was a somatic virtue. In "healthy human understanding," the German language—despite critiques by Kant, Hamann, Hegel, and Nietzsche—preserved something of this cosmotropic qualification. But since the seventeenth century, the attempt to master nature displaced the ideal of the health of a people.

This inversion gives the a-cosmic health created in this way the appearance of being engineerable. Under this hypothesis of engineerability, "health as possession" has gained acceptance since the last quarter of the eighteenth century. In the course of the nineteenth century, it became commonplace to speak of "my body" and "my health."

In the U.S. Declaration of Independence, the right to happiness is affirmed. The right to health materialized in a parallel way. In the same way as this happiness, modern-day health is the fruit of possessive individualism. There could have been no more brutal and, at the same time, more convincing way to legitimize a society based on self-serving greed.

Adaptation to the misanthropic genetic, climatic, chemical, and cultural consequences of growth is now described as health. Neither the Hippocratic-Galenic representations of balance, nor the Enlightenment utopia of a right to "health and happiness," nor any Vedic or Chinese notions of well-being have anything to do with survival in a technical system.

Health as function, process, mode of communication; health as orienting behavior that requires management—these belong with those postindustrial conjuring formulas that suggestively connote much but denote nothing that can be grasped. As soon as health is addressed, it has already turned into a sense-destroying pathogen, a member of the word family that Uwe Pörksen (1988/1995) calls *plastic words,* word husks that one can wave around, making oneself important, but that can say or do nothing.

The situation is similar with *responsibility,* although to demonstrate this is much more difficult. In a world that worships an ontology of systems, ethical responsibility is reduced to a legitimizing formality. The poisoning of the world is not the result of an irresponsible decision but rather of our individual presence, as when traveling by airplane or commuting on the freeway, in an unjustifiable web of interconnections. It would be politically naive, after health and responsibility have been made technically impossible, to somehow resurrect them through inclusion into a personal project; some kind of resistance is demanded.

Instead of brutal self-enforcement maxims, the new health requires the smooth integration of my immune system into a socioeconomic world system. Being asked for responsibility is, when seen more clearly, a demand for the destruction of sense and self. And this proposed self-assignment to a system stands in stark contrast to suicide. It demands self-extinction in a world hostile to death.

Precisely because I favor those renunciations that an amoral society would label suicide, I must publicly expose the idealization of healthy self-integration. To demand that our children feel well in the world we leave them is an insult to their dignity. Then to impose on them responsibility for their own health is to add baseness to insult.

Ironically, biological, demographic, and medical research of the last decade, focusing on health, has shown that medical achievements only contribute in an insignificant way to the medically defined level of health in a population. Even preventive medicine is of secondary importance in this respect. Furthermore, we now see that a majority of these medical achievements are deceptive misnomers, actually prolonging the suffering of madmen, cripples, old fools, and monsters.

Therefore, I find it reprehensible that the self-appointed health experts now emerge as caring monitors who, with their slogans, put the responsibility of suffering onto the sick themselves. In the last 15 years, propaganda in favor of hypochondria has certainly led to a reduction in smoking and butter consumption among the rich in the West and to an increase in their jogging. But throughout the world, propaganda for medically defined health coincided with an increase in misery for the many. In India, Banerji (1982) has demonstrated how the importation of Western thought undermined the hygienic customs of the majority and solidified advancement of elites.

Fifteen years ago, Hakin Mohamed Said (1981), the leader of the Pakistan Unani, spoke about medical sickening through the importation of a Western concept of health. What concerned him was the corruption of the praxis of traditional Galenic physicians, not by Western pharmacopeia so much as by a Western concept of health that sees death as the enemy. This hostility to death—which is to be internalized along with personal responsibility for health—is why I regard the slogan of "my body, my health" as indecent.

Studying the history of well-being, the history of health, it is obvious that with the arrival of discussions about life and its quality—which was also called health—the thread that linked what is called health today with health in the past was broken. Health has become a scale on which one measures an immune system's fitness for living.

The reduction of a person to an immune system corresponds to the deceptive reduction of creation to a global system, James Lovelock's *Gaia*. And in this perspective, responsibility ends up being understood as the self-steering of an immune system. As much as I would like to rescue for future use the word *responsible* to characterize my actions and omissions, I cannot do it. This is true, not primarily because through this slogan for self-regulation of one's own "quality of life," meaning is extinguished, management transfigured as beneficial, and politics reduced to feedback, but because God is thus blasphemed. And in saying this, I want to be understood as an historian, *not* as a theologian.

I have outlined my thinking. Longing for that which health and responsibility might have been I leave to romantics and dropouts. I consider it a perversion to use the names of high-sounding illusions that cannot fit in the world of computers and media for the internalization and embodiment of systems and information theory.

Only if one understands the history of health and life in their historical interconnection is there a basis for the passion with which I call for the renunciation of "life." With T. S. Eliot (1952), we can ask:

> Where is the Life we have lost in living?
> Where is the wisdom we have lost in knowledge?
> Where is the knowledge we have lost in information?
> The cycles of Heaven in twenty centuries
> Bring us further from God and nearer to the Dust. (p. 96)

The concept of a life that can be reduced to a survival phase of the immune system is not only a caricature, not only an idol, but a blasphemy. And seen in this light, desire for responsibility for the quality of life is not only stupid or impertinent, it is a sin.

THE ILLUSION OF RESPONSIBILITY

I can imagine no complex of controls capable of saving us from the flood of poisons, radiations, goods, and services that sicken humans and animals more than ever before. What sickens us today is something altogether new. What determines the epoch since *Kristallnacht* is the growing matter-of-fact acceptance of a bottomless evil that even Hitler and Stalin did not reach, but that today is the theme for elevated discussions of the atom, the gene, poison, health, and growth.

These are evils and crimes that render us speechless. Unlike death, pestilence, and devils, *these* evils are without meaning. They belong to a nonhuman order. They force us into impotence, helplessness, and powerlessness. We can suffer such evil, we can be broken by it, but we cannot make sense of it, cannot direct it.

There is no way out of this world. I live in a manufactured reality ever further removed from creation. And I know today what that signifies, what horror threatens each of us.

A few decades ago, I did not yet know it. At that time, it seemed possible that I could share responsibility for the remaking of this manufactured world. Today, I finally know what powerlessness is. I know that "responsibility" is an illusion.

In such a world, "being healthy" is reduced to a combination of the enjoyment of techniques, protection of the environment, and adaptation to the consequences of techniques, all three of which are, inevitably, privileges.

In order to live today, I must decisively renounce health and responsibility. *Renounce,* I say, not ignore or become resigned to. I do not use the word to denote indifference. What I mean is that I must accept powerlessness, mourn that which is gone, and renounce the irrecoverable.

Renunciation can free one from the powerlessness that robs me of my awareness, of my sense. But renunciation is not a familiar concept today. We no longer have a word for courageous, disciplined, self-critical renunciation accomplished in community. I will call it *askesis.*

I would have preferred another word, for askesis today brings to mind Flaubert and Saint Antony in the desert—turning away from wine, women, and fragrance. The renunciation of which I speak has very little to do with this.

The epoch in which we live is abstract and disembodied. The certainties on which it rests are largely sense-less. Their worldwide acceptance gives them a semblance of independence from history and culture. What I want to call *epistemological askesis* opens the path toward renouncing those axiomatic certainties on which the contemporary worldview rests. I speak of convivial and critically practiced discipline. The so-called values of health and responsibility belong to these certainties. Examined in depth, one sees them as deeply sickening, disorienting phenomena. That is why I regard a call to responsibility for my health senseless, misleading, indecent, and, in a very particular way, blasphemous.

HYGIENIC AUTONOMY: A MANIFESTO

Many people are confused today about something called health. Experts prate knowingly about "health care systems." Some believe that without access to sophisticated and expensive treatment, people will be sick. Everyone worries about increasing costs. One even hears talk of a "health care crisis." I would like to conclude with something about these matters.

First, I believe it necessary to assert the truth of the human condition: I suffer pain; I am afflicted with certain impairments; I will certainly die. Some undergo greater pain, some, more debilitating disorders, but we all equally face death.

Looking around me, I see that we—just like people in other times and places—have a great capacity to care for one another, especially in the moments of birthing, accidents, and dying. Unless unbalanced by historical novelties, our households, in close cooperation with their surrounding communities, have been wonderfully hospitable, that is, generally adequate to care for the real needs of living, celebrating and dying.

In opposition to this experience, some of us today have come to believe that we desperately need packages, commodities, all under the label of health, all designed and delivered by a system of professionalized services. Some try to convince us that an infant is born, not only helpless—needing the loving care of household—but also sick, requiring specialized treatment by self-certified experts. Others believe that adults routinely require various drugs and interventions in order to become old, while the dying need medical treatment.

Many have forgotten—or are no longer able to enjoy—those commonsense ways of living that contribute to one's well-being and ability to recover from illness. Many have allowed themselves to become dependent on a self-aggrandizing technological myth, against which they nevertheless complain, because of the impersonal ways in which it impoverishes many while enriching a few.

Sadly, I recognize that many of us are infected with a strange illusion: A person has a "right" to something called health care. Thus, one states a claim to receive the latest assortment of technological therapies, based on some professional's diagnosis, to enable one to survive longer in a situation that is often ugly, injurious, depressing, or just boring.

I believe it is time to state clearly that specific situations and circumstances are "sickening," rather than that people themselves are sick. The symptoms modern medicine attempts to treat often have little to do with the condition of our bodies; they are, rather, signals pointing to the disorders and presumptions of modern ways of working, playing, and living. Nevertheless, many of us are mesmerized by the glitter of high-tech "solutions"; we pathetically believe in "fix-it" drugs; we mistakenly think all pain is an evil to be suppressed; we seek to postpone death at almost any cost.

I appeal to the actual experience of people, to the sensibleness of the ordinary person, in direct opposition to professional diagnosis and judgement. I appeal to people's memories, in opposition to the illusion of progress. Let us look at the conditions of our households and communities, not at the quality of health care delivery; health is not a deliverable commodity, and care does not come out of a system.

I demand certain liberties for those who would celebrate living rather than preserve "life":

the liberty to declare myself sick

the liberty to refuse any and all medical treatment at any time

the liberty to take any drug or treatment of my own choosing

the liberty to be treated by the person of my choice, that is, by anyone in the community who feels called to the practice of healing, whether that person be an acupuncturist, a homeopathic physician, a neurosurgeon, an astrologer, a witch doctor, or someone else

the liberty to die without diagnosis

I do not believe that countries need a national health policy, something given to their citizens. Rather, we need the courageous virtue to face certain truths:

We will never eliminate pain.

We will not cure all disorders.

We will certainly die.

Therefore, as sensible creatures, we must face the fact that the pursuit of health may be a sickening disorder. There are no scientific or technological solutions. There is the daily task of accepting the fragility and contingency of the human situation. There are reasonable limits that must be placed on conventional health care. We urgently need to define anew what duties belong to us as persons, what pertains to our communities, what we relinquish to the state.

Yes, we suffer pain, we become ill, we die. But we also hope, laugh, celebrate. We know the joy of caring for one another. Often we are healed, and we recover by many means. We do not have to pursue the path of the flattening out of human experience.

I invite all to shift their gaze, their thoughts, from worrying about health care to cultivating the art of living—and today, with equal importance, to the art of suffering, the art of dying.

REFERENCES

Banerji, D. (1982). *Poverty, class, and health culture in India* (Vol. 1). New Delhi: Prachi Prakashar.

Eliot, T. S. (1952). Choruses from "The Rock." In *Complete Poems and Plays* (p. 96). New York: Harcourt Brace.

Ellul, J. (1977). *Le système technicien (The technological system.* New York: Continuum, 1980). Paris: Calmann-Lévy.

Merchant, C. (1990). *The death of nature: Women, ecology, and the scientific revolution* (2nd ed.). San Francisco: Harper & Row.

Pörksen, U. (1988). *Plastikworter: Die sprache einer internationalen diktatur.* (*Plastic words: The tyranny of a modular language.*) Stuttgart: Klett-Cotta. English translation: Pörksen, U. (1995). University Park, PA: Pennsylvania State University Press.

Said, H. M. (1981). *Main currents in contemporary thought in Pakistan.* Karachi: Hamdard Academy.

3 Deep Ecology From the Perspective of Ecological Science

FRANK B. GOLLEY

There is no need to describe the environmental problems we face at the end of the twentieth century. The literally thousands of environmental books, articles, and films produced in the past thirty years eloquently testify that the biosphere has been drastically disturbed by human activities. Although successes in environmental conservation and management can be observed, the global situation is serious (for an excellent summary, see Brown et al., 1994). Clearly, the conventional methods of managing human uses of the biosphere have not been adequate. A much deeper, different, even radical approach seems to be required. In developing such an approach, humans will have to reconsider their relationship with other living beings and with the nonliving environment. That is, we must examine the philosophical foundations of our relations with nature and reform our value systems (Callicott, 1984).[1] Such a theory must provide for the intrinsic value of both individual organisms and a hierarchy of higher-order organismic entities, such as ecosystems and regional biomes; it must be conceptually concordant with modern evolutionary and ecological biology.

One movement in environmental ethics that has proposed a nonanthropocentric value theory is called *deep ecology*. The phrase was coined by the Norwegian philosopher, mountaineer, and environmental activist Arne Naess in 1973. Naess contrasted his deep approach with a shallow environmental approach that accepts the extant social value system and works within it to solve environmental problems. Since 1973, deep ecology has developed into a substantial movement. For example, books titled *Deep Ecology* have been published, including two in 1985 (Devall & Sessions; Tobias), and deep ecology theory has contributed to such diverse organizations as the Green Party of Germany and Earth First! in the United States.

My intention in this chapter is to examine deep ecology from the perspective of scientific ecology. My justification for this exercise is twofold. First, a philosophy or movement with the name *deep ecology* must naturally attract the attention of an ecologist. What exactly is meant by the word *deep* when applied as an adjective to *ecology*? Second, as Callicott suggested, an environmental ethical system must be concordant with ecological knowledge.

In considering this second justification, it is important to point out that I do not mean that deep ecology should be derived from ecological principles. Indeed, Naess (1973, p. 98) explicitly denies this derivation for deep ecology. He states that whereas deep ecology was suggested, inspired, and fortified by ecological knowledge and the lifestyle of the ecological field-worker, the norms of deep ecology are not derived from ecology by logic or deduction. Rather, my purpose here is to examine the premises of deep ecology in the context of my understanding of ecological principles to determine if a concordance exists or not. I argue that if the premises of deep ecology contradict the principles of ecology, then we have a problem with this value theory.

DEEP ECOLOGY

Deep ecology refers to a rational, total-field image of life and nonlife in which diversity, complexity, autonomy, decentralization, symbiosis, egalitarianism, and classlessness are operative and which is clearly and forcefully normative. It involves both a philosophy, called an *ecosophy* by Naess (1973, p. 99), and a movement or program of action (Devall, 1980). These two activities are mixed in statements about deep ecology. For example, in his original presentation of his ideas, Naess (1973, pp. 95-98) characterized deep ecology as including the following:

1. Rejection of the man-in-environment image in favor of the relational, total field image
2. Biospherical egalitarianism—in principle

3. Incorporation of the principles of diversity and symbiosis
4. An anticlass posture
5. A fight against pollution and resource depletion
6. Complexity, not complication
7. Local autonomy and decentralization

In defense of the program, Naess described the tenets of the movement as follows:

1. The well-being of nonhuman life on Earth has value in itself.
2. Richness and diversity in life forms contribute to this value and have value in themselves.
3. Humans have no right to interfere destructively with nonhuman life except to satisfy vital needs.
4. Present interference is excessive and detrimental.
5. Present policies must therefore change.
6. The necessary policy changes affect basic economic and ideological structures and will be more drastic the longer it takes before significant change begins.
7. The ideological change is mainly that of appreciating life quality rather than enjoying a high standard of living.
8. Those who subscribe to the foregoing points have an obligation directly and indirectly to try to implement the necessary changes. (See also Naess, 1984.)

Clearly, the set of eight tenets differs from the set of seven points. This inconsistency characterizes statements about deep ecology generally. However, my objective in this chapter is not to consider the claims of the deep ecology movement in a formal way but rather to focus on the ecosophy that furnishes the premises that are the foundation of the programs of action. Naess presents two ultimate norms or intuitions that are the basis of ecosophy (Devall & Sessions, 1985, p. 66). These are self-realization and biocentric equality. These two norms are the target of my analysis.

SELF-REALIZATION

Under the theme of self-realization, Naess is discussing a comprehensive, broad concept of self, not the narrow ego self implied in the usual common usage of the word *self.* The comprehensive Self (Naess employs the capital *S* to identify this meaning) involves "me," defined by the boundary of the skin, or "mine," defined by the relations between me and others, *and* a larger set of beings and influences that might be called a *total field* of interaction. Self-realization occurs by a "process of ever-widening identification and ever-narrowing alienation" (Naess, 1985, p. 261). Thus, the Self is as comprehensive as the "totality of our identifications" (Naess, 1985, p. 261). Through identification, higher-level unities are experienced, from identifying with "one's nearest, through circles of friends, local communities, tribes, compatriots, races, humanity, life, and ultimately, as articulated by religious and philosophic leaders, unity with the supreme whole, the 'world' in a broader and deeper sense than usual" (Naess, 1985, p. 263). Thus,

> Self-realization in its absolute maximum is the mature experience of oneness in diversity. . . . The minimum is the self-realization by more or less consistent egotism—by the narrowest experience of what constitutes one's self and a maximum of alienation. As empirical beings we dwell somewhere in between, but increased maturity involves increase of the wideness of self. (Naess, 1985, p. 261)

The concept of widening identification and narrowing alienation is coupled with the idea that "we can make no firm ontological divide in the field of existence" (Fox, 1983). Warwick Fox terms this concept *the central intuition* of deep ecology. He states that "at the level of everyday life, the deep ecologist, as we have seen, intuits the same underlying structure of reality as does the 'new physicist' at the quantum level and the mystic at the transcendental level." In Bill Devall's (1980, p. 309) words, "Deep ecology begins with unity rather than dualism, which has been the dominant theme of Western philosophy." Like the mystic and the new physicist, the deep ecologist is drawn to a cosmology of wholeness, contradicting the classical view that analysis can divide the world into separate, independently existing parts. Thus, Self-realization grows across a network of organisms or a field of process and action involving human, nonhuman, and nonlife until it includes the universe.

As Fox points out, this concept of Self is not unique to deep ecology. Throughout human history, we have identified those who have progressed on the path of Self-realization toward identification with a wider field as mature and as wise. However, the idea that Self-realization unfolds in a total field in which individuals are knots in a biospheric network is different, being derived from ecological research, and will be a focus of our attention below.

BIOCENTRIC EQUALITY

The deep ecologist asserts that every living and nonliving thing has value. Every being has the right to live and flourish. And in some contexts, the right to exist is extended to rivers, mountains, and other landscapes. These rights and values have no connection with instrumental use; they are intrinsic within the biospheric net itself. Humans have rights to satisfy their vital needs but not the right to dominate and exploit other species, and, we must add today, not to cause them to become extinct. Yet conflicts of interest must occur. For example,

> Our vital interests, if we are not plants, imply killing at least some other living beings. A culture of hunters, where identification with hunted animals reaches a remarkably high level, does not prohibit killing for food. But a great variety of ceremonies and rituals have the function to express the gravity of the alienating incident and restore the identification. (Naess, 1973, p. 262)

Two rules seem to operate when we observe a value conflict. The more vital interest has priority over the less vital interest, in the sense of *vital* used above. And the near in time, space, culture, and species has priority over the more remote. The concept of vitality will be discussed more fully below.

THE PERSPECTIVE OF ECOLOGICAL SCIENCE

Do these premises accord with the observations of the natural world by the field ecologist? The concept of Self-realization is readily identified by the ecologist as calling for the self (the ego) to recognize its environment (all that is outside or beyond the self) through identification. Ecology was originally defined in 1869 by Ernst Haeckel, a German biologist, as the total relations of the animal to both its organic and its inorganic environment. One modern definition makes this even more general, by stating that ecology is the study of the structure and function of nature (Odum, 1971, p. 3). In the modern sense, organism and environment are understood to make up a system, called an ecosystem.[2]

There are two ecological concepts that follow from these definitions of ecology that are relevant to the deep ecology norm of Self-realization. First, the environment of an organism can be viewed hierarchically. The organism interacts directly with and acts directly on physical factors (such as the temperature of the air or water), chemical materials (nutrients), and biological organisms (competitors or food) (Patten, 1982). This immediate environment is in constant interaction with the individual. However, environment in this immediate sense is embedded in a hierarchy of larger environments. For example, periodic catastrophic events, such as hurricanes, affect organisms on an infrequent basis. Organisms evolve to cope with these irregular events, but the nature of the interaction is different from that of the immediate environment. Finally, there are even more remote environmental phenomena in time and space that indirectly influence the organism. These environmental events might include phenomena, such as glaciation, that were present in the history of the organism. This hierarchy of environment parallels the idea of widening identification of Self-realization.

Second, ecology has developed a quasi-field theory similar to that of physics (Callicott, 1986).[3] The concept of ecosystem implies flows of energy, matter, and information, with periodic storage (where the rate of flow abruptly changes) in organisms and physical structures. For example, as suggested by Morrowitz (1972, p. 156), individual organisms may be conceived as momentary formations of energy in an energy field. As long as there is a flow of energy, individuals exist as energy structures. However, as the energy flow ceases or the rate of flow changes, the organism is reformed, grows, or dies, and new individuals form that fit the new flow rate. Similarly, individuals experience a dynamic exchange of chemical elements from the cells of one body to the cells of another or to the physical environment. Such exchanges occur minute to minute, day to day, over the lifetime of the organism. The mental, perceptual, conceptual character of the organism is also affected at each moment by its sensory inputs. We are what we experience, and we constantly change our perspective as we experience new environments. Thus, all ecosystems are open to energy, materials, and information, and no individual is an isolated entity in any sense. All individuals are exchanging energy, matter, and information and are inherently linked to the other parts of the world.

The recognition of the temporality and interpenetration of the boundaries of organisms, lakes, and landscapes by the deep ecologist has strong resonance with the experience of the field ecologist and the ecosystem theorist. Self-realization reflects these insights and concepts, but it expresses them in a more personal way. The deep ecologist's premise begins from the self and expands through the environment. The ecologist's environment concept is objective and is applied to organisms and phenomena out there in the natural world. There is a close parallel between the two sets of concepts; one supports the other.

So far so good; the Self-realization intuition seems to fit closely the environment and ecosystem concepts of ecological science. What about biocentric equality? Biocentric equality appears to have two meanings in deep ecology. The statement "all living things have an equal right to live and flourish" may mean equality in a human political sense or equality of opportunity in an ecological sense (Naess, 1984, p. 266). The first meaning makes no sense ecologically, because the central phenomenon of existence is biological difference. Each individual, species, habitat, and ecosystem differs from each other. Nature seems seldom, if ever, exactly the same. Mutation; gene insertions, deletions, and rearrangements; and sexual recombination all create change in genotype. Natural selection acts upon these differences at the individual level, producing adaptation and evolution. The field ecologist observes selection of such differences in subordinance-dominance relations, in competition, predation, feeding, cooperation, and other interaction. Clearly, organisms have no equality in the human political sense.

However, in another sense, biocentric equality does find support from the ecological sciences. Biocentric equality can mean that all species and individuals have the right to play those roles that they have evolved. Ecosystems have a recognizable character because the individuals and species that compose them have, over time, evolved networks of interaction and exchange that are persistent and predictable. Survival of the ecosystem, with its complement of species, depends on these species being allowed free opportunity to organize and operate within the environmental constraints. Species in such systems respond to natural disturbance in recognizable patterns of response. Although one cannot say that species or ecosystems are stable, individuals, species, and ecosystems do exhibit consistent behavior. Biocentric equality asserts that these systems should be permitted to display these behaviors.

This interpretation of the premise of biocentric equality may also be understood as a proscription of human meddling and manipulation in order that a human design may be imposed upon nature. Management of the natural world is best accomplished by working with nature. Ecological knowledge is insufficient to design and manage ecosystems as if they were engines or machines. For example, there may be a thousand species and a million individuals in a single small patch of forest. With this complexity, it is an unending task to understand all the flows and interactions within the ecosystem as we would in a machine.

Biocentric equality admonishes us to keep our hands off and let the individuals and species function according to their evolutionarily selected patterns. Biocentric equality requires that humans be part of the system and not a separated, godlike environmental force that acts upon nature.

THE ETHICAL PERSPECTIVE

In this brief analysis we have discovered that the two ultimate norms or intuitions of deep ecology coincide with ecological understanding. The language in which these premises are presented is misleading. *Self* and *equality* are employed in unconventional ways but, with interpretation, the meanings of these words can be understood in an ecological context. Thus, I conclude that these premises of deep ecology do not conflict with the observations and conclusions of the field ecologist.

However, the analysis raises a series of questions. The first question concerns the form of the biosphere in which we live. Naess recognizes the biosphere as a relational, total field in which there is no ontological divide between object and environment. This insight is supported by ecological science, which finds numerous physical connections between objects and objects and between objects and the physical environment. The objects we recognize in the world, such as individual trees and lakes, are linked to other objects through flows of energy, materials, and information. Trees have connections between their root systems (root grafts) that couple different trees together to allow exchange of nutrients between apparent individuals. Lakes are a part of watersheds that furnish water, sediment, and nutrients to the lake. Thus, although objects are convenient for human purposes, in another sense they are momentary entities in energy, matter, and information fields. Ecological science treats natural phenomena in both ways, as objects and as nodes in interaction fields.

The second question involves the value of ecological objects. Value is an attribute of an object, but it assumes a *valuer,* which may be the object itself or another object. Ordinarily we would expect an object to have value for another object when it is used by that other object. A seed, for instance, has value to the Savannah sparrow, which may eat the seed as food. Rolston (1981) has discussed seven levels of meaning of value for wildlands. These meanings are individual preference value, market price, individual good value, social preference value, social good value, organismic value, and ecosystemic value. In addition, Rolston recognizes twelve types of value: economic, life support, recreational, scientific, genetic diversity, aesthetic, cultural symbolism, historical, character building, therapeutic, religious, and intrinsic. The first eleven types are ultimately anthropocentric; they involve value to humans. The last form, intrinsic, may be interpreted to recognize or reflect the biospheric network, the lack of a division between organisms and environment, and the relational, total-field theory of the ecosystem. In this context, all entities we recognize in the biosphere have some form of value; these values are instrumental when they derive from the specific vital needs or desires of objects, and they are intrinsic when they contribute to the performance and maintenance of the ecosystem through the biospheric field of interaction.

We are left with one final question. What do we mean, in an operational and theoretical sense, by the phrase "to satisfy vital needs" in the context of the sentence "all species and individuals have the right to act out their natural, evolved roles in ecosystems free of human disturbance, except where humans must satisfy their vital needs?" I propose that there are two kinds of criteria for determining vital needs. First, there are criteria concerned with performance of individual organisms. For example, vital needs might involve the capacity to reproduce, grow, maintain one's self, and survive. This is a familiar form and is the basis of adaptation and evolution of the individual. Second, there are those criteria that concern the ecosystem. These criteria include maintenance of the well-being of keystone species, primary producing species, those species whose role in the flows and influences are poorly understood, and those who have an additive or synergistic impact on system function. For example, cutting old-growth forest destroys the trees that dominate the entire forest. Old-growth trees are very rare and unusual; they serve as a comparative basis for human understanding of forests; they support species that cannot live in young forests; they are a source of inspiration. Wood can be obtained so easily elsewhere that there can be no excuse for this type of destruction. The trees and the deadwood of old-growth forest are so vitally important, such a key element in the forest, that it is of highest priority to maintain them (Harmon et al., 1975). It does not matter that trees will regrow; destruction of old trees destroys a fundamental aspect of the forest that cannot be re-created within our lifetime. These definitions are not rigid but rather are comparative, requiring understanding of the context in which value is defined. This is a very important point because it moves from a lawlike, abstract system to a real-life, relative system of value.

Contrary to the assertion of some critics of deep ecology, a capacity to be practical exists in this approach. The deep ecologist requires that action be based on knowledge, especially on knowledge of the context or the indirect effects of the action. As Gandhi showed us, with knowledge we can weigh the impacts of an action and determine if vital needs are in jeopardy (Naess, 1965). When there is inadequate information, the deep ecologist argues for no action. Organisms and the environment have the right to be free of ill-informed meddling by humankind.

More information about the relational, total-field, biospheric network is obviously needed for ethical as well as scientific reasons. There needs to be a free interplay between field investigation and philosophy. As Callicott (1986) has observed, science and ethics seem to be moving in the same direction, and this common focus gives us reason for confidence in a time when the environment and the human race seem to be in serious trouble indeed.

Summarizing, in one sense it appears that Naess presents us with a self-centric, equalizing value theory to replace an anthropocentric, abstract theory. The self in this theory is defined as an entity in a biospheric network of energy, matter, and information relationships. Naess's theory is eminently practical, because it begins with the ego and then extends outward through identification to encompass a larger and larger part of the environment of the self. As the self begins this journey of identification, it encounters what it defines as objects. The norm of biocentric equality, as I've interpreted it, tells us not to order these objects by some abstract system of value, but to order them according to vital needs, considering both the vital needs of the individual and the ecosystem.[4] Thus, Naess presents a theory that recapitulates our field experience of the life processes of birds or mammals. For example, the fox leaves the den and is alert to each event in its environment. No smell, sound, or item seems to be uninteresting. Then an object signifying food is encountered. This object is attacked and eaten. The next food item may be ignored because hunger has been satisfied and the vital need of feeding fulfilled.

This theory is set in a larger context—the total field of biospheric relationships. Objects are recognized as momentary configurations, as artifacts of human perception. What is fundamental is the unity of life and nonlife in a widening circle of relationship, leading ultimately to the planet and the universe. Self-realization leads us to identify with this unity. This fundamental intuition answers the question one must raise about the desire of humans to satisfy vital needs by building dams and nuclear bombs. All life and nonlife is linked into patterns of energy, matter, and information flow. It is a vital need for any organism to fit into this system and to maintain it, to the degree an individual can, in a predictable state so that in the next instant of time, the individual can satisfy its other vital needs. A radically oscillating system or a chaotic system is less predictable, and an individual can easily lose its way and die. Thus, to maintain life, it is essential to maintain the system in which one has evolved, developed, and was born. All individuals have this conservative tendency. Biocentric equality is a theory that strengthens this tendency.

NOTES

1. Richard A. Watson (1983) delivers a criticism of this type of theory. Watson defines *anthropocentric* as the position "that considers man as the central fact, or final aim, of the universe and generally conceives of everything in the universe in terms of human values" (p. 245).
2. The term *ecosystem* was coined by Sir Arthur Tansley (1935). The concept developed from Tansley's interest in the plant ecological community but with the community as an analog of a physical system.
3. Callicott (1986) presents the history of ecological concepts and the linkage of modern ecology with modern theoretical physics.
4. George Sessions, in a March 1986 letter commenting on this point, emphasizes that biocentric equality tells us not to order objects at all.

REFERENCES

Brown, L., Chandler, W. U., Flavin, C., Pollock, C., Postel, S., Stark, L., & Wolf, E. C. (1994). *The state of the world.* New York: Norton.

Callicott, J. B. (1984). Non-anthropocentric value theory and environmental ethics. *American Philosophical Quarterly, 21,* 299-309.

Callicott, J. B. (1986). The metaphysical implications of ecology. *Environmental Ethics, 8,* 301-316.

Devall, B. (1980). The deep ecology movement. *Natural Resources Journal, 20,* 299-322.

Devall, B., & Sessions, G. (1985). *Deep ecology.* Salt Lake City: Peregrine Smith.

Fox, W. (1983, August). *The intuition of deep ecology.* Paper presented at a conference on Environment, Ethics, and Ecology at Australian National University.

Harmon, M. E., Franklyn, J. F., Swanson, F. J., Sollins, P., Gregory, S. V., Lattin, J. D., Anderson, N. H., Cline, S. P., Aumen, N. G., Sedell, J. R., Lienkaemper, G. W., Cromack, K., Jr., & Cummins, K. W. (1975). Ecology of coarse woody debris in temperate ecosystems. In A. MacFadyen & E. D. Ford (Eds.), *Advances in ecological research* (Vol. 15, pp. 133-302). London and New York: Academic Press.

Morrowitz, H. J. (1972). Biology as a cosmological science. *Main Currents in Modern Thought, 28,* 156.
Naess, A. (1965). *Gandhi and the nuclear age.* Totowa, NJ: Bedminster.
Naess, A. (1973). The shallow and the deep, long range ecology movement: A summary. *Inquiry, 16,* 95-100.
Naess, A. (1984). A defense of the deep ecology movement. *Environmental Ethics, 6,* 265-270.
Naess, A. (1985). Identification as a source of deep ecological attitudes. In M. Tobias (Ed.), *Deep ecology* (pp. 256-270). San Diego: Avant Books.
Odum, E. P. (1971). *Fundamentals of ecology* (3rd ed.). Philadelphia: W. B. Saunders.
Patten, B. C. (1982). Environs: Relativistic elementary particles for ecology. *American Naturalist, 119,* 179-219.
Rolston, H., III. (1981). What sorts of value does nature have? In R. C. Schultz & J. D. Hughes (Eds.), *Ecological consciousness* (pp. 351-369). Washington, DC: University Press of America.
Tansley, A. (1935). *Introduction to plant ecology.* London: George Allen & Unwin.
Tobias, M. (Ed.). (1985). *Deep ecology.* San Diego: Avant Books.
Watson, R. A. (1983). A critique of anti-anthropocentric biocentrism. *Environmental Ethics, 5,* 245-256.

4 Beastly Questions

MICHAEL W. FOX

As a former animal researcher myself, I am no stranger to the altruistic rationalizations of the vivisector, one being that the suffering of the few for the benefit of the many is justifiable. Yet, the only animal model for human disease is the human being, and the vivisector is one such. Vivisection is in itself symptomatic of a diseased attitude that no amount of animal research and suffering and killing will ever cure. Metaphysically, our "dis-eased" condition in part reflects the state of mind and the social consensus that accepts terrorism and war (the killing of human beings), on the one hand, and vivisection (the infliction of suffering and killing of animals), on the other.

The similarity between terrorism and vivisection warrants some reflection. Both entail a deliberate, indeed calculated transgression of the doctrine of *ahimsa* (nonviolence) and of the Golden Rule, inflicting suffering and death to achieve some purportedly greater good.

And just as the antiterrorist does violence in the name of peace, so too the vivisector does violence in the name of medical progress. Both are accepted by society, if not as altruistic acts to further some greater good, then as necessary evils. Even though the deliberate infliction of harm is an evil in itself, in both instances the absolute ethic of ahimsa, avoiding harm to all living things and to the natural environment, is overridden by situational ethics, which condone evil means for purportedly just ends. The circle of violence is completed when, like the

---

AUTHOR'S NOTE: Adapted with permission from The Hasting Center Report, March/April, 1989, pp. 40-42, a publication of the Hastings Center, Briarcliff Manor, New York.

antiterrorist, the antivivisectionist engages in threats and acts of terrorism (as distinct from destruction of property and assuming protective custody of animals) against biomedical researchers in the name of animal liberation.

In vivisection there are innocent victims; these are the animals that have been variously bred and captured and that are regarded as inferior, even as our own creations. In the secular if not profane world of medical science, animals are not generally seen as manifestations of divine creation: as belonging to God and therefore "ours" only in sacred trust, to be treated with respect and love. Under the perceived threat of disease, suffering, death, and loss of our loved ones, we devalue the lives of animals, violating the sanctity of life by valuing our own kind over our fellow creatures.

This attitude of mind fears death and suffering and, by objectifying certain other sentient fellow beings, human or nonhuman as the case may be, becomes empathetically disconnected from them and sees them as being inferior, less important than they are.

This anthropocentric disconnectedness becomes generalized in sociopathic, biopathic, and zoopathic behaviors that collectively lead to the desecration of nature and the destruction of Earth. Collective biopathic behavior is exemplified by industrialism's destructiveness of the natural environment and by values that place material gain over ecological sensibility and inevitably lead to economic instability and environmental disease.

Institutionalized zoopathic behavior, as in vivisection, factory farming, and the wholesale harvesting of wildlife species, underlies the cultural and ethical disintegration of industrial society by way of materialism and secular humanism.

Recent developments in genetic engineering biotechnology, which entails considerable animal experimentation and suffering, will only serve to hasten the demise of industrial society, if this technology is not integrated with a more healthful, ecologically sound, and humanely sustainable agriculture; and with a more holistically, environmentally, and ecologically oriented medical paradigm. The modern medical paradigm is inadequate insofar as it barely addresses the environmental health problems associated with industrial pollution and agrichemical poisons (and it will remain so in the absence of appropriate political involvement). Applying new developments in medical science and genetic engineering biotechnology to help us adapt to an increasingly pathogenic, disease-enhancing environment is a massive denial and a waste of public resources and good minds, sowing seeds of false hope.

It is from this perspective that vivisection should be abolished. Although it has contributed to the advancement of medical knowledge, it now stands in the way of any further significant medical progress that will benefit humanity in these times of environmental degradation and cultural and spiritual crisis.

Indeed, vivisection contributes to the failure of medical science to prevent human disease and alleviate human sickness and suffering. So often this is the consequence of harmful treatment side effects, of a false reductionistic and mechanistic orientation; or it may arise out of false hopes and promises of recovery based on animal models that, for many human diseases, are of poor fidelity and scientifically invalid. The aphorism "physician do no harm" has been preempted by the reductionistic and mechanistic approach of drug-dependent allopathic medicine and, with it, dependence upon vivisection and laboratory animal experimentation for the "good" of society.

A reverential attitude of heart and mind automatically precludes vivisection because one's own self is felt to be of equal significance and sanctity as the life of any other being. Animal research would then be limited to the care and study of animals that are already sick and injured, for their benefit and the possible future benefit of their kind. Coincidental but nonetheless significant benefits in the advancement of human health would arise naturally from the knowledge and skill gained in treating such animals.

A reverential attitude toward all life would preclude the use of normal, healthy animals in psychological research: in stress, pain, and trauma studies; in toxicity and cosmetics testing; in military weapon and biological warfare testing. Genetic engineering and selective breeding of sick and mutant creatures would also be unthinkable. But reproductive, nutritional, genetic, and other studies of endangered species to facilitate their viability and reintroduction into restored and protected natural habitats would be accepted because the animals themselves would be the beneficiaries of such research.

Research on farm animals to enhance their productivity, efficiency, and adaptability to factory farming conditions would be something of the past, because the ethic of *ahimsa* mandates vegetarianism, or at least a dramatic decrease in consumption of animal products by all industrialized nations. Concern for wildlife, both terrestrial and aquatic, necessitates such a shift toward vegetarianism and a sustainable agriculture to protect natural habitats and wild species displaced and exterminated by overfishing and by the conversion of natural habitats to provide feed for farm animals.

Few people in the United States realize that some farm animal produce, meat (notably beef), and livestock feed are imported from the Third World. In this way, U.S. consumer habits contribute indirectly to deforestation—especially in Central and South America—and to disenfranchisement, poverty, and malnutrition of native peoples and peasant farmers in many parts of the world.

Masanobu Fukuoka (1978), a Japanese farmer-philosopher and author of *The One Straw Revolution,* said "the ultimate goal of farming is not the growing of crops but the cultivation and perfection of human beings" (p. 68). Unfortunately, there is little compassion and understanding in modern agriculture, which has been appropriately renamed *agribusiness* by the food-production industry itself. We rarely hear the term *animal husbandry,* which implies a kind of marriage, or mutually enhancing symbiosis, based on compassion and understanding, between the farmer and animals. Instead, we have the term *animal production science,* and we are on the threshold of witnessing genetic-engineering biotechnology transform farm animals into even more productive biological machines. The hidden price of this technocratic attitude toward nature and sentient life is surely great, in terms of the ethical and spiritual stature of our Western civilization.

Now, informed consumers, outraged by government's complicity in these matters, are beginning to "eat with conscience," eating lower on the food chain and supporting organic farmers and a more humane, sustainable agriculture that is good for people, good for the animals, and good for the planet. It is ironic that the petrochemical-pharmaceutical and food industry complex should profit from pesticides and from tax-subsidized agriculture that makes people sick from agrichemical residues and a diet too high in animal fat and protein—and then profits further from selling cures (often based on animal experiments) when consumers get sick from cancer, obesity, arteriosclerosis, and other chronic degenerative diseases.

We cannot expect the terrorist to kill the terrorist within or lay down the gun. Nor can we expect the dedicated vivisector to lay down the needle, the scalpel, the electrode, or the laser. Without increasing public awareness, legislative pressure, and consumer boycotts of all companies and industries whose products and services have entailed animal suffering, coupled with educational reforms that foster an empathetic and compassionate respect and a reverence for all life, the unjust and unnecessary suffering of animals in biomedical laboratories around the world will continue.

The abolition of vivisection should be seen as part of the healing process of a humanity that has become so disconnected from reality that it is still at war with itself and condones the killing of human beings in the name of justice, security, and peace while the planet we inhabit is dying. This is not an overstatement, and to contend otherwise, or to believe that more animal research and new technological and legislative correctives will suffice, is a denial of reality.

Denial and fear are two great obstacles to human progress, along with ignorance, arrogance, and greed. The end of vivisection could herald a new beginning, in which all policies and decision making at the personal, corporate, and political levels alike are based on the three principles of a humane, planetary society: namely, obedience to the Golden Rule, *ahimsa,* and reverence for all life. The integrity of creation and the future of humanity itself may then be better ensured. In the final analysis, animal liberation and human liberation are one and the same, because they are consonant and complementary with the ethics and morality of a truly civilized society.

REFERENCE

Fukuoka, M. (1978). *The one-straw revolution: An introduction to natural farming.* Emmaus, PA: Rodale Press.

5 Transgenic Animals and "Wild" Nature

A Landscape of Moral Ecology

STRACHAN DONNELLEY

Animal biotechnology and the fashioning of transgenic animals, along with biotechnology in general, are potent new tools in the arsenal of modern, postindustrial societies. They promise to transform scientific and biomedical research, medical therapies and health care, economic markets and agribusiness, if not the rest of our lives. They augur a new era of human existence and well-being. Yet, animal bioengineering in particular confronts a curious cultural stumbling block. It faces a cacophony of ethically ardent supporters and passionate opponents alike, animated by equal moral zeal (Dresser, 1988; Krimsky, 1991).

We do not live in a morally harmonious world, undergirded by some one or coherently few ethical values that neatly organize our moral life and coordinate our practical activities. Rather, the opposite seems to be true. With respect to humans, animals, and nature, we confront an ineradicable moral plurality: a bewildering variety of values and ethical obligations, each claiming attention and not readily coordinated with the others (Brennan, 1992). How can we make philosophic sense of this

AUTHOR'S NOTE: Adapted with permission of the Hastings Center, Briarcliff Manor, New York from Strachan Donnelley, Charles R. McCarther, and Rivers Singleton, Jr., "The Brave New World of Animal Biotechnology (Section 2, Philosophic Challenges of Animal Biotechnology) Special Supplement, *Hastings Center Report 24,* 1 (1994), pp. 514-524.

moral disjointedness? And how ethically and practically do we deal with this plurality with respect to animal biotechnology?

Historically and logically, there seem to be two basic strategies for dealing with the pull of opposing values or obligations. One is to subsume the moral many under some one grand monistic scheme: to establish a hierarchy of values and obligations under the hegemony of one ultimate value. The other possible strategy is to face the plural values and obligations squarely and somehow attempt to give each its proper due in conjunction with the others.

The monistic strategy may serve the peace of the soul by reducing internal moral conflict. Perhaps it is possible in relatively small and homogenous communities, but it is not an option for us. In any case, it invariably is bought at the price of the variety and richness of human experience and significant cultural activity. In this sense, it impoverishes the soul.

To effectively face plural obligations, we need to recognize that there are several relatively autonomous yet mutually interacting spheres of human activity. This means that there are always specific or "provincial" contexts of human activity. Thus, the coordination of obligations must always be contextual. Moreover, given that the many spheres of human activity can and do influence one another, there must be a coordination of values both *within* and *among* particular spheres of activity (Norton, 1991). Contextually coordinating our plural obligations requires a decision-making art of moral ecology, applying judicious mutual weighting of the several obligations in the various contexts at hand, be they narrower or wider.

PHILOSOPHIC AND ETHICAL CHALLENGES

From the early days of biotechnology and the fashioning of transgenic organisms, a major ethical concern has been the purposeful introduction or unintended escape of bioengineered organisms into natural habitats and ecosystems (Krimsky, 1991). Will the novel organisms wreak ecological havoc, threaten the dynamic stability of habitats, and set off destructive chain reactions throughout resident populations of animals and other organisms? The fear is of negative systemic effects that would undermine the well-being of both humans and the natural world.

The immediately relevant critical questions are: Do we know the effects of such introductions? Can we predict them? Can we control them? Reasonable doubt on any of these questions counsels practical and ethical caution. Only the most weighty obligations to humans would justify countering this caution, if the risks are truly considerable and systemic. The Achilles' heel of ethical decision making is our endemic ignorance of causes and effects when it comes to the flourishing of natural ecosystems. Yet, in this context, the ethical weight decidedly should be with concerns for nature and the multiple significance of nature for humans, rather than more parochial and marginal human interests.

Take the case of experimentally designing transgenic fish—for example, carp, trout, and salmon (Rowan, 1992). The motives for such interventions might be complex: economic, recreational, or preservationist. The practice might serve fish farming (faster growing fish, with a better and more standard quality of meat). Beyond entrepreneurial aspirations, the technology might answer the pressing nutritional requirements of local human communities or the protection of rapidly dwindling, if not endangered wild fish stocks. (This is a worldwide crisis already upon us.) Or, the transgenesis might produce fish better adapted to polluted or regional aquatic habitats than their wild counterparts and with qualities attractive to sport fishermen (gullibility, size, or fighting ability).

Here, long-range, morally ecological thinking is crucial. We may easily dismiss the putative "needs" of sport fishermen and entrepreneurs. It is less easy to counter genuine nutritional requirements of human populations and the protection of wild fish stocks and aquatic food chains. Yet, issues of escape and exotic species introduction haunt the moral ecology. The genetic or behavioral qualities of transgenic fish introduced or escaped into the wild might undermine the very wild stocks and habitats that they were meant to preserve, to the long-term detriment or impoverishment of both humans and nature (Allen & Flecker, 1993). This is not to mention the problems of environmental pollution engendered by fish farming.

But this is not all. There is the more elusive, less urgently practical, but fundamental cultural issue for which we need the ethical reservations of natural preservationists, philosophers, and theologians. By practicing transgenesis in the wild, do we or do we not break into natural processes that are goods in themselves and that hold an ultimate significance (cultural, religious, ethical) for many, if not most of us? This is nature engendering its own, more or less well-adapted biological creations—individuals, species, and ecosystems—the animate and animal issue of evolutionary and ecological processes. How important is it for us humanly, culturally, and ethically to protect, within the overall mandates of plural moral obligations, original nature and its still originating or creative dynamism? (Rolston, 1991). All these pragmatic and moral factors, human and natural, must be relatively weighted in deciding the role that animal biotechnology ought to play in the wild.

TRANSGENIC ANIMALS, BIOMEDICINE, AND SCIENTIFIC RESEARCH

The plural values and obligations relating to humans, animals, and nature that arise in ethically considering animal biotechnology in the wild also surface in scientific and biomedical laboratory settings. But in shifting the scene of scrutiny, the constellation and relative weightings of the values and obligations may change significantly as well. Typically, practical ethical concerns for nature—for wild animal populations, habitats, and ecosystems—fade into the moral background. We may still be seriously concerned with the genetic (genomic), bodily, and behavioral intactness of individual animals, but these concerns are now dominantly conjoined with issues of animals' experiential welfare and the possible benefits of the biotechnological interventions for basic science and fundamental human welfare, particularly the alleviation of suffering.

All things considered, we might allow biotechnological interventions in "controlled" laboratory settings that we would deny in the wild. This shift, beyond pragmatically determined considerations, is due to the dominant values and moral imperatives of scientific and biomedical activity: human (and animal) welfare, the relief of suffering and physiological distress, and the pursuit of basic knowledge about ourselves and the natural world. Thus, we might ethically condone the transgenic production of Oncomouse, Cystic Fibrosis mouse, and Memory mouse (undertaken to facilitate the study of fundamental memory and learning processes). The decision would depend on the importance of the scientific project's purpose, amid all other things that need to be considered.

Further considerations involve the legitimate stakes of the other realms of human activity, with their own ethical mandates, in biomedical and scientific research. From our participation in private life and webs of intimate personal relations involving both humans and animals comes an insistence on attention to the welfare of individual animals, with a minimization of suffering in research protocols and care settings as is appropriate to legitimate scientific goals. From public political ethics comes the ethical demand that there be a just and fair proportion between the overall benefits to be gained and the harms (especially suffering) to be inflicted, with a maximization of the former relative to a minimization of the latter. From the cultural and natural preservationists and others responsible for protecting ultimate values comes a serious questioning of the admissibility of intervention and research: whether it is ethically out of bounds with regard to violating the animal's individual or species integrity or inflicting significant suffering, no matter what the benefits envisioned (Donnelley & Nolan, 1990).

These are the characteristic demands that are placed on animal care and use committees in their review of research and educational protocols. The scrutiny is only exacerbated by animal biotechnological innovations. The chief "novel" issues concern animal welfare and animal integrity. How can researchers, laboratory technicians, and animal caretakers know their animals and promote their well-being or welfare if a new strain or species of animal has been created with altered and perhaps unprecedented behavioral habits? And how is animal integrity—that which might be inadmissibly violated—to be understood? Is it the intactness of the animals' genetic or genomic structure and functionings, or bodily structure and functionings, or behavioral, social, and "worldly" habits? Or are these all dimensions of animal integrity, however difficult to define adequately?

These particular hazards of animal research ethics and protocol review are only highlighted by animal biotechnology and transgenic innovations. They do not change the fundamental nature of an ethical decision making that must be contextual. In particular, no ethical value or obligation can have an absolute or final precedence over the others. Given the plurality of ultimate and fundamental values, there can be no principled "trumping" of one value over the others. Rather, there must be a contextually defined and proportionate coordination of obligations.

For example, religious objections to tampering with natural creation cannot by themselves block the creation of Oncomouse or CF mouse, with the anticipated benefits to human welfare and scientific knowledge. On the other hand, given deeply ingrained cultural or religious habits (which themselves may change over time), what might be ethically tolerable or even mandated in one local human community with respect to science and biomedicine may be inadmissible in another (Balk, 1991). Presumably one would not transgenically manipulate a sacred animal or plant of an indigenous culture, for example, cows in the more traditionally Hindu regions of India. This only underscores the cultural and social embeddedness of all scientific research and medicine, and the fact that human welfare concerns and a thirst for knowledge do not always take precedence over other humanly or naturally important values.

ANIMAL BIOTECHNOLOGY, ECONOMIC MARKETS, AND AGRIBUSINESS

The domains of scientific and biotechnological research, biomedicine, and economic activity increasingly overlap and shade off into one another. The creation of mice, goats, and other animals that produce easily retrievable pharmaceutical products such as human insulin or t-PA at once serve significant human welfare needs and economic entrepreneurial goals. We move away from such immediate health care concerns and attendant ethical obligations when we come to potentially lucrative bovine somatotropin (BST)-boosted cows, growth hormone-primed pigs, and the aquatic factory farming of transgenic fish (Evans & Hollaenher, 1986; Rowan, 1992). As we traverse this spectrum, pressing human welfare obligations often recede, and the morally ecological analyses of animal biotechnological practices significantly change. Animal welfare and human social/cultural factors come more to the fore.

The Beltsville pig, genetically fashioned for cost-efficient growth rates and feed consumption and for the leaner quality of its meat, proved to be severely compromised by arthritis and multiple other diseases. All parties, including the scientific animal production community, consider this an unfortunate ethical misadventure. There remains, however, the biotechnologists' expectant hope that the animal welfare issues can be overcome and that a new generation of engineered "food animals" will be more ethically acceptable (but at what ethical harm?). Similarly there are animal welfare concerns for the BST cows, although immediate animal suffering or harm seems much less acute, and ethical attention is more on the effects of intensifying factory-farming practices.

Beyond heightened concern for animal welfare and unjustifiable suffering, the economic boosters of animal biotechnology, whether from agribusiness or pharmaceutical industries, meet an interesting and complex social and cultural resistance. Small dairy farmers complain that the "big business" of BST-boosted cows will hasten the demise of family farms and local rural traditions. Others object to the pollution of milk with the bovine growth hormone. Still others challenge the patenting and economic commodification of animals: the conceptual reduction of their status as genuine living beings, aboriginally the creation of nature and unowned by humans, to mere configurations of living matter instrumentally at the disposal of humans for their own self-interested purposes, economic or other (Dresser, 1988; Verhoog, 1992).

Obviously, whatever the actual saliency of these ethical charges and critiques, fundamental social, cultural, and religious values are at stake, arising out of broad cultural traditions and interests. Animal biotechnology, coupled with the engines of corporate economics, is felt to threaten fundamental and traditional moral, religious, and cultural orientations.

Again this poses an important challenge to a morally ecological analysis of animal biotechnologies, in the context of economic activity and elsewhere. There may be certain human communities or cultures in which animal biotechnological practices, even for the best human welfare reasons, are considered morally inadmissible. This raises important social or cultural justice issues on an international scale as biotechnology's province becomes increasingly global. Arguably, local cultural communities ought to decide whether they wish to participate in the enterprise and benefits of animal and wider biotechnology, regardless of the insistent pressures of global economic markets and more narrowly defined international issues of economic justice (Balk, 1991; Johnson, 1991). (For example, who should benefit economically from the genetic resources, natural or "artificed," that are swept up into international biotechnological-economic activity?)

On the other hand, what should the moral ecology be when cultural or religious objections come from a minority within a wider and culturally diverse community, such as the United States and many other countries? Granted, social, cultural, and community considerations ought to receive serious attention, especially in relation to optional or peripheral economic practices. But again, with a plurality of moral obligations, no sphere of human activity and no ethical interest group can be allowed to override the legitimate ethical interests of the plural others. What then should be done? How do we reach an ethically adequate accommodation between rival values and ethical obligations and their human advocates? This question remains at the core of moral ecology's unfinished business.

MORAL ECOLOGY'S LANDSCAPE: THE OUTSTANDING ISSUES

We have been arguing that the ethical consideration of animal biotechnologies defies any easy solution or subsuming under a "mono-valued" ethical system. There are too many different interventions in too many different contexts involving too many different motives, values, and ethical obligations (Russow, 1991). Yet the call for a contextual consideration of plural obligations and moral ecology decidedly implies a coordination of disparate and perhaps conflicting values and obligations within and between specific contexts. We require systematic ethical responses that genuinely recognize the plural value and ethical dimensions of our worldly existence. How do we square this circle, which is demanded by our overall responsibilities to humans, animals, and nature? How should such practical decisions be substantively guided? This is an outstanding and unsettled issue.

Yet we may begin to see our way. The first clues come from the sheer plurality of practices, contexts, values, and obligations themselves. This constitutes concrete and experientially incontestable evidence of the plural and complex goodness of human existence. Moreover, the goodness of both humans and nature is vulnerable to change and various harms. We must become ethically committed, as an overarching and fundamental moral duty, to this plurality itself: to upholding and promoting the various abiding and culturally significant spheres of human activity amid the ecosystemic life and animate world in which they are embedded (Jonas, 1984; Norton, 1991).

Herein is the second set of clues: The spheres or domains of human activity interpenetrate one another, and there are contexts within wider contexts within still wider contexts of activity and moral significance. Ethical atomism or provincialism is practically impossible and ethically irresponsible. Rather, we must concurrently pursue the human, animal, and natural good. We must fashion an ethically and publicly responsible life that is broadly cosmopolitan.

Such a cosmopolitan ethics cannot be rationalist or universalist in a traditional sense, that is, they cannot involve principled logical arguments from first moral premises. Rather, its "reasonable connections" must be more ethical-aesthetic. Its modes of thought must be more in keeping with the informal reasoning and moral art of the private realm of intimate relations, which must take in whole webs of life and multiple moral considerations at once. In short, moral ecology deals with complex wholes.

Even if we could adequately see our way through the methodological and epistemological problems of establishing priorities of ethical concern and obligation, we face another problem. Is this commitment to the coordination of plural activities, values, and obligations practically realistic or an impossible dream, given the aggressive disharmony inherently spawned by ethical and political pluralism itself and the dynamic nature of humans' worldly life? History, recent or not, is sobering. Yet the world's dynamic becoming, which will not be rationally, technologically, politically, or ethically subdued, presents a way out of such impasses. Different cultures and different domains of human activity can over time grow together, at least in understanding if not also in practice. This requires both mutual appreciation and mutual criticism as a way of moving toward a more adequate and ethical flourishing within and between particular spheres of activity and human cultures.

THE GOODNESS AND SIGNIFICANCE OF NATURE AND ANIMAL LIFE

Given our newly emerging and insistent responsibilities for biological life, ecosystems, and the environment, nowhere is mutual appreciation and criticism more globally and regionally needed than in trying to ferret out the meaning, significance, and goodness of animate life and evolutionary and ecological processes (Norton, 1991; Rolston, 1989). (As we have seen, this is crucial to the various contextual ethical analyses of animal biotechnologies.) For such an understanding, we need to bring together thinkers from various spheres of scientific and cultural activity: evolutionary biologists, animal researchers, anthropologists, philosophers, theologians, and others with a central stake in the multileveled significance of nature. A serious mutual confrontation of these plural areas of disciplined thought and activity promises philosophical and ethical advances.

For example, more traditional philosophers or theologians, committed to long-dominant modes of essentialist thinking, might see the significance of nature and animal species as arising from (or grounded in) atemporal and unchanging Platonic *ideas* (for example, the archetypal form "horse"). Or they might appeal to Aristotlean *substantial forms* (the "formal plan" of development into an adult horse, perhaps an unintended adumbration of genomic information) or a once-and-for-all creation ex nihilo by a transcendent deity. This is how traditional modes of thinking typically account for the definite character, integrity, and goodness of nature's animate beings. Such traditional Western perspectives might (or might not) ethically counsel against modern forms of genetic tinkering, transgenesis, and the confounding of the eternal order of creation.

But contemporary molecular and evolutionary biologists would unite in contending that an essentialist explanation and interpretation of the animal and animate world is fundamentally flawed (Mayr, 1982). Biological species arise and pass in dynamic evolutionary and ecological processes. Thanks to random genetic variation (via genetic mutation and sexual reproduction) and natural selection, species diversify and evolve out of their biological predecessors, sharing and reconfiguring genetic information. Moreover, nature is no realm of essentialist perfection. Rather, our biosphere is an extraordinary, historically particular, and "chaotically orderly" realm of dynamic and systematically related "imperfections": individual organisms more or less well adapted to worldly life; populational species of such individuals more or less well adapted to ever-changing ecological niches; and ecosystems themselves more or less internally robust and dynamically viable, while changing in evolutionary/ecological time.

This by now well-founded and incontestible general evolutionary and ecological perspective does not annihilate the questions of natural goodness and integrity posed by philosophers and theologians. It only defeats and renders obsolete essentialist modes of naturalistic thinking and philosophic interpretation. The natural goodness and integrity of biological individuals and species, as well as ecosystems, only need a new and more philosophically nuanced interpretation. Individual organisms still present themselves as having a lively integrity, intactness, or "oneness" that encompasses bodily, subjective, behavioral, and outwardly social functionings that are more or less flexibly adapted to an active, if vulnerable, life in the world. Species as populations of biological individuals exhibit a spatio-temporally bounded and flexible integrity relative to some ecological niche, also changing. Moreover, species evolve in a creative, though orderly fashion, according to relatively few generic organic or bodily *Bauplane* (Mayr, 1988). Finally, the habitats and ecosystems themselves evidence a flexible and dynamic intactness with respect to internal stability and species diversification, more or less vulnerable to outside, wider ecosystemic processes or forces (Rolston, 1991).

No doubt these several senses of integrity—individual, species, and ecosystemic—require further and careful conceptual and philosophic articulation and systematic coordination. Moreover, we will need further collaborative efforts in appreciating the full significance and goodness of the individuals, species, and ecosystems of the animate realm. But such an enterprise should only ethically and practically serve us well. It would further and more clearly reveal the complex meanings of "nature natural" for us humans. It would help us discern what the limits of our biotechnological and other human interventions in the wild ought to be and what needs to be ethically protected in scientific and biomedical research and economic activity.

Moreover, we would better understand ourselves and our embedded existence in an animate nature that is ultimately significant, yet imperfectly good: that we and animate nature are not to be perfected, but that the world's evolving complex and finite goodness—the various dimensions of activity and value realized by humans and other organisms—is to be unequivocally affirmed and ethically protected.

In conclusion, a speculative, disciplined advance in our understanding and assessment of the multileveled worth of nature would help us in the ethical coordinations required by our contextual plural obligations. Although, in themselves, such an understanding and assessment do not uniquely determine the outcome (positive or negative) of moral deliberations in different contexts, they would better inform us when it is ethically appropriate to move forward biotechnologically and when it is appropriate to take ethically protective stands. We would better know how to integrate our cultural, technological, and natural selves and how practically to fit our human communities within the wider natural and animate world.

REFERENCES

Allen, J. D., & Flecker, A. S. (1993). Biodiversity conservation in running waters. *BioScience, 43*(1), 32-43.

Balk, R. (1991, Spring). Moral issues in animal biotechnology. Paper presented at the Animal Biotechnology Project Meeting, The Hastings Center, Briarcliff Manor, NY.

Brennan, A. (1992). Moral pluralism and the environment. *Environmental Values, 1*(1), 15-33.

Donnelley, S., & Nolan, K. (Eds.). (1990). Animals, science, and ethics [Special supplement]. *The Hastings Report, 20*(3), 1-32.

Dresser, R. (1988). Ethical and legal issues in patenting new animal life. *Jurimetrics Journal, 28*(4), 399-435.

Evans, J. W., & Hollaenher, A. (Eds.). (1986). *Genetic engineering of animals: An agricultural perspective.* New York: Plenum.

Johnson, N. (1991, Spring). Biotechnology: Justice and biodiversity. Paper presented at the Animal Biotechnology Project Meeting, The Hastings Center, Briarcliff Manor, NY.

Jonas, H. (1984). *The imperative of responsibility.* Chicago: University of Chicago Press.

Krimsky, S. (1991). *Bioethics and society: The rise of industrial genetics.* New York: Prentice Hall.

Mayr, E. (1982). *The growth of biological thought.* Cambridge, MA: Harvard University Press.

Mayr, E. (1988). *Toward a new philosophy of biology.* Cambridge, MA: Harvard University Press.

Norton, B. (1991). *Toward unity among environmentalists.* New York: Oxford University Press.

Rolston, H., III. (1989). *Philosophy gone wild.* Buffalo, NY: Prometheus.

Rolston, H., III. (1991). Environmental ethics: Values and duties to the natural environment. In F. H. Bormann & S. R. Kellert (Eds.), *Ecology, economics, and ethics* (pp. 73-96). New Haven, CT: Yale University Press.

Rowan, A. N. (1992, Spring). Biotechnology case studies: A discussion of issues in animal biotechnology. Paper presented at the Animal Biotechnology Project Meeting, The Hastings Center, Briarcliff Manor, NY.

Russow, L. (1991, Fall). Biotechnology: A perversion of Mother Nature's design. Paper presented at the Animal Biotechnology Project Meeting, The Hastings Center, Briarcliff Manor, NY.

Verhoog, H. (1992). The concept of intrinsic value and transgenic animals. *Journal of Agricultural and Environmental Ethics, 5,* 47-60.

6 Politics, Spirituality, and Environmental Healing

DAVID J. HUFFORD
MARIANA CHILTON

Many alternative health systems[1] define health and healing in ways that dramatically reduce distinctions between the health of individuals and the health of their environment. As a result, many such systems value environmental conservation and connect the healing of humans with the healing of the world in which they live. This is in sharp contrast to biomedicine,[2] where the differences among clinical medicine, social policy, public health, and environmental protection are clearly demarcated. In many alternative health systems, the linkage among personal, social, and environmental health is strongly associated with a spiritual understanding of the world. These spiritual views powerfully integrate humans with the rest of the natural world as "relatives" rather than adversaries and provide motivations that transcend material self-interest. This presents an even sharper contrast to biomedicine, which seems to owe its greatest accomplishments to a materialistic ideology that governs medical science, even for those physicians and scientists who hold strong spiritual beliefs. In this chapter, we describe some of these ecological orientations in alternative healing and suggest some of the reasons for them. Our purpose here is not neutrally descriptive; we believe strongly that the environmental and spiritual dimensions of alternative health traditions are genuine insights that serve all aspects of health, and that biomedicine's environmental and spiritual shortcomings constitute a grave weakness that can undercut healing.

DEFINING ALTERNATIVE MEDICINE

In April 1995, the Office of Alternative Medicine of the National Institutes of Health held its second conference on research methodology. At this meeting, a working group, chaired by Bonnie O'Connor, Ph.D., developed the following definition of the field:

> The broad domain of complementary and alternative medicine (CAM) encompasses all health systems, modalities, and practices other than those intrinsic to the politically dominant health system of a particular society or culture. CAM includes all practices and ideas self-defined by their users as preventing or treating illness or promoting health and well-being.

This definition is intentionally political in scope, referring to the power to allocate resources but open with regard to conceptual content. Even those scholars and activists most critical of medicine have generally taken medical knowledge for granted in their political analysis. But biomedicine wields its cultural authority most powerfully in the establishment of widely accepted knowledge claims. A narrow focus on questions of access to standard biomedical care or of government's adequate use of biomedical knowledge in formulating environmental health policies, avoids serious questions about the completeness and validity of that knowledge. For doctors, the politics of medicine follows inevitably from the truth of medical knowledge, whereas some critics see medical knowledge claims as mere shams that support the profession's privileged position in society. Highlighting the relationship of political and epistemological processes regarding health prevents this common reduction of politics and epistemology to one another by opposing sides. If biomedical science and practice were all politics, then proper goals would be entirely social, such as the right to be free from the intrusion of biomedicine either individually or as a society. But such take-it-or-leave-it choices obscure the fact that even many of those who feel most oppressed and abused by biomedicine do want access to some of what it controls. It is the terms of access and the choices among biomedical and alternative health resources that are at issue. For example, in Oklahoma recently, a Native American World War II veteran had his foot amputated because of complications from diabetes. He understood the medical issue and accepted the surgery. But he also asked to take his amputated foot home with him. He intended to keep it and one day have it buried with him in his coffin, believing this to be important for him in the next life. The physicians refused. (This example is from Mariana Chilton's current fieldwork in Oklahoma. The same problem, with other surgically removed organs and other ethnic groups, has been observed in Philadelphia [Bonnie O'Connor, private communication], and is probably widespread.) This is not a question of preferring *either* biomedical care *or* traditional practices. Although one can imagine some health-related arguments in such a case, they certainly do not apply universally—and the methods of the anatomy lab and the mortuary solve such problems when solutions are genuinely desired. Such instances show the cultural values of medicine competing with the cultural values of the patient "as if" the medical values were all scientifically necessary and culturally neutral.[3]

Ironically, the wholesale deconstruction and dismissal of biomedicine as a hegemonic fiction, which radical critics sometimes suggest, actually serves medical hegemony by creating a forced choice between biomedical care as presently constructed and forfeiture of all biomedical resources. That forced choice has long operated to protect the institutions of biomedicine in the context of patient care. That is one reason, for example, that the medical literature has so often used Christian Science as a favorite example of "alternative medicine," even though it involves a very small fraction of potential patients, or that alternative birthing practices are often discussed as a complete rejection of biomedical resources at the same time that midwives and women who choose home birth have been prevented from obtaining access to the medical backup that they desire. The same thing occurs when environmental activists are assumed to oppose all technology and development. Organic farmers were long criticized as romantic know-nothings, at the same time that they were conducting agricultural experiments, developing biological controls, and making deliberate and careful choices among the resources of agricultural technology to construct an approach to food production that served both individual health and environmental conservation. Alternative healing traditions are simultaneously knowledge claims about health and models of cultural and social organization, arising outside the entrenched institutions of biomedicine and the related domains of science and government. As such, they are rich sources of information and ideas about health and the world, from the perspective of ordinary people.

When the pathophysiologically based definitions of biomedicine dominate discussions of alternative health systems, environmental sources and effects are largely omitted. For example, through the medical lens, questions about natural diet are restricted to whether a particular regimen, such as macrobiotics, can halt a particular disease process. But although the effect of the diet on this patient at this time is important, from the natural healing perspective that issue cannot be separated from the global effects of diets that are low on the food chain. For example, there is now growing awareness in orthodox medicine that a reduction of red meat in the diet may reduce some people's risk for certain kinds of cancer. From the natural healing point of view, such a reduction can also help to reduce global warming (the high value of rangeland to produce beef for North American and European markets is a major factor in the destruction of the rain forest in South America); help save the Chesapeake Bay by reducing nitrogen-rich runoff from feedlots, which is contributing to eutrophication; help reduce the suffering of animals raised in unnatural conditions; and reduce starvation throughout the world because meat production is such an inefficient way to produce food. These other good results are not accidental "side effects"; they all constitute healing. In fact, many advocates of alternative health systems reject the notion of primary effects and side effects altogether, insisting instead on recognizing that all events arise from and produce multiple complex effects (Weil, 1983). This is part of what is meant by the *holistic* character of many alternative health traditions.

Holism constitutes a fundamental difference between many alternative health systems and the categories of biomedicine. Although biomedicine recognizes environmental causes of disease, its pathophysiological viewpoint locates disease within the individual; in alternative health traditions, "dis-ease" is generally situated in the larger systems of which the individual is a part, so that sicknesses of persons are symptomatic of processes in their environment or of their relationship to that environment. Healing, then, is the reestablishment of the proper state of the environment and the sick person's place in it. In alternative health systems, a healing is not necessarily a cure and may have no effect at all on pathophysiology. The successful healing may be found in emotional growth, deepened relationships, a more intense and aware perception of the environment, spiritual awakening, or a more graceful cooperation in the natural processes of the world—of which death is one. Each such healing engages the individual in processes and meanings in the social, natural, and spiritual environment. Conversely, "successful" biomedical treatment sometimes leaves patients alienated from their social environment (as when the side effects of medication destroy sexual functioning or the financial and emotional burdens of care destroy families) and from their physical environment (as when the side effects of medication interfere with the patient's sensory world or energy level).

NOT ALL ALTERNATIVE HEALTH SYSTEMS ARE EXEMPLARY

Holism, spirituality, a rich understanding of costs and benefits, and a great variety of other valuable characteristics are often found in alternative traditions. But they are also missing in many, and in some cases, where found, they are superficial rhetorical devices rather than substance. We do not mean to idealize alternative health traditions, any more than we mean to dismiss the value of biomedicine. The great value of alternative traditions is their extreme diversity and their location outside the vested interests of biomedicine and the industrial world responsible for so much environmental degradation. As with free speech, an understanding of this value requires the recognition that not all of what is said and done is good, but that the value of openness to alternative views requires both tolerance and judgment.

Some alternative health practices actually bring pressure on endangered species, as in the use of rhinoceros horn or bear gall bladders in several Asian healing traditions. And the pharmaceutical industry has often appropriated the plant knowledge of other cultures with no apparent regard for the impact of their work on the people and environments they exploit. But by applying the common issues of individual health to a much larger context, alternative health traditions have now gone beyond the question of whether the people of the Amazon rain forest know something about plants that would be helpful in treating the diseases of North Americans to the broader issue of what obligation outsiders incur when seeking and making use of such information (Plotkin, 1993).

NATURAL HEALING

The use of plants in healing is one aspect of what is often called *natural healing*. Because it uses materials from the natural environment and requires biological diversity, natural healing has some obvious relevance to ecological issues. In the United States, the health food movement has had the greatest influence in developing and disseminating natural healing ideas throughout the twentieth century (Hufford, 1971, 1988). It has provided an accessible model within which herbalism, nutritional therapy, environmental protection, a variety of lifestyle factors including exercise, and spiritual concerns could be integrated and explored. Today the widespread availability of health food stores and the appearance of health food language in supermarkets both reflect and continue to advance public attention to natural healing ideas.

Critics often disparage the idea that some human practices are more "natural" than others as naive and meaningless. However, most alternative traditions do use an understandable definition of *natural* that has shown the ability to evaluate likely health effects on principle, without waiting for the elucidation of mechanisms or the support of quantitative studies. In most healing traditions, *natural* simply refers to the extent to which a practice resembles events found in nature without the technological intervention of humans. Whole grain is more natural than refined flour, because it uses less technology. Breast-feeding is more natural than formula feeding for the same reason. Natural healing advocates assume that things are in nature for good reasons and that technological interventions are, therefore, likely to have unpredictable costs. On the basis of this principle, natural healing proponents in the late nineteenth century were already advocating diets high in fiber and low in animal fats. Biomedicine did not reach the same conclusions about diet for one hundred years.

In the 1960s, breast-feeding, for which the La Leche League was the primary advocate, was highly regarded in the natural health movement. Although the La Leche League is now widely accepted, and medicine has now officially endorsed breast-feeding (Simopoulos, de Olivera, & Desal, 1995), there remains substantial tension between pediatricians and nursing mothers on the topic. This tension can be readily understood in terms of medicalization. A mother may need medical advice if her nursing baby fails to gain weight or if illness reduces her supply of milk, but that does not make breast milk a medicine nor breast-feeding a medical activity. The giving of food is a complex social interaction, not merely the provision of the chemical building blocks of tissue. Many mothers were far ahead of medicine in recognizing the biological advantages of breast-feeding, and mothers do not need behavioral medicine research to tell them that bonding occurs during nursing. As with many health-related ideas and practices, we see here the tendency of medicine to seek administrative control—based on technical knowledge—over all activities relevant to health. But because alternative health traditions reach beyond technical interventions to lifestyle practices, efforts at medical control are often intrusive and unwelcome.

WOMEN'S HEALTH, ALTERNATIVE MEDICINE, AND THE ENVIRONMENT

The La Leche League example illustrates an important point regarding the culture and politics of alternative healing ideas. Because the history of women's health in the era of biomedicine has been one of constant struggle, women's interests and experience have been fundamental sources of energy and insight in alternative healing. Over a little more than a century, the development of a powerful, male-dominated obstetrics and gynecology profession has led to a great variety of cultural constructions about health, many of them very disadvantageous to women. The medicalization of such natural female processes as menstruation and menopause, as well as most aspects of reproduction, has interrupted the traditional basis for woman-to-woman knowledge and sought a radical monopoly (Illich, 1976) over knowledge and control of women's bodies (Apple, 1990; Martin, 1987). Ironically this medical control serves both intrusive treatment, as in hormone replacement for menopause constructed as a disease, and dismissal of women's claims of sickness when diagnosis or treatment are difficult. "Menstrual problems" are the default diagnosis of choice until menopause serves the same function. Coupled with the trivialization of common problems such as urinary tract infections and *candida* vaginitis, this situation has guaranteed that women persistently seek more effective, alternative health ideas for specific sickness problems.[4] A reconstruction of the values and social organization of health culture was also ensured.

In addressing women's health in the context of alternative healing and the environment, it is crucial not to fall back on the stereotypes of women as inherently more connected to nature. Such naive and romantic notions merely bring a different set of factors to bear on the dismissal of women's voices. Women's concerns about health and the environment arise specifically and directly out of the negative impacts they experience as a result of the activities of powerful segments of society that neither value nor consider the interests of women as understood by women. The near destruction of the traditions of midwifery and woman-to-woman knowledge of pregnancy and childbirth by medical obstetrics is a well-known example of this (Leavitt, 1986).

In its dealings with the natural processes of the female body, biomedicine still sees nature as capricious and requiring constant technical intervention. Even more important, the knowledge of women, both as received from other women and as a reflection of personal experience, continues to be dismissed as merely subjective—along with such knowledge of patients generally. From the orthodox medical viewpoint, such knowledge has something to do with patient satisfaction, but it is not seen as valid or even comparable to technical medical knowledge. The hegemony of this male-dominated medical ideology has consistently led the women's health movement, like women's healing traditions of all sorts, to fiercely retain a sense of authority and validity that does not rely on a medical imprimatur. This is one reason that the women's health movement has been so influential within the alternative health movement.

As women have increasingly questioned the effect of environmental degradation on their health and the health of their children, the same set of tensions and political forces has engaged women in an environmentalism linked to health. For example, there are Mohawk and Inuit women who can no longer safely breast-feed their babies because of the PCBs from industrial pollution that have entered their bodies through contaminated groundwater and fish. As Katsi Cook, a Mohawk woman put it, "We as women and mothers are our children's first environment. . . . The analysis of Mohawk mothers' milk shows that our bodies are, in fact, a part of the landfill" (LaDuke, 1994, p. 45). The national concern of women over the apparent link between environmental pollution and the regional distribution of breast cancer is another source of personal-environmental linkage and growing resistance to the freedom of industry to continue to degrade the environment until "scientific proof" can connect particular cases to industrial practices. This is one place where biomedicine colludes with polluters by clinging to standards of evidence and explanation that guarantee immense damage will be done before intelligent policies can be put into place. Natural healing, in contrast, asserts that the history of technology and the environment demonstrates that the policy approach needs to be reversed; we should assume that each major human environmental impact has important health costs until good science shows that it does not. The women of northern Mexico and the southwestern United States who associated the increased prevalence of anencephaly and other severe birth defects with industrial pollution have a shared interest with the natural healing tradition in basing policy on a coherent set of philosophical principles about health and its relationship to the world, rather than reacting individually to crises after they have been exhaustively documented by the patient observation of enormous human costs.

COOPERATION VERSUS CONTROL OF NATURE

The natural healing movement's values practically obliterate the distinction between individual and environmental health. The natural healing alternative in both human and environmental health involves locating naturally occurring defenses with which humans can cooperate, as opposed to the development of powerful interventions to overwhelm natural processes. This is the most basic difference between biomedicine and most alternative traditions: the choice between a cooperative or an adversarial relationship to the environment. The medical assumption that nature must be subdued has great historical depth. For example, John Harley Warner says the following about Benjamin Rush, a highly influential medical practitioner and educator at the time of the American Revolution and in the early nineteenth century:

> Nature, Rush believed, acted capriciously in disease, generally to the patient's detriment. "In all violent diseases nature is like a drunken man reeling to & fro & occasionally stumbl[ing] against a door with so much violence as to break it through," he told his students. "Always treat nature in the sick room as you would a noisy dog or cat[;] drive her out at the door & lock it upon her." (p. 18)

More recently, Joseph B. DeLee (1920), M.D., stated, in *The American Journal of Obstetrics*, "Labor has been called, and still is believed by many to be, a normal function. It always strikes physicians as well as laymen as bizarre, to call labor an abnormal function, a disease, and yet it is a decidedly pathological process" (pp. 39-40). Many of the values of biomedicine are associated with this outlook on nature, such as the suppression of symptoms with anti-inflammatory and antipyretic drugs, or the emphasis on prompt action and simple (that is "pure") active principles. Natural healing tends instead to accept limits and seek harmony in a self-correcting world that has purposes and goodness inscrutable to human investigation and that rewards cooperation.

ALTERNATIVE MEDICINE AND SPIRITUALITY

Until recently, scholars sharply distinguished natural healing from *metaphysical* or *magico-religious* healing. Even today, natural healing that involves herbs, diet, and physical practices such as setting broken bones is treated as empirical and rational, the direct predecessor of pharmacological medicine and surgery, whereas spiritual healing ideas are taken as naive psychology or as metaphor. This distinction, however, reflects the culture of scholars rather than the categories of traditional alternative healers. In fact, the inextricable association of spiritual and natural ideas is one of the strongest overall characteristics of alternative health traditions. In contrast, many histories attribute the technological successes of biomedicine to its radical separation from religion. Contemporary biomedicine is the only major health tradition that explicitly contains no spiritual elements (except where *spiritual* is used as a proxy for *psychological*).

Spirituality in alternative traditions serves as a powerful link between the individual and larger domains. For example, herbalists have often assumed that humans and plants relate to one another in a variety of deep ways reflecting spiritual realities. As herbalist Norma Meyers said,

> After 15 years of observing the plants, I have come to believe that herbs work not so much because of biochemistry and nutrition as because of energy fields. . . . I have two beliefs that have grown out of feeling the energies of the herbs. The first is that these plants were made by the same Creator that made you and me. I was not a religious person when I first came into contact with the plants. But because of their influence on me I have now become a religious, spiritual person. (Quoted in Conrow & Hecksel, 1983, pp. 193, 195)

Such a belief that the natural world is saturated with spirituality is a feature of many traditions. For example, in many Native American religions, the world is imbued with spirits, and people have a family relationship with their natural environment through these spirits. This bond is so deep and provocative that one can only feel great sadness at popular culture's trivialization of such images as Mother Earth as mere metaphor. The significance of such a relationship between persons and environment is sharply focused by comparison with the popular metaphor of spaceship Earth. The spaceship image suggests our self-interest in maintaining a machine needed to fulfill our demands. But no one ordinarily thinks of their mother as a tool for self-gratification. The personalization of the natural world that comes with an immanent spirituality leads beyond immediate self-interest. After all, people make sacrifices and may even die willingly for those they love.

We do not intend to suggest that a personal and affectionate relationship with nature is universal among alternative health traditions, or that this spiritual dimension has only positive implications. As already noted, some Asian health traditions have an adverse impact on endangered species, despite their spiritual underpinnings. Also, the willingness to die for loved ones sometimes means a sacrifice in the service of ethnic cleansing, justified by claims of spiritual attachment to a "fatherland." Spiritual ideas about humans and the world, and the experiences from which they arise, are powerful. And like anything powerful, they can be used for good or for evil. Nonetheless, belief in a world imbued with spirit is more congenial to the constructive integration of personal healing with care for the environment than are the forms of spirituality that have become increasingly dominant in the West since the Enlightenment.

During the past several hundred years, official religion in the West joined the academic process of secularization, a process associated with enormous social and economic change (Weber, 1963). Modern Christian theology has moved away from a worldview within which the natural and supernatural interact constantly, toward what has been called *radical transcendence*. In this process, the view of the supernatural and the scope of its interactions with the natural, temporal world have become increasingly sparse. The world came to be seen as a useful machine, and whatever ideas of spiritual relation persisted had to do only with the long ago, the far away, or the not yet. As in Deism, the Creator built the place, but now it was entirely for humans to control it and select from among possible futures based on their own self-interest.

The spiritual revivals of the late twentieth century reflect a disillusionment with the results of decoupling the spiritual from the natural world. For some, this has meant a renewed interest in the traditional religions of Native Americans and other cultures around the world. Some of these responses seem shallow and superficial, and some of them do at least as much damage as good. For example, some white, middle-class Americans have naively appropriated rituals—and the pipestone and eagle feathers involved—in a way that many custodians of those traditions call cultural genocide. Unwilling to subject themselves to the authority of the peoples whose beliefs and practices they claim to follow, they decorate an unchanged life with sacraments they do not understand and cannot honor. But although it is easy to sneer at New Age superficiality, we should remember the difficulty of reconstructing a rich and integrated religious understanding of the world in contemporary society. Those who try and have only modest success are at least making an effort. Neither should we underestimate the amount of energy and desire that are being poured into this attempt, an attempt that goes back at least to the nineteenth century and that has been very influential throughout the Western world since the 1960s.

CONCLUSION

Health, environmental conservation, and spirituality cannot be disentangled. Repeatedly the sources of a host of human problems are being found in the disintegration of these domains. The interests of women and ethnic minorities in bringing about dramatic changes in these aspects of contemporary society are powerful sources for change. The healing of our world cannot be accomplished through ever finer analysis, scientific rigor, and technological interventions—although proper scientific work and technology are indispensable to the process. The *propriety* of solutions can only be reformed by new voices, new points of view, and new interests. Alternative healing traditions and their current popularity provide a great opportunity for such social change. But that change can only happen so long as alternative health traditions avoid assimilation into the powerful institutions of biomedicine. Honoring, listening to, and selecting leaders from those groups in society who have been consistently disempowered is one crucial key to retaining the independence and radical possibilities of the alternative healing movement.

NOTES

1. There are many problems in current terminology in this field. We prefer alternative health *systems* to alternative *medicine*, because *system* suggests the complexity of the ideas and practices involved and avoids the assumptions associated with the word *medicine*. We use *alternative health tradition* to mean the same thing and as a reminder of historical depth—although the word does not require any minimum number of years.

2. As with alternatives, terms for the medicine taught in medical schools and tested on medical board examinations are all problematic. In this essay we have adopted the common term biomedicine because of its widespread usage. This does *not*, however, suggest that all such medical thought and practice is biologically based in a direct way, nor does it suggest that alternatives have no biological basis.

3. For another example, many natural healing advocates whose children are forcibly treated for cancer and even placed in foster homes because of parental noncompliance

actually want initial chemotherapy but balk at the follow-up that physicians consider crucial in raising the chances of a cure (Frohock, 1992).

4. Two recent examples of medical research documenting the effectiveness of natural, alternative treatments for common female health problems involve eating yogurt to treat or prevent candidal vaginitis (Hilton, Isenberg, Alperstein, France, & Borenstein, 1992), and drinking cranberry juice to prevent and treat urinary tract infections (Avorn, 1994). Both clinical studies, published in major medical journals (*Annals of Internal Medicine* and *Journal of the American Medical Association*), drew skeptical reactions from doctors and calls for caution in endorsing such "panaceas" (e.g., Drutz, 1992; Podolsky, 1992).

REFERENCES

Apple, R. D. (Ed.). (1990). *Women, health, and medicine in America: A historical handbook.* New York: Garland.

Avorn, J. (1994, March 9). Reduction of bacteriuria and pyuria after ingestion of cranberry juice. *Journal of the American Medical Association, 271*(10), 751-754.

Conrow, R., & Hecksel, A. (1983). *Herbal pathfinders: Voices of the herb renaissance.* Santa Barbara, CA: Woodbridge.

DeLee, J. B. (1920). The prophylactic forceps operation. *American Journal of Obstetrics,* 39-40.

Drutz, D. J. (1992). *Lactobacillus* prophylaxis for *candida* vaginitis. *Annals of Internal Medicine, 116,* 419-420.

Frohock, F. M. (1992). *Healing powers: Alternative medicine, spiritual communities, and the state.* Chicago: University of Chicago Press.

Hilton, E., Isenberg, H. D., Alperstein, P., France, K., & Borenstein, M. (1992). Ingestion of yogurt containing *lactobacillus acidophilus* as prophylaxis for candidal vaginitis. *Annals of Internal Medicine, 116,* 353-357.

Hufford, D. J. (1971). Natural/organic food people as a "folk group": Nutrition, health system, and worldview. *Keystone Folklore Quarterly, 16*(4), 179-184.

Hufford, D. J. (1988). Contemporary folk medicine. In N. Gevitz (Ed.), *Unorthodox medicine in America* (pp. 228-264). Baltimore, MD: Johns Hopkins University Press.

Illich, I. (1976). *Medical nemesis: The expropriation of health.* New York: Pantheon.

LaDuke, W. (1994, Winter). Breast milk, PCBs, and motherhood: An interview with Katsi Cook, Mohawk. *Cultural Survival Quarterly.*

Leavitt, J. W. (1986). *Brought to bed: Child-bearing in America, 1750-1950.* New York: Oxford University Press.

Martin, E. (1987). *The woman in the body: A cultural analysis.* Boston: Beacon.

Plotkin, M. J. (1993). *Tales of a shaman's apprentice: An ethnobotanist searches for new medicines in the Amazon rain forest.* New York: Viking.

Podolsky, S. (1992). Yogurt for candidal vaginitis. *Annals of Internal Medicine, 117,* 345-346.

Simopoulos, A. P., de Olivera, J. E. D., & Desai, I. D. (1995) *Behavioral and metabolic aspects of breast-feeding: International trends.* Freiburg: Karger.

Weber, M. (1963). *The sociology of religion* (4th ed.). Boston: Beacon.

Weil, A. (M.D.) (1983). *Health and healing: Understanding conventional and alternative medicine.* Boston: Houghton Mifflin.

7 Birth in the Technocracy

Body Image and Worldview

ROBBIE E. DAVIS-FLOYD

Through the act of controlling birth, we disassociate ourselves with its raw power. Disassociation makes it easier to identify with our "civilized" nature, deny our "savage" roots and connection with indigenous cultures. Birth simultaneously encompasses the three events that civilized societies fear—birth, death, and sexuality.

—Holly Richards (1993, p. 28)

Childbirth, on which the perpetuation of the human species depends, is a powerful reminder of our dependence on nature. As Richards points out, our Western cultural attitude toward birth is fear-based. Since the dawn of the Industrial Revolution, Western society has sought to dominate and control nature, a right that was chartered early on in Genesis when God gave man "dominion"—but could only be fully carried out with the emergence of modern technology. The more able we became to control nature, including our natural bodies, the more fearful we became of the aspects of nature we could not control.

AUTHOR'S NOTE: Parts of this chapter are abridged from *Social Science and Medicine,* Volume 38, No. 8, pp. 1125-1140, with the kind permission of Elsevier Science Ltd., The Boulevard Langford Lane, Kidlington 0X51GB, United Kingdom.

The industrialization of the West has led, in the United States, to the emergence of the *technocracy*—a hierarchical and bureaucratic society organized around an ideology of technological progress—and of a phenomenon that anthropologist Peter C. Reynolds (1991) has labeled the "One-Two Punch." Take a natural process that is working well—say, a river in which salmon annually swim upstream to spawn. Punch One: "Improve" it with technology—build a dam and a power plant, generating the unfortunate by-product that the salmon can no longer swim to their spawning grounds. Punch Two: Fix the problem created by technology with *more* technology—take the salmon out of the water with machines, let them spawn and grow the eggs in trays, feed the babies through an elaborate system of pipes and tubes, then truck them back to the river and release them downstream.

Reynolds's (1991) brilliant insight is that, although most people see Punch Two as an accidental by-product of Punch One, the deeper truth is that *Punch Two is the point.* We in the West have become convinced that culturally altering natural processes makes them better—more predictable, more controllable, and therefore safer. For example, when the U.S. Army Corps of Engineers lined the banks of large sections of the waterways of the Everglades and installed floodgates, most people thought of this as an improvement. No matter that the effect has been to lose huge portions of this natural resource to soil erosion.

It is not hard to see how this One-Two Punch of mutilation and prosthesis applies to birth. We fear the birth process—like the waterways of the Everglades with their frequent floods, it seems to us to be chaotic, uncontrollable, and therefore dangerous. So we improve it with technology. First, we take it apart—deconstruct it—into identifiable segments. Then we control each segment with the obstetrical equivalent of dams and floodgates (electronic fetal monitors, pitocin, drugs). When the unfortunate by-product of this technological reconstruction of birth is a baby in distress from a now-dysfunctional labor,[1] we rescue the baby with more technology (episiotomy, forceps, cesarean section). Then we congratulate ourselves on saving the baby, just as the builders of the salmon hatchery Reynolds visited in California put a plaque on the wall to congratulate themselves for "saving the salmon."

As is evident in this One-Two Punch of birth in the technocracy, the core values of our technocratic society center around science and technology and the institutions that command them. In every society, core cultural beliefs and values are most highly visible in the rituals that accompany important life transitions such as birth, puberty, marriage, initiation into a religious or occupational group, parenthood, and death.

Rituals at the most basic level are enactments of these core cultural values and beliefs. Thus it is not surprising that the core values of the technocracy would be most visible in the rituals with which we surround the birth process.

Basic to initiation rites across cultures is the removal of the initiate from normal social life (Turner, 1969, 1964/1979). Once so removed, initiates are stripped of their individuality—their heads are often shaved or their hair clipped short, their clothes and adornments are taken away, and they are dressed in identical gowns or robes. Then they are subjected to a hazing process designed to break down their normal ways of thinking. Once this cognitive breakdown is well under way, the initiate is bombarded with messages about the core values of the culture. These messages are conveyed through powerful symbols. Symbols operate through the right hemisphere of the brain—their messages are emotionally felt, not intellectually analyzed, and their impact is often very powerful (d'Aquili & Laughlin, 1979, pp. 173-177; Lex, 1979, pp. 124-130; Luria, 1966). These symbolic messages serve to build up the belief system of the initiates in accordance with the dominant beliefs and values of the group or society into which they are being initiated.

It is not difficult to see the strong parallels between this cross-cultural initiation process and hospital birth. In an earlier work (Davis-Floyd, 1992), I present a detailed analysis of hospital birth as technocratic initiation. Here I will summarize. Birthing women are removed from the realm of normal social life and taken into the hospital—a powerful institution organized to express our culture's supervaluation of science and technology. Their clothes are taken away, they are dressed in uniform hospital gowns, and their pubic hair is shaved or clipped—symbolically desexualizing the lower half of their body and marking it as institutional property. Labor itself is a natural process—the pain of contractions leaves women disoriented and wide open to internalize the symbolic messages they are sent. The powerful cultural symbols that convey these messages are the intravenous tube (IV), the electronic fetal monitor, the pitocin drip, and all the other myriad technological procedures through which most birthing women in the United States must pass during their rite of passage into motherhood. Exactly what messages do such procedures convey?

The IV is the symbolic umbilical cord to the hospital. It makes a birthing woman appear to be dependent on the institution for her life, just as the baby in the womb depends on her for its life. This, of course, is a perfectly accurate mirror of technocratic society—in fact, we *are* dependent on institutions for our lives. The frequent examinations of the cervix to see if it is dilating fast enough (and the pitocin drip administered if it isn't) convey strong and accurate messages about the importance of time in the technocracy and about the importance of on-time production by our body-machines. The electronic fetal monitor is there to warn of possible malfunctions—like the IV, it powerfully symbolizes the woman's dependence on the institution and its technology. The flat-on-the-back (lithotomy) position keeps the woman "down" in relation to the medical staff's "up," enacting our cultural value of hierarchy and reinforcing women's structural subordination at the moment of birth. Forceps and cesarean sections allow the physician to be the birth giver; they clearly express our culture's insistence on restructuring natural processes and on shifting creative power from women to men. The all-too-brief bonding period allowed in many hospital deliveries conveys the message that society gives the baby to the mother, then has the authority to take the baby away. (Most newborns are whisked off to the nursery shortly after birth.)

The separation of self from body, mother from child, which begins in the hospital is continued in countless American homes. Babies are constantly put into their separate cultural spaces—carried in rockers or strollers, put down to play in playpens, put to sleep in cribs surrounded with toys—and fed with plastic bottles. In no other culture is there so much separation between parents and child. It is no wonder—no cultural accident—that our babies bond to technology and grow up to be voracious consumers. Their constantly increasing levels of consumption drive our economy, and so the technocracy feeds itself.

As a medical anthropologist, I have a long-standing research interest in how the technocracy symbolically transforms the natural processes of pregnancy and birth and in how that transformation affects women's own perceptions and experiences of these biological events (Davis-Floyd, 1987, 1990, 1992). In the remainder of this chapter, I present, in abridged form, the results of a study I carried out on the correspondences between women's individual body images and the wider social values and beliefs described above (Davis-Floyd, 1994). This study explores the body images and worldviews of 32 professional, career-oriented women who gave birth in the hospital and 8 women who made the alternative choice of giving birth at home. I suggest that body image can provide a microcosmic mirror of worldview, and that this mirror also reflects implications for medical care and environmental relationships.

THE TECHNOCRATIC BODY AND THE PROFESSIONAL WOMAN

> When it came time for Susan Blume to deliver her baby, she was blessedly calm. No sweat soaked her brow, no pain lined her face. She uttered not a sound. As the baby squeezed down the birth canal, Blume [anesthetized by an epidural] lay placidly on her side, reading *People* magazine and robbing the gods of one more woman bringing forth children in sorrow.
>
> —Elaine Herscher, *San Francisco Chronicle*[2]

The 32 professionals who chose hospital birth hold a wide range of occupations, from college professors to managers to chief executive officers (CEOs) of their own companies. Most of them make as much or more money than their husbands. During our hour-long interviews,[3] it quickly became apparent that one of their overriding concerns is control. They hold the strong belief that life is controllable and that to be strong and powerful in the world, one must be in control. They achieve control over their lives through careful planning and organization of their time and activities, over their bodies through regular exercise, and over their own destinies through reaching positions of independence and importance in the wider society. Interestingly, those who admitted to wanting and enjoying power insisted that it was not power over others that appealed to them, but power to make things happen in the world. Lina said: "I didn't want to be like my mother. . . . I didn't want to be picked on by my husband at the time, and be powerless." When I asked her what she did to be powerful, she replied, "I got a Ph.D. and a job."

These professional women seemed to judge every situation by the degree of control they felt they could maintain over it. Even their pregnancies were usually carefully controlled, planned to occur at just the chosen time in their careers. But once those processes were set into motion, they became uncontrollable, and thus presented these women with a division within their most treasured notions of self, between the cultural, professional parts within their control and the personal, biological processes outside of it. Lina experienced this division so intensely that she could hardly believe it when she became pregnant:

> Deep down inside of me I believed that I had desexed myself by being the successful professional and that I would have to pay [for that success by having] a hard time getting pregnant. . . . A couple of my male faculty colleagues, when they would see me with the baby, would constantly say,

"I can't believe you are a mother." . . . What they were really saying to me is, "I thought you were a guy."

This separation of self from biology is clearly reflected in the body concepts held by many of these women. I asked each one, "How do you think about your body? What is your body?" Most immediately expressed the belief that the body is both imperfect (Lou said, "It's fat around the middle, and my boobs are too small") and separate from the self:

> My body is a vehicle that allows me to move around, a tool for my success in the world. (Joanne)

> My body is the recipient of the abuse from the lifestyle that I choose. . . . It's my weakest link. You have to pay the price somewhere—I'm out of shape, overweight, and not eating right—my body to me is what has paid the price for this career. [Question: Can you describe your relationship with your body?] Abusive. (Beth)

Predictably, then, the physical state of pregnancy was problematic at best for some of these women. For intrinsic to the notion of the body as vehicle are the corollary notions that the body is worth less than the self it houses, which, being worth more, should control the body, should be "in charge." Concomitantly, most of these women experienced the bodily condition of pregnancy as unpleasant because it was beyond the control of the self, or, as they put it, "out of control." As Linda said,

> I think there are a lot of women who love being pregnant, and they would say that. My sister, the Earth Mother, did. Especially before I got pregnant, I thought, "Maybe I'll get into it." I felt bad and large and awkward and nauseated. And oh, I love having the baby, but I wish there were an easier way.

Asked how she felt about her body while she was pregnant, Lina responded,

> I didn't like it. It just overwhelmed me, the kinds and the variety of sensations, and the things that happen to your body because of the pregnancy. I didn't like it at all. I felt totally alienated from my body.

And even Leah's positive experience of pregnancy was expressed in terms of separation and a feeling of lack of control: "It was . . . so curious. I was watching all this happening. It was something taking control all over me and it was all good." Joanne added,

> I was real apprehensive about going into labor. It kind of terrified me, mostly because I like to be in control . . . and you don't have any control when that happens. I used to have nightmares about standing in front of the president and making a presentation and having my water break.

Here is how Beth experienced birth:

> I mean, it's like a demon to me. There's another being in your body that has to get out and it's looking for a way to get out. And all of a sudden, it's like my center of control left my brain and went to this, this thing in my body. And I had no control. . . . That was the thing I liked the least.

As they viewed the body as a vehicle for the mind or soul, so these women tended to see the pregnant body as a vessel, a container for the fetus (who is a being separate from the mother) and to interpret its growth and birth as occurring through a mechanical process in which the mother is not actively involved. (Sarah flatly stated, "You're just a vessel. That's all you are, just this vessel.") These beliefs were behaviorally expressed in myriad ways during pregnancy. For example, the evidence these women relied on for proof of the baby's health and growth was objective, coming primarily from ultrasound photographs and electronic amplification of the fetal heart rate. They understood the importance of nutrition and knew that they had to eat well so the baby would be well-nourished. They tended to see this in terms of a simple, mechanical cause-effect relationship. If they ingested good foods, the necessary nourishment would travel to the baby through the placenta, enhancing overall development and especially brain growth. Excessive ingestion of alcohol or junk food, however, might result in a child with less-than-optimal brain capacity. Thus, eating well was a mother's duty to her unborn child and one of the most important things, along with ultrasound and amniocentesis, that she could do to ensure optimal growth conditions. Although most of these women experienced giving up alcohol and junk food as something of a burden, to them it was also a logical necessity, something they did as a matter of course. But it did not, conceptually speaking, entail their active participation in growing the child. It merely made them into the best possible vessels.

In keeping with these attitudes, most of these women did not view the processes of labor and birth as intrinsic to their feminine natures.

Said Linda, "If my husband could do it the next time instead of me, that would be just fine." Joanne added,

> Even though I'm a woman, I'm unsuited for delivering . . . and I couldn't nurse. . . . I've told my mother—I just look like a woman, but none of the other parts function like a mother. I don't have the need or the desire to be biological. . . . I've never really been able to understand women who want to watch the birthing process in a mirror. . . . I'd rather see the finished product than the manufacturing process.

Emergent in Joanne's words we see the technocratic notions that birth is a mechanical process and that there is no intrinsic value in giving birth "naturally," because technology is better than nature anyway. Thus we can understand when Joanne says that she enjoyed her cesarean birth because her anesthesiologist explained what was happening step by step, and because she felt no pain and was able to be so *intellectually* present to the birth that she could watch the clock, to see which of her many friends who had placed bets on the time of the birth would win the $18 in the pot. She stated,

> [I liked that because] I didn't feel like I had dropped into a biological being. . . . I'm not real fond of things that remind me I'm a biological creature—I prefer to think and be an intellectual emotional person, so you know, it was sort of my giving in to biology to go through all this.

Here Joanne expresses a view held by most women in this group: The ideal, whole woman is intellectual and emotional, but not necessarily biological.

Like Joanne, Katie preferred the sense of control provided by cesarean delivery and in no way saw this as a disempowering loss, but only as an empowering gain because it was something *she* had caused to happen. When her baby was two weeks overdue and labor had not begun, she told her doctor, who was urging restraint,

> "I am really getting sick of this. Please schedule [the cesarean]." [Question: How did you feel about yourself after the birth?] "I felt pretty special. Proud . . . I felt as if I had accomplished quite a bit."

Kathy, who also described her cesarean as personally empowering, said,

> I don't feel like I missed out on anything. With my first two, I was put to sleep. With my third, Bryan, I was given an epidural. Heaven! I would never do it any other way. A cesarean with an epidural. I was awake,

> everything. Ah, it was just wonderful. . . . I would have to say, hey, I participated in it. I was awake and I felt the pulling and the tugging. I did not push or anything. But I was definitely a part of what was going on.

Elaine summarized,

> They induced labor and I wasn't very good at my relaxation techniques and my breathing and after about four hours of labor I decided I would prefer to have a cesarean and so that's what we did. . . . I know some women get all uptight about that, that it wasn't a normal delivery, but I didn't feel the least bit cheated. . . . I was very happy when I heard [my children] cry. It was a very pleasant experience.

In their words, we hear again the value these women place on control, as well as their strong belief that the mind is more important than the body, that as long as their minds are aware, they are active participants in the birth process. We hear this expressed even in Clara's recounting of her rapid and unmedicated vaginal delivery:

> Travis came in a little over an hour and that was just not enough time to get mentally prepared. I felt . . . my body pushing me into having this baby. My mind was not there to work with it. I needed more time to be able to get on top of it and be there.

As a corollary of the idea that technology is better than nature, most of the hospital birthers in this study felt rather strongly that labor is naturally painful, that pain is bad, and that not to have to feel pain during labor is good and is their intrinsic right as modern women. Asked what she wanted out of the birth experience, Joanne responded, "Out of the birth experience itself I wanted no pain. I wanted it to be as simple and easy and uncomplicated as most everything else has been for me." Said Leah, "I made the decision—I had two hits of Demerol in the IV. I controlled the pain through that." Beth, who "had planned for but did not end up with natural childbirth," was nevertheless very pleased to feel that she also was in control of the decisions that were made. She had expected a long labor with little pain. When the pain became severe, she asked for relief, "and you know, even though I hadn't planned on an epidural, they were very responsive when I said I wanted one." The next time around, Beth planned for an epidural:

> When I got there, I was probably about five centimeters, and they said, "Uh, I'm not sure we have time," and I said, "I want the epidural. We must go ahead and do it right now!" So we had an epidural.

And Elaine stressed that

> ultimately the decision to have a cesarean while I was in labor was mine. I told my doctor I'd had enough of this labor business and I'd like to . . . get it over with. So he whisked me off to the delivery room and we did it.

In keeping with the high value they placed on making their own decisions, the major discontents these women expressed with the medical handling of their labors and deliveries resulted not from the administration of anesthesia, but from its withholding.

Kay reported,

> I [asked] for an epidural at one point, but they said they didn't have time to do it. [Question: Was that OK with you?] Not really! I . . . remembered how wonderful it was [with my first birth] and that I had instantly felt terrific. . . . I was mad that I was in so much pain, and then they would tell me something like "we don't have time," you know—that just drove me wild. . . . I wanted to have it when *I* wanted to have it.

Another woman expressed outrage that a friend of hers in advanced labor had been denied anesthesia for the same reason as Kay, saying earnestly, "no one has the right to tell you that you have to go through that kind of pain." In spite of their awareness of existing evidence on the depressive effects of analgesia and anesthesia on the baby during labor and birth, most of these women felt very strongly that they had an absolute right to the mind-body separation offered by such drugs, especially the epidural. Lina spoke for the majority when she said,

> I read all this stuff that told me I would be a complete asshole to have an epidural and I revolted. [The books were saying that] I would be able to see that it's [sarcastic tone] "much better for the baby" and "it's a natural experience," and there's just all this pressure. . . . I quit smoking, ate meat, drank milk for months and months—I had been such a good girl. A couple of hours of whatever an epidural was going to do to me, tough. You can put up with it, kid.

Hand in hand with their intense desire for control—for not dropping down into biology—goes a lack of interest (on the part of most of these women) in breast-feeding for any extended length of time. To breast-feed is to be out of control—the milk comes unbidden and runs down your blouse; you must drop what you are doing and attend to the child's hunger. Bottle-feeding, on the other hand, enables someone else to do that for you and frees you from enslavement to biology as surely as does an epidural. With good reason, a woman in a novel of the 1930s tells her daughter, "The bottle was the war cry of my generation!" (McCarthy, 1954, p. 247). That cry is echoed in 1991,

> I really thought I wanted to breast-feed, but I didn't. I wanted my body back. (Lina)

> Yes, it's good for the baby, but if you're uncomfortable with it, for any reason, don't do it. It just isn't worth the trauma. This time I'm not going to do it at all, uh-uh. Part of it goes back to not having the need or the desire to be biological. The other is the confinement of nursing. You know, I wanted to be able to get up and go, and let somebody else feed the baby, and the idea of expressing just nauseated me. (Joanne)

About leaving her six-week-old baby at a day care center, Linda the pediatrician noted,

> Possibly [it would be better for my baby to be with me]. On the other hand, I also feel like I probably wouldn't be very happy. I'd probably start climbing the walls, and in a way that would be a bad thing to do to him, to say well, alright, I'm going to throw away 20 years of education to stay home with you so that you can be the perfect child.

Thus we arrive at a central question for most of these women: Where are they going to put their bodies, carriers of their selves, in relation to their children? The answer in general is, at some distance. The majority of these women work ten-hour days, and so they see their children only for a maximum of an hour and a half or two hours per day. To rationalize the time differential between parenting and work, most hung their hats on the popular notion of quality time. Although some were beginning to question the wisdom of this arrangement, Carolyn spoke for the majority:

> My husband and I just do the best we can every day to be terrific parents and terrific professionals. And if the kid gets left on the street corner for three hours because we each thought the other was supposed to pick him up—yes, that happened once!—we know better than to burden ourselves with guilt. We are giving him all we can—those two hours a day when we are with him are spent in close physical proximity. We don't waste time on the house or other stuff—we just focus on him.

HOME-BIRTHERS AND THE ORGANIC BODY

> The contractions kept coming. Each one of them pushed. . . . I tried joining in, very carefully. I pushed with my stomach muscles, just a little . . . but whoa, my uterus grabbed me and drove me along with itself. I couldn't push just a little. It had to be a lot. . . . It was so powerful and uncontrollable. I might push myself inside out if I went too far. But who cares? I didn't try to hold back any more. I pushed hard. I grabbed onto Vic, onto the folds of his clothes. I held my breath and pushed as hard as I could and it felt good. It felt better. The contractions didn't hurt as much any more. It was exciting. I'm pushing!
>
> —Janet Isaacs Ashford (1984), p. 76

A number of the beliefs about self and body held by the professionals are immanent in the American middle-class worldview—most obviously the Cartesian notion of mind-body separation, which has been a fundamental principle of technocratic life. This principle is consciously rejected by the eight home-birthers in my study, who see self and body as One; they say "I am my body," or "My body is the physical expression of me." In belief and behavior, these women stress the body's organic interconnectedness with both mind and environment and view the female body as normal, beautiful, and healthy. (Said Susan, "I feel great, and I like the way I look.") They feel deeply and strongly that female physiological processes, including birth, are healthy and safe:

> Well this one friend—she said, "Sandra, are you still thinking about having this baby at home? . . . I think you're absolutely insane. What if something happened?" My friends think I'm crazy. But I think *they* are. I mean really, they are—they're the ones that have missed the whole birth experience, not me.

In dramatic contrast to the high value placed on control by the hospital-birthers, these home-birthers felt that giving up control was far more valuable in birth and in life than trying to maintain it—a philosophical position again arrived at through lived experience. Said Liza,

> I was brought up in the mainstream, and I used to knock myself out trying to control everything. Then I got sick, and I realized that I actually can't control anything or anyone. As soon as I let go of trying, and just began to surrender to what is, everything in my life started to work. I got well, I got married, I had a baby. And if the lesson needed reinforcing, labor did it. That is a force beyond control, a powerful wave that will drown you if you

> fight it. Better then to dive into it, to relax, let it carry you. Whenever I tried to control my labor or myself during labor, I was in agony. But when I let go and surrendered to the waves, they carried me.

As we might expect, the home-birthers enjoyed pregnancy's constant changes and came to value their lack of control over these changes. Tara declared, "I loved all of it. I liked looking at my body in the mirror. I couldn't wait to see what would happen next." Susan said, "I was in awe. . . . Being pregnant was fascinating. . . . It isn't when you're barfing in the toilet bowl every morning, but when that part is over, you feel good. You feel better than you ever had in your life."

To the direct question, "Other women I have interviewed experienced their body changes during pregnancy as being out of control, meaning that they didn't have control. Why didn't you?" Susan responded,

> Whenever anything like that happened to me, I had already read up or talked to midwives and I knew it was coming. I knew that that was going to happen next, and it was all part of this wonderful experience of getting pregnant. One step closer to having that baby there.

This response and others like it show that these women value not only the intellect but also the synergy of body-with-mind.

Like self and body, the home-birthers conceptualized mother and baby as *essentially One*—an integrated system that can only be harmed by dissecting into its individual parts. Much more than a passive host or vessel, the mother saw herself as actively growing the baby. Susan said,

> Especially when you're actually actively doing all the exercises you're supposed to be doing and you're actively eating and drinking what you're supposed to be eating and drinking, then you really feel like you are feeding and nourishing and growing the baby.

This belief in the oneness of mother and child makes possible the experience of active communication with their unborn babies that these women often reported. Kristin said,

> When I was about two months pregnant I was lying on my waterbed one night in the dark, not sleeping, but also not really thinking, just drifting along, when suddenly, from somewhere inside of the front of my head I

> heard these words, "I'm here, I'm a girl, and my name is Joy Elizabeth." . . . One night [much later on], I had a Braxton Hicks contraction and I heard a voice inside say "I'm scared." I told her I was scared, too, and that everything would be OK because we were partners—we would do this thing together.

Elizabeth experienced this sort of active communication and sense of partnership with her unborn in a rather dramatic way:

> Two weeks before he was born, he was still breech. My midwives felt confident about a breech delivery, but I . . . wanted him to turn. I went to a therapist who, several people had told me, was really good at visualization, and asked her to help me get in touch with him. She helped me see myself as tiny, and to travel through my nose down to my stomach, and then to see a little window opening into my uterus, which got bigger until I could step through. I swam over his body, past his genitals, which I could clearly see were male, and up to his face. I told him I loved him and couldn't wait to hold him in my arms, and then I asked him please to turn. I told him it was really important to me. He looked right at me and I suddenly felt that if I would show him what to do, he would do it. So I started swimming down, toward my cervix, motioning for him to follow me. . . . By the time I woke up the next morning, he had completely turned, and he stayed that way until he was born!

For the home-birthers (as, in their very different way, for the hospital-birthers), this active, agentic role was key. Near the beginning of her first pregnancy, during her first interview with an obstetrician, Susan became very angry because his response to her questions was, "You don't need to worry about that. I'll take care of that." She said, "He thought he knew more about it than I did!" When I asked her why she didn't assume that he *did* know more, she replied,

> Well, I didn't consider having a baby something I wasn't supposed to take part in. That I was just there to grow this baby, and he was going to take it out of me, but I couldn't do that on my own. I knew better than that. I knew . . . that it was me 100% that was going to get this baby through the birth canal and out into the world . . . and I wanted somebody who would work with me to do the best job I could [so I went out and found a midwife].

Just as these home-birthers see themselves as actively growing their babies, so they also see labor and birth as hard work that a woman does.

This holistic view, which does not separate the woman from the process of labor, accepts pain as an integral part of that process. To eliminate that one part would interfere with the systemic whole and would begin a cycle of interference that might have unforeseen results. When I asked whether the pain had any meaning for her, Tara responded,

> Oh yes. . . . Even though during labor I remember feeling it was almost unbearable, it never entered my mind to wish I had "something for the pain." . . . [There is] wonderful physical and emotional stuff going on at the same time as the pain. If you took drugs for the pain, you would change all the rest of it, too.

In the technocratic worldview, not only are mother and baby viewed as separate, but the interests of each are often perceived as conflicting. In such circumstances, the mother's emotional needs and desires are almost always subordinated to the medical interpretation of the best interests of the baby as the all-important product of this "manufacturing process." Individuals who see the world this way often criticize home-birthers as selfish and irresponsible for putting their own desires above their baby's needs. But the holistic worldview of these home-birthers insists that, just as mother and baby form part of one integral and indivisible unit until birth, so the safety of the baby and the emotional needs of the mother are also one. The safest birth for the baby will be the one that provides the most nurturing environment for the mother.[4] Said Tara, "The bottom line was that I felt safer [at home], and I think that's what it boils down to for most people. . . . It seemed strange to me that people feel safer with the drugs and machines." Elizabeth noted, "My safest place is my bed. That's where I feel the most protected and the most nurtured. And so I knew that was where I had to give birth." And Ryla added,

> I got criticized for choosing a home birth, for not considering the safety of the baby. But that's exactly what I *was* considering! How could it possibly serve my baby for me to give birth in a place that causes my whole body to tense up in anxiety as soon as I walk in the door?

In the hospital, the uterus is viewed as an involuntary muscle that labors mechanically in response to hormonal signals. In contrast, all of the home-birthers were attended by midwives who see the uterus as a responsive part of the whole, and who therefore believe that the best labor care will involve attention to the mother's emotional and spiritual—as well as her physical—needs:

> Nikki [the midwife] kind of got worried about it toward the afternoon. Because it just kept going on and nothing was changing. And she took me to the shower and said, "Just stay in there till the hot water goes away." . . . And then Nikki asked my friend Diane, "What's the deal with Susan? . . . Is she stressed out about work?" And Diane said, "Well, yeah, I think she's afraid . . . that once she's had the baby . . . she's not going to be able to go back to her job." So when I came back out, Nikki started in on me about it. She said, "Right now your job is not important. What you have to do right now is have this baby. This baby is important." And I just burst into tears and was screaming at her and started crying, and I could feel everything when I started crying just relax. It all went out of me and then my water broke and we had a baby in 30 minutes. Just like that.

Just as the principle of separation governs many domains of life for the hospital-birthers in this study, so the principles of integration and interconnectedness govern the lifestyles of these home-birthers.[5] Many of them work in family enterprises centered around the home, and some of them also home-school their children. Susan, a newspaper editor, reports that she is learning to put the principle of giving up control to use in the office and is finding that the results include lowered stress levels and improved relationships with subordinates, who feel freer to innovate and take on more responsibility as she becomes less controlling. She uses her experience of birth to conceptualize more concretely her link to all of life:

> Birth is what ties us to other forms of life, creates a bond between human women that goes back hundreds of generations, and bonds us to other species as well. The more technological birth becomes, the more it differentiates us, and the more unlike other species—and other members of our own species—we become.

Tara's vision of the future makes an explicit connection between the ecological principles of the environmental movement and home birth:

> Mother Earth has historically been seen as feminine. If we get back to caring about the Earth, being caretakers, it would be difficult not to translate that into other parts of our lives. Sooner or later people will ask themselves how they can give birth drugged and hooked up to machines, when they are trying to stop treating their own Mother Earth that way.

BODY IMAGE AND SOCIETY

In the 1920s and 1930s, many American women eagerly sought hospital birth because of the freedom it provided from their regular household work cycles (Wertz & Wertz, 1989). Hand in hand with this freedom went a redefinition of the roles of women in American society. Formerly, a woman's place was in the home. Her primary duties were childbearing, nursing, and childrearing. Longing to be emancipated from these burdens, women found the beginnings of that emancipation in the removal of the birthplace to the hospital. For accompanying this shift in birthplace was a shift in society's definition of women's bodies, reflecting a cultural reconstruction of femininity and the female role. As long as women gave birth exclusively in the home, that home remained their exclusive domain, excluding them by definition from participation in the wider world and its challenges. To reconceptualize birth as a mechanical process best handled by trained technicians and machines was to remove its feminine mystique, and, in so doing, to remove the mystique from the feminine. When separated from the biological "earthiness" that had so long kept them down, women were to be freer than they had been for countless centuries in the West, finally given license to seek equal opportunity with men in the nonbiological arena of the workplace.

Pursuing this trend to its logical conclusion, we might well expect that today's highly competitive professional women would wish to identify with their earthy biological selves and the confines of the domestic realm even less than their turn-of-the-century sisters who paved the way for them. Although today's holistically oriented birth practitioners make earnest and sincere efforts to help their clients both desire and achieve self-empowering natural childbirth—an ideal still highly valued by many—the professional women in this particular study do not want such services. They want plenty of education and personal attention, but not when it is framed under a holistic paradigm; in fact, they perceive the holism of the home-birthers described above as frightening, irresponsible, limiting, and, *dis*empowering. Whereas home-birthers see the hospital as out-of-control technology running wild over women's bodies, these professionals experience the hospital and its technology as liberating them from the tyranny of biology and empowering them to stay in control of an out-of-control biological experience; for them, Punch Two is indeed the point.

Some social scientists suggest that such feelings of being empowered and in control are illusory, and that losing control in birth "can mean having one's body physically penetrated [by] cesarean section" (Martin, 1990, p. 309). But for these professional women (one of whom scheduled her cesarean to take place between conference calls), having a cesarean is not losing control but gaining it—given the models of reality they individually hold. Regardless of how they came to believe in the value of technological control over their imperfect, mechanistic bodies, the fact that they do believe in and value such control is not an illusion, and their feelings of empowerment when they achieve such control through the agencies of the professionals they have hired for that purpose—their physicians—are not illusions either. It is a cultural reality that those who participate most fully in a society's hegemonic core value system, as these women do, are most likely to be empowered by and to succeed within that system, as these women have.

The dichotomies between mind and body, mother and child, that provide so much structural tension in the lives of the pregnant professionals in this study constitute a fulcrum for the swirlings of cultural change. Most of that change seems to be heading in the direction of intensified separation between these categories, including the phenomena of surrogacy, test-tube babies, and similar directions in reproductive research. But a vast cultural movement, which includes home-birthers and unnumbered others concerned with holistic health, is organizing around the alternative concept of mind-body integration. In the oppositions between self and body that define the lives of the professional women in this study, we can read, writ small, the paradigmatic struggles that are defining opposing movements and trends within American society. We would do well to recall that not only the lifestyle and worldview, but also the defining values and environmental relationships of an entire society are often encapsulated in the self- and body images of its individual members.

NOTES

1. For a full analysis of obstetrical procedures and their often-detrimental effects on labor, see Chalmers, Enkin, & Keirse, 1989; Davis-Floyd, 1992, pp. 76-150; Goer, 1995.

2. This quotation is published with permission of the *San Francisco Chronicle*. The article appeared in *The Chronicle* on September 22, 1988.

3. Eleven of these interviews were conducted and transcribed by the following students: Kim Durham, Melody Hatsfield, Courtney Hollyfield, Mark Thompson, and Erin Rogers. I wish to express my appreciation to these students for their hard work and enthusiasm.

4. For a thorough review of recent studies on the safety of planned, midwife-attended home birth, see Goer, 1995.

5. For the sake of brevity, I use the labels *professionals* and *home-birthers* in this chapter. But it is important to keep in mind that this simple dichotomy is misleading: four of the home-birth mothers in my study have professional careers. For a more complete discussion of the overlap between these groups, see Davis-Floyd, 1994.

REFERENCES

Ashford, J. I. (1984). Doing it myself. In J. I. Ashford (Ed.), *Birth stories: The experience remembered*. New York: The Crossing Press.

Chalmers, I., Enkin, M., & Keirse, M. (1989). *Effective care in pregnancy and childbirth*. Oxford: Oxford University Press.

d'Aquilli, E. G., & Laughlin, C. D. (1979). The neurobiology of myth and ritual. In E. G. d'Aquilli, C. D. Laughlin, & J. McManus (Eds.), *The spectrum of ritual: A biogenetic structural analysis* (pp. 152-182). New York: Columbia University Press.

Davis-Floyd, R. E. (1987). Obstetric training as a rite of passage. *Medical Anthropology Quarterly, 1*(3), 288-318.

Davis-Floyd, R. E. (1990). The role of American obstetrics in the resolution of cultural anomaly. *Social Science and Medicine, 31*(2), 175-189.

Davis-Floyd, R. E. (1992). *Birth as an American rite of passage*. Berkeley and London: University of California Press.

Davis-Floyd, R. E. (1994). The technocratic body: American childbirth as cultural expression. *Social Science and Medicine, 38*(8), 1125-1140.

Goer, H. (1995). *Medical myths and research realities*. New Haven, CT: Bergin & Garvey.

Lex, B. (1979). The neurobiology of ritual trance. In E. G. d'Aquilli, C. D. Laughlin, & J. McManus (Eds.), *The spectrum of ritual: A biogenetic structural analysis* (pp. 117-151). New York: Columbia University Press.

Luria, A. R. (1966). *Higher cortical functions in man*. New York: Basic Books.

Martin, E. (1990). The ideology of reproduction: The reproduction of ideology. In F. Ginsburg & A. L. Tsing (Eds.), *Uncertain terms: Negotiating gender in American society*. Boston: Beacon.

McCarthy, M. (1963). *The group*. New York: Harcourt Brace Jovanavich.

Reynolds, P. C. (1991). *Stealing fire: The mythology of the technocracy*. Palo Alto, CA: Iconic Anthropology Press.

Richards, H. (1993, May). Cultural messages of childbirth: The perpetration of fear. *International Journal of Childbirth Education, 7*(3), 28.

Turner, V. (1969). *The ritual process: Structure and antistructure*. Chicago: Aldine.

Turner, V. (1979). Betwixt and between: The liminal period in rites de passage. In W. Lessa & E. Z. Vogt (Eds.), *Reader in comparative religion* (4th ed., pp. 234-243). New York: Harper & Row. (Original work published 1964)

Wertz, R. W., & Wertz, D. C. (1989). *Lying-in: A history of childbirth in America* (2nd ed.). New Haven, CT: Yale University Press.

8 The Caretakers of Suffering

JANICE MORSE
HELEN WHITAKER
MARITZA CERDAS TASÓN

> Nurses who work in the hospital work with patients who have ongoing, irreversible, irretrievable suffering. Physical suffering, emotional suffering, mental suffering—anguish beyond belief.[1]

Earlier in this century, the responsibility for providing such care moved from the home to the hospital, and the responsibility for caring for the sick shifted from the extended family to the nurse. This trend is now reversing. With the increasing costs of hospitalization the care of the chronically, terminally, and less acutely ill is once more being returned to the family. However, with the disintegration of the extended family and neighborhoods, family caring has been irrevocably altered. No longer is a multigenerational, extended family living in close proximity, so that care may be provided within the context of a supportive kin network. Rather, the caregiving responsibilities are now the responsibility of one person, usually a spouse, a parent, or an adult child of the ill person, with the support, guidance, and limited assistance of professional services, nursing, social work, and organizations in the community, such as day care for Alzheimer's patients. A backup system of community houses, such as homes for care of those with AIDS, or terminal care, such as hospice, also compensates, in part, for care previously provided by the hospital.

The transference of the dependent ill from homes to hospitals, occurring prior to 1950, placed the suffering of the ill beyond the awareness of the family and the visibility of the community and into the purview of nursing. Family members were often excluded by hospital regulations from witnessing the patient's suffering, and perhaps they accepted this without guilt, believing that their loved ones were "in good hands." Family members became visitors to those who were in pain or dying—transitory companions—rather than managing the daily (and nightly) pain and incontinence: the feeding, bathing, monitoring, and orienting of their relative.

This shift of care to the hospital created profound ethical and moral dilemmas for nursing. As a profession, nursing does not have control of treatments for the ill. A nurse, for example, can request an analgesic to be ordered, but the type of analgesic, the dosage, and how often it may be given—even if it is prescribed or not—is in the control of physicians who are not actual witnesses to the suffering of the patients. The dilemma of the nursing profession is that it does not have control—or has only limited control—over the alleviation of suffering, yet nurses are required to observe and are mandated to relieve the suffering.

Nurses' work and witness have remained silenced, concealed "behind the screens" (Lawler, 1991)—silenced by legal and professional regulations designed to ensure patient confidentiality, muffled by societal norms of what constituted "polite" and appropriate topics of conversation, and constrained by the reluctance of the populace to hear the unpleasant, even horrifying, aspects of illness. Hollywood has portrayed death by illness as a quiet "slipping away," rather than something that is possibly an agonizing, air-hungry experience that distorts one's body and removes one's control of bodily functions. Dying is often a tumultuous experience with distress that assaults all of the senses. It may occur noisily or quietly. And it may occur with uncertainty and ambiguity, for there is often no definite moment demarcating its onset, and the coldness and stiffness seem disconcertingly unreal to relatives.

Unlike the nurse, medical practitioners are removed from observing unrelenting suffering. They remain at a patient's bedside and view patient suffering for only a few minutes each day, as they transiently move through their rounds, monitoring the patient's progress by reviewing laboratory reports and nurses' records, the only contact with patients being brief, physical examinations. Although this system enables physicians to provide care to the maximum number of patients, this style of care also removes physicians from observing patients' suffering. It is the nurse who spends hours, days, and sometimes weeks with the patient.

The changing family structure, as well as the loss of a generation of caregivers in the home able to provide competent care, will not permit the nature of caregiving to return to the norm earlier in this century. Rather, the pattern and nature of care in the home will be dramatically altered, and nurses will continue to be primarily responsible for care of the suffering in the homes and for teaching comforting measures. However, with the return of the suffering to the home, the suffering experience will no longer be silenced. As suffering is an experience that is shared with the caregiver, the return to home care will once more bring suffering into the awareness of the family and the community. Suffering will again be visible, all day and every day. We argue that this renewed awareness—and social responsibility for suffering—will bring profound moral and legal changes in care. Nursing care provided in the community will be increased, both in coverage and in the nature of support provided to families. Community support to relieve the family of care, such as day care and hospice hostels, will become commonplace. But most dramatically, needless suffering will not be tolerated; new methods to control pain will be given research priority, new social responsibility for the support of caregivers will eventually arise, and the recent emerging trends of assisted suicide and euthanasia as methods of alleviating suffering will increase.

WHAT IS SUFFERING?

Suffering has been defined as the emotional response to that which was being endured (Morse & Carter, 1996). It requires acceptance of one's condition. Those who are suffering are aware of their condition and the ramifications of their suffering for the future.

Suffering may be caused by the illness itself, by the illness experience, by pain, or by other symptoms. Alternatively, suffering may be caused by the *meaning* that the illness has for the person (Cassell, 1991); the meaning of the prognosis (such as the fear of dying); or the ramifications of the illness (such as the loss of mobility or the change of lifestyle resulting from the disease or injury) (Morse & Carter, 1995). Suffering may also be experienced by those close to the ill person, as they witness that person's suffering. Suffering is visible in the ill person's expressions and posture, and it is transmitted through empathetic association, so that others accompanying the suffering person experience a similar affect.

Caregivers may experience suffering as they observe another, even if the afflicted person is not suffering, per se. Caregivers may suffer as they mourn loss and death, observe the changes that illness has brought, or watch the daily struggle against pain and disability. For example, with some conditions, such as advanced Alzheimer's disease, the afflicted people may be unaware of their condition and may even forget the identity of their own family. This does not exempt their caregivers from suffering; caregivers mourn the loss of the person and experience immense suffering for the loss of the past, the lost present, and the lost shared future. The critical factor is that the experience of suffering is communicated to others and shared. Because suffering is an emotional response, suffering is manifest emotionally in the expression, the voice, and the posture of the sufferer. Thus, the degree of suffering is visible to others and may be assessed by another.

THE RAMIFICATIONS OF SUFFERING FOR NURSES

In the conduct of their daily work, nurses in hospitals perform many tasks that bring comfort to patients, are necessary for their survival or recuperation, and bring satisfaction to both nurse and patients. Other tasks may be accomplished routinely, with little, if any, emotional investment by the nurse—tasks that have little significance to the patient or of which the patient may not even be aware. Other tasks demand an enormous emotional investment on the part of the nursing staff. These include instances that involve the infliction of pain; the inability to relieve excruciating or prolonged pain; involvement in extraordinary medical procedures that have little, if any therapeutic gain; and feelings of impotence about the course of the nurse's own involvement in carrying out a perceived useless or unnecessary medical order.

Rushton (1992) notes that nurses describe "intense emotional responses in relation to their clinical encounters" (p. 30). Not only do nurses respond to their patients' physical plight, but they also identify with the patients' responses as a *person*—to the

> indignity of being seriously ill, the damage to their self-image, the depletion of their financial resources, the stress of loved ones who desperately

hope for recovery, and the anxiety resulting from the overwhelming sense of powerlessness over a situation beyond their control (p. 303).

MODES OF CONTROLLING CAREGIVER SUFFERING

It's almost essential to get through your daily task, that you dehumanize the person in the bed. Otherwise, you can't do those things that are inhumane.

Since Nightingale, nurses have been trained to develop a paradoxical stance toward their patients. They must be simultaneously detached, yet caring (Reverby, 1987); they must serve as a patient advocate without becoming involved (Morse, 1991). And while *caring* for the patients, they are often required to inflict pain and provide care that, to the patient, does not appear to be in the patient's best interest. In these instances, the patient may try to resist care or become angry and abusive toward the nurse, further adding to the nurse's conflict.[2]

Nurses resolve this apparent contradiction of caring for a patient while maintaining or increasing the patient's suffering by dehumanizing and objectifying the patient (Gadow, 1990). If nurses "forget" that the patient is a person, that the patient is human, the process of caring for the patient becomes easier. If the patient does not respond normally or if the patient does not respond at all, he or she may be treated as an object, without the nurse's awareness.

A second technique nurses use in order to be able to inflict pain is to focus on the immediate task, for example, as illustrated in the next quotation, to focus on the dressing, thereby ignoring the ramifications of their actions. This technique may unexpectedly fail:

In the burn unit, we had a man with 90 percent burns, and facial burns, and he had a suture through his eyelid. Both eyelids. And, we would do his full face dressing, and then what we would do would be gently pull the suture to pull the lid down over totally unseeing eyes and then finish, finish the dressing. And, I worked with one of the most talented, skilled burn unit nurses . . . and she pulled the suture to pull that eyelid down gently and it flaked off in her hand.

[The whole eyelid?] Yeah. And, uh, she had a blink, blink experience. Only hers involved having to sit down, put her head between her knees, *because she had not seen him as a person who could see.* She saw him as a set of dressings that needed to be done, and, and so, when the, when the lid came off, and she saw an eye, and she said later, "I just never thought of him as seeing. So why on earth am I doing dressings on a person who's never going to see again?"

And then she said, "He's never going to have an erection again because he had his leg and his genitals burnt off." She went on, she said, "Well, there you are from one end to another." Now, we, we did lose her out of nursing. She won't nurse anymore.

When the nurse is performing tasks, fulfilling physicians' orders in the course of providing care, these tasks are much more difficult to do if the patient responds, or is responsive:

We had a lady who had a plate that had been implanted in her skull, [and it] became infected and then they removed it. And—the process of disease caused her brain to expand and explode through her skull, so that when we did her dressing, we actually were wiping up brain tissue, and, yet her eyes were open and would sometimes follow you.

In the next quotation, a nurse tells how the process of depersonalization was complete for some members of the staff. When a nurse realized that "there was a *person* in the bed," she was so shocked that, without the special support of her peers, she would have left nursing:

One day, I took this patient—she smelled so gross, and she was just, sort of really decomposing, like—bladder tissue was coming out into her urine. [It was] not just urine. And, it was of a color and a consistency that was so gross that, that you or I, if you wanted to project quality of life onto her . . . you, that you would not wish this ever. And, when you looked at the picture at her bedside, and you saw this gracious elegant lady with beautiful long hands, playing the piano. . . . I always called her Jane, I always spoke with her, I've always done that, regardless of whatever we knew their *Glasgow Coma* score to be. And she smelled so, so dreadful that we put her in a semi-private room, alone, because we couldn't put another patient in with her.

And, one day I was bathing her and turning her and talking to her, and one of the nurses came into the room and said, "Who are talking to?" And I said to her, "Jane, I'm talking to Jane," and she sort of went, blink, blink—you know—my God! And that's a nurse who had worked a long time on that floor, you know. [She thought] "My God. There's a person in that bed?" Yeah. . . . She just had a—insight, an instantaneous insight that she hadn't thought of this person in the bed as a person. She asked me, "Who was I talking to? Did you think someone was in the room with you?" You know. And, certainly we did laugh about it. But she wept. She was

> horrified. She was so distressed, she didn't work for two weeks. She didn't work for two weeks. And I knew that we were in danger of losing her [from nursing].

Nurses are often involved with the providing of extraordinary care—treatments and procedures—to patients. These tasks require commitment and strength and involve personal cost. Nurses observe suffering and cause suffering in their daily work, yet these roles are poorly understood by the public and overshadowed by the image of the nurse as an *alleviator* of suffering. Hospitals have served to silence suffering, to conceal suffering from families and from the public, and nurses have played a significant role in this silencing.[3]

WHY HAS SUFFERING BEEN HIDDEN?

It is an ethical and professional requirement that nurses do not speak of patients outside of the hospital. Patient care is confidential, and nurses are taught that, when discussing incidences, even if they omit patients' names, such chatter jeopardizes patient confidentiality and places the hospital at risk. As a result, nurses cannot "debrief" when they leave the hospital. And, in spite of some hospital-based programs for debriefing and supporting staff after, for example, a serious accident, most nurses obtain emotional release informally. Nurses talk to one another on breaks and during quiet moments on the floor or cry quietly alone. The extent of the suffering remains unrecorded, in a pact of silence between the nurse and the patient.

Informal mechanisms for the expression of suffering are, for the nurses, largely inadequate and unsatisfactory. All nurses have haunting nightmares, imprinted within their consciousness. A nurse who had worked in the burn unit spoke of these horrors—of doing burn dressings for inadequately sedated patients and having the patients "screaming personal invectives at the nurses. Screaming in excruciating pain, and blaming the dressing do-er for it. . . . must tell you, I would never go back to *that* nursing." These incidents leave "incredible visual[s] to this day"—nightmares that reoccur. Nurses feel the weight of their involvement in the provision of such care and the suffering inflicted. In an interview, a nurse noted that the informal policy appeared to be: "To save a life, no matter what. . . . If there was a scrap of life . . . we preserved what we believed to be life, and what was promoted as hope."

But not all of the responsibility for maintaining the silence around suffering falls on the shoulders and the conscience of nursing. Other factors include the societal value of the maintenance of life at any cost, the maintenance of the medical myths that research may change the prognosis at any time, the maintenance of the "condition comfortable" myth, the devaluing of the experiential component of illness, and the Christian value on the maintenance of life. Each of these other contributing factors will be discussed briefly.

1. *Societal value of the maintenance of life at any cost.* Society at large has condoned and has conferred to the courts and to the medical establishment the right to force the maintenance of life at any cost (see, e.g., Birnie & Rodriguez, 1994).

2. *The maintenance of the medical myth of the power of research to cure.* A persuasive argument for the continuance of life is the hope of a "miracle cure" at any time, preferably as soon as possible. There is a disproportionate amount of research funding that is provided for research of cures and relatively little funding for the other components of care: prevention and care for the afflicted. AIDS is an excellent example of such a disease; after more than a decade, medical researchers have still not identified a vaccine to prevent AIDS. The only mode of prevention is through the use of education and prevention programs, such as the provision of free condoms or a needle exchange program. The most important contribution to care is through the provision of palliative care in the late stages. Despite this, government funding continuously focuses on medical research, while the epidemic reaches pandemic proportions.

3. *The condition-comfortable myth and minimizing of the illness experience.* What is *condition comfortable*? Does it mean that the patient no longer is in pain? Not necessarily. Does it mean that the patient is comfortable? Not necessarily. Condition comfortable is a euphemism for public disclosure that the patient is, perhaps, not about to die (is not critical) or may die (condition serious). It is, therefore, a system of rating and communicating patient morbidity to the public.

4. *The devaluing of the experiential component of illness.* Suffering and pain are frequently not objectively measured, and the amount of pain, or the degree of suffering experienced, must be verbally described by the patient to the physician or the nurse. These verbal descriptions may not be considered valid, and the onus remains with the patient to convince the caregivers that the pain is legitimate.

5. *Suffering for the continuance of life.* The Christian ethic values noble suffering. Suffering is not considered something that should necessarily be alleviated, and life is valued as sacred.

Thus suffering, and the work of nurses in concealing and managing it, is condoned by society at large. Although nurses have all the responsibility for the care of suffering, they have no control over the nature of the treatment but must defer to physicians; they are actually acting on behalf of physicians in carrying out the medical orders. Individuals in such situations have been described by Wolgast (1992) as "artificial persons"—a person who "acts in the name of someone else" (p. 1). Wolgast notes that the use of the artificial person introduces moral conflicts, because it prevents us from assuming individual responsibility. In this case, suffering becomes embedded in an institution, constrained but not understood by the medical profession at large.

THE EVOLVING DEINSTITUTIONALIZATION OF SUFFERING

> Because the health care system intrinsically obscures the fact of suffering, nurses have a moral obligation to speak out about the suffering they witness. (Kahn & Steeves, 1994, p. 260)

The first movement toward deinstitutionalization came in the 1970s with the rapid deinstitutionalization of psychiatric patients into the community to organized and less formal community-living arrangements. The movement was so extensive that large institutions were vacated. Despite criticism that this move led to increased numbers of homeless people and to lack of care for former patients because of inadequate community resources, there has been no effort to return to the former level of institutionalization for the mentally ill.

Citing the escalating cost of the health care system, the patient length of stay has been steadily decreasing (U.S. Department of Health and Human Services, 1994). Postoperative stays are being reduced and preoperative stays shortened, with most of the preoperative tests performed on an outpatient basis. Sick care in the home is now being provided to increasingly sicker family members, and acute care in hospitals is correspondingly increasing. In addition, while patients are remaining in their homes with increasingly serious conditions, home care is becoming more complex. For example, thousands of children on respirators are being cared for in the home. More of the frail elderly are remaining in their homes, and frailty has now been labeled a national epidemic (National Institute on Aging, 1992); those with terminal illness such as cancer and AIDS are dying at home (Carney, 1990; Kelly, Chu, Buehler, & The AIDS Mortality Project Group, 1993).

Gerontologists have been quick to note that passing care onto the family is not simple. The first problem is to identify the family, so that appropriate support and referrals can be made (Keating, Kerr, Warren, Grace, & Wertenberger, 1994). Keating et al. (p. 271) note that the rhetoric of "family caregiving" is simply a euphemism for the care provided by female family members, often one member. Secondary caregivers may provide informal support, but the burden of care invariably and disproportionally falls on one person.

THE RESPONSES OF FAMILY CAREGIVERS

Regardless of the actual training of family caregivers on how to do actual caregiving tasks (such as monitoring medications, lifting, bathing, or giving injections), the vigilance required for the consistent monitoring and continuous observing of the suffering eventually becomes unbearable. "Caregiver burnout" is a disease of the 1980s and 1990s; the provision of respite care and the increase of assistance provided by secondary caregivers will not eliminate it (Motenko, 1989). The witnessing of suffering—the 24-hour suffering in the home—has removed the silence imposed on nurses and introduced new and important social and legal issues of euthanasia—often conducted by the caregiver out of mercy and desperation—and assisted suicide, with the involvement and permission of the primary caregiver.

The witnessing of suffering is provided as reason for the mercy killing of those who are provided care in the home. Despite the knowledge that the legal ramifications of the action will be a charge of first-degree murder, these killings continue to occur at a significant rate. For example, a 75-year-old retired electronic engineer shot his wife of 51 years. It was reported that she had Alzheimer's disease and osteoporosis, and he would not allow her to live her life as "a suffering animal" (Rosenblatt, 1985). He was convicted and sentenced to twenty-five years in prison.

Not all of these mercy killings occur among the elderly. In a rural Saskatchewan case, a man was found guilty of second-degree murder for killing his 12-year-old daughter with carbon monoxide fumes in the cab of his truck. The girl was severely mentally retarded and physically disabled by cerebral palsy. She required constant and complete care; either he or his wife had to be with her constantly, taking turns to sit with her throughout the night—in addition to caring for their other three children and running the farm. The girl's life was being sustained by medical science; she had a feeding tube through her abdomen into her stomach and had undergone repeated surgeries. She was in constant pain and had been scheduled for another surgery when her father decided that his daughter has "suffered enough" (Jenish, 1994).

THE RESPONSE OF THE COMMUNITY

The response of the community to alleviating suffering through assisted suicide is divided (Jonsen, 1993). However, in the nursing and medical communities, there is some direction, both formal and informal, toward the right to die, thus easing the responsibility of the staff. The conflict still may occur in crisis situations, such as a "code," and the development of legal means to avoid extraordinary measures in the maintenance of life.

Stringent guidelines have been developed for ceasing resuscitative efforts; "Do not resuscitate" orders appear with more frequency on patient charts, and when they do not appear, the staff have developed an informal system of a "slow code" (of walking, rather than running) when responding to monitor alarms from a patient who has little opportunity for life. However, once life-maintenance measures have been instituted, they remain difficult to remove, even with the full support of the family or at the plea of the patient (Birnie & Rodriguez, 1994).

When life-maintenance measures have not been instituted and when suffering is overwhelming, the role of the caregiver is most conflicted. In the medical and nursing community, the dilemma has been brought to the fore with the Kevorkian cases. What is legal in the Netherlands (Pollard, 1991; van der Sluis, 1989)—physician-assisted suicide—is being challenged case by case by Dr. Jack Kevorkian, in defiance of court orders. Internationally, organizations such as the World Federation of the Right to Die Societies; The Hemlock Society, founded in the United States in 1980; and, in Canada, the Toronto-based Dying with Dignity Society and the Right to Die Society of Canada in Victoria, provide support and information for individuals and caregivers and lobby for changes in legislation. Nevertheless, the medical establishment appears pessimistic that the legalization of euthanasia will resolve the needs of people who are suffering interminably, and many believe it will create unforeseen dilemmas. Burgess (1983, p. 268), for example, argues that the caregivers' cost "to assist suffering persons to make their continued suffering tolerable" will cast doubts on the choice of active euthanasia.

NURSING'S EVOLVING ROLE IN ALLEVIATING SUFFERING

The present trend of dehospitalization is again returning those who are suffering to the care of the family—but to a family that is not prepared to provide care for the sufferer. Caregiver research has demonstrated that home care is not "cheap" if the care is to be both adequate and appropriate. Yet today, most of the responsibility for the provision of home care falls on a single individual—usually female (Logue, 1993). A salary for the caregiver frequently is not considered in the caregiver costs, and the bombardment of constant care without respite, the lack of support from others, and the lack of professional support from nurses result in rapid burnout.

The trend toward dehospitalization continues, and a void for the care of the suffering in the home and the community continues to exist. This gap must be filled quickly and responsibly by nurses. With renewed role maturity and independent practice, nurses may participate in the care and alleviation of suffering, in decision making, and in strategies for the alleviation of suffering.

NOTES

1. The quotations used in this chapter are from interviews conducted from 1991 to 1994 on suffering and the nurse's role in providing comfort. The research is supported by NIH NINR 2R01 NR02130-07 to Dr. Morse. The views expressed in this article are the authors' own.

2. From Hinds (1992), it is evident that this problem is not confined to nurses as caregivers or to acute care.

3. Kahn and Steeves (1994) suggest it is the moral responsibility of nursing to give voice to suffering, and the primary mechanism for this will be through the use of narrative inquiry.

REFERENCES

Birnie, L. H., & Rodriguez, S. (1994). *Uncommon will: The death and life of Sue Rodriguez.* Toronto: Macmillan Canada.

Burgess, M. M. (1983). The medicalization of dying. *Journal of Medicine and Philosophy, 18*(3) 269-279.

Carney, K. L. (1990). AIDS care comes home: Balancing benefits and difficulties. *Home Health Care Nurse, 8*(2), 32-37.

Cassel, E. J. (1991). *The nature of suffering and the goals of medicine.* New York: Oxford University Press.

Gadow, S. (1990). The advocacy covenant: Care as clinical subjectivity. In J. Stevenson & T. Tripp-Reimer (Eds.), *Knowledge about care and caring* (pp. 33-40). Kansas City, MO: American Academy of Nursing.

Hinds, C. (1992). Suffering: A relatively unexplored phenomenon among family caregivers of noninstitutionalized patients with cancer. *Journal of Advanced Nursing, 17,* 918-925.

Jenish, D. (1994). What would you do? *Maclean's, 107*(48), 16-20.

Jonsen, A. R. (1993). Living with euthanasia: A futuristic scenario. *Journal of Medicine and Philosophy, 18*(3), 241-251.

Kahn, D. L., & Steeves, R. H. (1994). Witness to suffering: Nursing knowledge, voice, and vision. *Nursing Outlook, 42*(6), 260-264.

Keating, N., Kerr, K., Warren, S., Grace, M., & Wertenberger, D. (1994). Who's the family in family caregiving? *Canadian Journal on Aging, 13*(4), 268-287.

Kelly, J. J., Chu, S. Y., Buehler, J. W., & The AIDS Mortality Project Group. (1993). AIDS deaths shift from hospital to home. *American Journal of Public Health, 83,* 1433-1437.

Lawler, J. (1991). *Behind the screens: Nursing, somology, and the problem of the body.* Edinburgh: Churchill Livingstone.

Logue, B. J. (1993). *Last rights: Death control and the elderly in America.* New York: Lexington Books.

Mor, V., & Kidder, D. (1995). Cost saving in hospice: Final results of the National Hospice Study. *Health Survey Research, 20,* 15.

Morse, J. M. (1991). Negotiating commitment and involvement in the patient-nurse relationship. *Journal of Advanced Nursing, 16,* 455-468.

Morse, J. M., & Carter, B. (1995). Strategies of enduring and the suffering of loss: Modes of comfort used by a resilient survivor. *Holistic Nursing Practice, 9*(5), 33-58.

Morse, J. M., & Carter, B. (1996). The essence of enduring and the expressions of suffering: The reformulation of the self. *Journal of Scholarly Inquiry for Nursing Practice, 10*(1).

Motenko, A. (1989). The frustrations, gratifications, and well-being of dementia caregivers. *Gerontologist, 29,* 166-172.

National Institute on Aging. (1992). *Physical frailty: A reducible barrier to independence for older Americans* (NIH Publication No. 91-397). Washington, DC: Department of Health and Human Services, Public Health Service.

Pollard, B. J. (1991). Medical aspects of euthanasia. *Medical Journal of Australia, 154,* 613-616.

Reverby, S. M. (1987). *Ordered to care: The dilemma of American nurses: 1850-1945.* Cambridge, MA: Cambridge University Press.

Rosenblatt, R. (1985, August 26). The quality of mercy killing. *Time, 126,* 74.

Rushton, C. H. (1992). Caregiver suffering in critical care nursing. *Heart & Lung, 21*(3), 303-306.

U.S. Department of Health and Human Services. (1994, May). *Health, United States, 1993* (DDHS Pub No. PHS 94-1232). Hyattsville, MD: Centers for Disease Control & Prevention, National Center for Health Statistics.

van der Sluis, I. (1989). The practice of euthanasia in the Netherlands. *Issues in Law and Medicine, 4*, 455-465.

Wolgast, E. (1992). *Ethics of an artificial person: Lost responsibility in professions and organizations*. Stanford, CA: Stanford University Press.

9 Aboriginal Healing and Its Relevance for Nonaboriginals

DAVID E. YOUNG

Shamanism is associated, by many, with indigenous peoples living at a hunting and gathering level in non-Western societies. It should be remembered, however, that at one time, some form of shamanism[1] was practiced by nearly everyone around the world. Therefore, shamanism is part of the legacy of both Western and non-Western cultures. Moreover, it is still a vital force in the world today. It is practiced by a variety of aboriginal groups on every continent, and it is undergoing a revitalization in many aboriginal communities. Shamanism also has growing appeal for individuals living in industrial, urbanized settings. Suffering from various forms of alienation, many urban dwellers are searching for healthier ways to relate to themselves, to others, and to the environment. It is for these people that this chapter has been written.

Because Canadian aboriginal people do not use the terms *shaman* or *shamanism,* in the remainder of the chapter, I will use the terms *aboriginal healer* and *aboriginal healing practices.* It should be emphasized that this chapter is based on my experiences with aboriginal healers in the prairie provinces of Canada over the past ten years[2] and therefore should not be generalized to all North American aboriginal groups. The chapter will proceed from observations about the North American aboriginal worldview to a discussion of various aspects of aboriginal healing, and finally, to a discussion of the relevance of aboriginal healing for nonaboriginals.

NORTH AMERICAN ABORIGINAL WORLDVIEW

The Source of Life, referred to with terms such as *Great Spirit*, the *Great Mystery*, or *Wakan Tanka*, is so holy that many people believe it cannot be approached directly. There is, however, a sacred realm, referred to by many groups as the Grandfathers and Grandmothers, which is more accessible. It consists of the spirits of those individuals who have gone before, spirits associated with the primordial forces of nature (such as thunder, wind, and lightning), spirits associated with natural elements that have been present from the beginning (such as rocks); spirits associated with animal, bird, fish, insect, and plant species; and a variety of other spiritual forces. Collectively, this sacred realm is a repository of power and knowledge that can be revealed to individuals who "stay on the sweetgrass trail" (lead a good life) and cultivate a sacred attitude by participating in rituals such as fasting, meditation, and sweat lodge ceremonies. Power and knowledge from the sacred realm are conveyed to humans by spirit messengers who appear in dreams and visions as people and animals, or other recognizable forms. Spirit messengers are not really separate from the Great Mystery. Words like *spirits* are used to describe how humans experience the sacred realm, but the reality itself cannot be captured by such concepts. The sacred realm is timeless and spaceless—a dimension that, although hidden, is eternally present in each of us and in all of nature.

Any object from the natural world, such as a rock, tobacco, pipe, or eagle feather, can be dedicated for use in ceremony. After being dedicated, it serves as a bridge between us and the sacred realm. For example, in the sweat lodge ceremony, rocks are dedicated, heated, and placed in a pit in the center of a domed structure. From time to time, water is sprinkled on the hot rocks to release steam. Those who participate in the ceremony with the right attitude enter an altered state of consciousness in which visions can occur.

Power from the sacred realm can be used for both good and evil purposes. For example, power can be used to heal, or it can be projected as a curse to bring harm to others. As individuals mature in their spiritual practice, they are less tempted to use power in harmful ways. Those individuals who have attained the wisdom to use knowledge and power for the welfare and guidance of the group as a whole are referred to as *elders*. Elders are a priceless gift, without which aboriginal cultures would be lost. Healers, who frequently are also elders, are those who have embarked on a special path (usually involving apprenticeship) that involves learning how to use ceremonies and/or medicines to facilitate interaction with the sacred realm. Although healers may be selected as a result of demonstrating unusual abilities or charisma, they do not perform the healing themselves. They are conduits of knowledge and power from the sacred realm.

HOLISTIC NATURE OF ABORIGINAL HEALING

Aboriginal healing emphasizes that illness occurs when the natural equilibrium of the body is thrown out of balance by poor food, immoderate drinking and sex, emotions such as hatred or jealousy, lack of exercise and fresh air, or intrusive agents such as bacteria or "bad medicine." Therapy is designed to bring the body back into balance with the mind, emotions, and spirit. Therapy also involves helping individuals establish a healthy relationship with their family, community, and environment. Because therapy involves treating the entire person, the healer combines the roles of physician, psychologist, priest, and social worker.

THE HEALER AS PHYSICIAN

After an appropriate ritual (which in many areas of Canada involves presenting the healer with tobacco, a piece of colored cloth, or a colored ribbon, as well as a gift), the patient explains his or her problem and asks the healer for help. If the healer is familiar with the problem and knows that it can be alleviated, he or she may agree to assist. If the healer is not familiar with the problem, he or she may pray, meditate, or fast in order to achieve spiritual insight concerning the cause of the problem and how it should be treated. The initial goal of this spiritual diagnosis is to determine whether the patient is suffering from some kind of internal imbalance or whether an intrusive agent is involved. If the latter, the healer must determine if the agent is natural (such as a virus or bacteria) or sent by another human (as in the case of bad medicine). The two are not necessarily contradictory in the sense that the immediate cause may be a strain of bacteria, but the ultimate cause may be a human being who has caused the victim to be susceptible to the infectious agent.

If bad medicine is involved, a special ceremony may be performed to counteract its effect. If a natural cause is involved, the healer may use a variety of medicines, often in conjunction with special healing rituals, to treat the condition. One healer with whom I worked had a repertoire of at least forty herbs and a number of animal parts that he combined in numerous ways, depending on the condition being treated (Young, Ingram, & Swartz, 1989). Learning to identify the herbs, when to harvest them, how to process and preserve them, and how to combine them requires many years of learning and practical experience.

It is important to note that healers frequently refer a prospective patient to another healer, tell the patient to see a medical doctor, or advise the patient to go to a hospital for emergency treatment. Although aboriginal healers deal with a variety of problems, some healers are well-known for treating certain kinds of illness and may attract referrals from other healers on a regular basis. Most healers are reluctant to treat highly infectious diseases (which they recognize may require a modern drug) or advanced cases of a disease such as cancer. They frequently deplore the fact that aboriginal healing is often seen, even by aboriginal people, as a last resort—after everything else has failed.

THE HEALER AS PSYCHOLOGIST

Aboriginal healers recognize a close relationship between mind and body. It is recognized that an emotion such as guilt can cause an individual to fall ill or prevent the immune system from functioning at full capacity. Likewise, a physical ailment may lead to depression or other mental conditions that prevent an individual from leading a productive life. For this reason, a healer spends a good deal of time talking to patients, learning about their background, and finding out about their fears and aspirations. Treatment involves continual reinforcement—assuring patients that the Great Spirit has the power to heal, especially if a patient has faith.

The psychological sophistication of aboriginal healers can be illustrated by the principles employed in the sweat lodge ceremony (Swartz, 1988; Wilbush, 1988). The sweat lodge is a dome framed with willow saplings and covered with tarps to create a dark interior. Participants sit around a central hole into which are placed heated rocks. During the ceremony, herbs and water are sprinkled on the rocks to create a blast of medicated steam. The darkness, rhythmic chanting, and singing help induce an altered state in which participants are susceptible to suggestion and are encouraged to set aside rational thought for a more intuitive and spiritual mode of knowing. Patients are encouraged to verbally express their problems and needs, to confess misdeeds, and to ask forgiveness from the Great Spirit. Because of the heat, patients are forced to focus and ignore distracting thoughts; otherwise they could be burned. The combined effect of these techniques is a sense of physical, mental, emotional, and spiritual cleansing. In some cases, the altered state produces a vision in which a spiritual messenger brings special knowledge or healing.

THE HEALER AS PRIEST

An aboriginal healer attempts to bring about healing not only of the mind, body, and emotions but also of the spirit. The spirit of a person might be conceived as a part of the Great Spirit that dwells in everything—a part of the mind described above as the sacred realm of the Grandfathers and Grandmothers. Because the Great Spirit is part of us and we are part of the Great Spirit, we have a natural yearning for the sacred. But we become so engrossed in the pursuit of worldly affairs that this link with the sacred is forgotten. The role of the aboriginal healer is to help restore the sacred link. The healer performs this priestly function by conducting the sacred ceremonies passed down from previous generations.

THE HEALER AS SOCIAL WORKER

Aboriginal healers frequently deal with drug and alcohol abuse, as well as assisting in the rehabilitation of those convicted of crimes. An important aspect of therapy in such situations is to educate clients about the importance of regaining a balance between mind, body, emotions, and spirit, and the necessity of dispelling negative emotions and behaviors that cause disruption with loved ones, the community, and the environment. This kind of work takes aboriginal healers into a variety of institutions, such as schools, jails, and hospitals, and provides them with the opportunity to educate administrators and other officials on how to bring about change in behavior and attitude and how to help clients reintegrate into their communities following treatment or incarceration. In addition, aboriginal healers frequently work with the families of patients and clients as a social support system that is regarded as an important aspect of healing.

COMPARISON OF ABORIGINAL AND BIOMEDICAL TREATMENT STRATEGIES

Modern biomedicine is one of the greatest contributions of Western culture to the rest of the world. Created by the scientific revolution, biomedicine has led to significant breakthroughs in the control of infectious diseases, organ replacement, genetic engineering, and many other procedures beyond the scope of traditional therapies. Traditional therapies, on the other hand, appear to be more successful than biomedicine in treating some forms of chronic, stress-related diseases, mental illness, substance abuse, and psychosomatic illnesses. This generalization is controversial in that there has not been sufficient research done to provide conclusive support. Even so, increasing numbers of people appear to be turning to alternative and traditional therapies for help. Why is this the case? I will address this issue in terms of aboriginal healing, but the following suggestions apply to many other forms of alternative and traditional healing techniques as well.

GENERAL ORIENTATION

As argued above, aboriginal healing is holistic (directed at the entire person) whereas modern biomedicine is particularistic (directed at a specific disease). Specialization is useful if the source of the problem lies with a specific organ, such as the heart; but if illness is the result of an imbalance in the system, knowledge of specific parts of the body may be inadequate. Many physicians are not trained to diagnose and treat illness for which they can find no organic basis. Aboriginal healers, on the other hand, know that many illnesses can be alleviated only when the underlying emotional, spiritual, or social cause is addressed. Modern biomedicine is based on the faith that the most intractable diseases can be cured if more money is invested in basic research and technological innovation. Sometimes this is the case, but often a sympathetic ear and a little counseling can achieve a good deal.

INTERACTION WITH PATIENTS

Aboriginal healers maintain a normal interaction distance with patients, provide continuous verbal support, and engage in physical contact with patients (such as massage and application of lotions), whereas the physician maximizes physical distance while minimizing contact (Morse, Young, & Swartz, 1991). If contact is essential, the doctor usually wears gloves. The message communicated to patients differs accordingly. The aboriginal healer attempts to inspire self-confidence in the belief that a sense of self-worth and positive thinking play an important role in healing. The physician, perhaps knowingly, communicates a desire to distance himself or herself from patients and a belief that patients may be "dangerous." In addition, interaction with a physician tends to be brief, whereas interaction between patients and an aboriginal healer tends to be prolonged. Patients are given ample opportunity to list their symptoms, explore their feelings, and ask questions of the healer. This kind of personal interaction can bring a sense of profound relief to patients, who may be reluctant to discuss the problem with family or friends.

IS COLLABORATION POSSIBLE?

The purpose of the above comparison was not to suggest that aboriginal healing and other forms of alternative and traditional healing are superior to modern biomedicine. The point I have attempted to make is that although there is a good deal of overlap in conditions treated, biomedicine does some things better than aboriginal medicine and vice versa. This suggests the possibility of a collaborative model in which physicians and aboriginal healers work together to provide better care for patients. There are many types of collaborative models currently under study in Canada. To take three examples, Anishnawbe Health in Toronto, Ontario, is an inner-city clinic administered by aboriginals, whose mandate is to help meet the health needs of the numerous aboriginal people living in the Toronto area. Treatment is provided by aboriginal healers, assisted by biomedical personnel. The Royal Alexandria Hospital in Edmonton, Alberta, hired an aboriginal healer and his wife to conduct workshops on aboriginal culture for hospital staff who routinely deal with aboriginal patients. The hospital is also experimenting with a program that would see aboriginal healers, upon request, collaborate with biomedical personnel in the treatment of patients. A new hospital in White Horse, the capitol of the Yukon Territory, has a special room where aboriginal healers can conduct ceremonies and treat aboriginal patients. Such experiments indicate a growing tolerance on the part of the biomedical profession for alternative and traditional healing practices and a growing willingness on the part of aboriginal healers to cross cultural boundaries.

THE RELEVANCE OF ABORIGINAL HEALING FOR NONABORIGINALS

Growing collaboration between aboriginal healers and biomedical personnel may be beneficial for aboriginal people, but how can non-aboriginals benefit from aboriginal healing? One possibility is that physicians will begin to refer their patients to aboriginal healers in cases where aboriginal healing has been demonstrated to be superior to biomedicine. For example, a doctor friend of mine has referred patients to an aboriginal healer who has demonstrated success in treating psoriasis. Such referrals will undoubtedly become more common if aboriginal healing is legally recognized. An increasing number of people are not waiting for referrals but are seeking out aboriginal healers on their own, a trend that will increase as nonaboriginals learn more about aboriginal culture and the strengths of aboriginal healing.

But Canada is somewhat unique in the size of its aboriginal population and abundance of aboriginal healers. There are many areas in North America, as well as in other countries, in which indigenous populations have been eliminated, moved, or absorbed. In these areas, direct contact with an indigenous healer is unlikely for most people. Even in Canada, many aboriginal healers are worried about a major influx of nonaboriginal patients because interaction is time-consuming, and participation in rituals such as sweat lodge ceremonies is limited to a few people.

It is reasonable to assume that the major impact of aboriginal healing upon the broader society will be indirect rather than direct. For example, as biomedical personnel become better educated concerning the efficacy of aboriginal healing techniques, as well as other alternative therapies, they are beginning to adopt more holistic practices. This trend is being encouraged by the holistic health movement on the part of consumers who are demanding more broadly trained physicians and less reliance upon modern drugs and surgery.

Perhaps more important, many individuals are turning to traditional cultures for a more holistic set of values. There is a widespread prophesy among many North American aboriginal groups that eventually non-aboriginals would turn to them for knowledge about how to heal themselves and the planet. Some aboriginals feel that this prophesy is now being fulfilled; they believe that this is possible because aboriginal culture, long overlooked and even despised by many, is the repository of an ancient healing wisdom that the world once depended on and now needs again.

10 Yoga for Health and Freedom

B. K. S. IYENGAR
Compiled by DEAN LERNER

Ecology is concerned with both the individual and the environment. It is an intimate relationship. One cannot change without affecting the other. In the same way, Yoga is concerned with the individual developing and evolving personally, and within society and the world. Yoga touches a person's life at every level: physical, mental, and spiritual. It brings a dynamic state of health, vitality, and balance and a benevolence of mind for the yoga practitioner to be a positive example in the family, society, and world.

Yogacharya Shri B. K. S. Iyengar, world-renowned master of Yoga and author of the classic texts *Light on Yoga, Light on Pranayama, Light on the Yoga Sutras of Patanjali,* and numerous other books, expresses his thoughts on the subject of natural health in terms of the philosophy of life that he follows and practices, which has its roots in the ancient subject, Yoga. Iyengar states his view on health and life, "that it is a dynamic process like fire which goes on engulfing until there is space for the fire not to spread. Both health and life are like water of a river, which is ever new and fresh."[1]

What follows is an overall view and explanation of Yoga for true health adapted by Lerner from works by Iyengar, published with his permission.

A TRIUNE OF BODY, MIND, AND SOUL

Whether one wants to follow the science of duty, to earn a livelihood, or to enjoy life or to seek liberation, health is a *must,* as health is the *wealth* of everyone. The *Upanishads* proclaim that a weakling cannot enjoy the pleasures of the world nor become a master of the self.

It is said that man is a triune of body, mind, and Soul. The outer cover of the inner man is the body. This body is called the field, and the inner man, the dweller of the body. Not only for the sake of convenience but to convey the depth of the body, our sages of lore divided this body into three tiers with five sheaths or *kosas*. The three tiers are known as the core of the body—the self, the mental body, and the gross body. In these three tiers are the five cases known as the anatomical body, the physiological body, the psychological or mental body, the intellectual body, and the spiritual body. These three bodies with five sheaths interpenetrate from the skin to the self as well as outerpenetrate from the self to the skin as one single unit.

Yet, it is not easy, nay, it is impossible to pinpoint where the body ends and the mind begins, or where the mind ends and the self begins. They are all woven together through the string of intelligence.

By nature, the body is dull and sluggish, the mind active and dynamic, and the self, illuminative. Practice of Yoga destroys the sluggishness of the body, and it becomes equal to the active mind. Then both body and mind are transcended to the level of the illuminative self, with perfect health in body, stability in mind, and clarity in intellect.

If the mirror is clean, it reflects the object clearly. Practice of Yoga removes the impurities of the body and reflects like the mirror in man the light of knowledge and wisdom, so that his body, mind, and self work in unison.

Fortunately, nature provides this precise instrument—the body—to adjust to its rhythm with the turmoil of day-to-day pressures. It is also astonishing that in spite of imbalances created by the possessor of the body, through overindulgence in satisfying his or her greedy wants, it maintains its balance. When these imbalances are overstepped, physical, physiological, and psychological diseases set in, and doubts and fears occupy the seat of the mind, creating emotional disorders that are termed psychosomatic diseases.

Generally, health is understood as freedom from illness, but it is more than that. Health is a perfect state of equilibrium, balance, and harmony with the whole body—joints, tissues, muscles, cells, nerves, glands, respiration, circulation, digestion, and elimination. Also, it is a perfectly happy disposition of mind toward sorrow and joy, pain and pleasure, evil and good, inspiration and expiration, respiration and resplendence.

Life is a combination of conscience, consciousness, intelligence, mind, senses of perception, and organs of action. Health is a tremendous communication with each and every part of the individual, so that each cell communes with the other. This cannot be purchased in the bazaar; it has to be earned by inspiration and toil. Does Yoga do that? Yes. Yoga starts from the health of the body and makes one climb the Everest of happiness, poise, and peace.

Yoga also helps in avoiding the hidden, unknown diseases that may surface later in life. Hence, it works not only as a therapeutic science but also as a preventive art. Yoga can be practiced regardless of whether one is young or old, male or female, healthy or unhealthy, valid or invalid, poor or rich, undernourished or overnourished. This is its beauty.

An aggressor annexes a nation when it is weak, and a thief burgles when the owner is careless; so, also, the body becomes a breeding ground for diseases if one is careless. Like the farmer who ploughs the uncultivated fallow land, removes the weeds, provides water and manure, sows the best of seeds, tends the crops, and enjoys the best of harvests, *yama* and *niyama* (moral and ethical principles) plough the body, *asanas* (yoga postures) remove toxins and symptoms of diseases, and *pranayama* (yoga breathing) irrigates with energy and tends the mind like a crop, to enjoy the harvest of health, peace, and happiness. Then it becomes a heaven on earth, both for the body and its dweller, the self.

INTRODUCTION TO YOGA

The term *Yoga* comes from the root *Yuj*, meaning to join, to bind, to associate with. Yoga means union, the union of the individual soul with the universal spirit. Yoga is a discipline that removes all dualities and divisions. It integrates body with breath, breath with mind, mind with intelligence, and intelligence with the Soul. Yoga makes one penetrate from the outer skin toward the inner core of being, as well as from the core of being toward the periphery. Yoga is both an evolutive path (onward journey) and involutive path (inward journey) in the quest of the Soul.

According to Patanjali, author of the *Yoga Sutras*, Yoga is the restraint of the fluctuations of the mind. When the fluctuations cease, the Soul is uncovered. These fluctuations are summarized in five categories: real knowledge, contrary knowledge, imagination, sleep, and memory. This raises the questions, why do fluctuations and modifications in the mind arise, and how are they to be restrained? Fluctuations and modifications arise because of afflictions. Surprisingly, Patanjali also summarizes five afflictions. They are lack of spiritual wisdom, egoism, attraction toward attachment, aversion to pain, and passionately clinging to life. The afflictions are subliminal impressions, and they are the roots of fluctuations in consciousness. These afflictions, fluctuations, modifications, and modulations are partly inherited and partly acquired.

Patanjali speaks at cognizable levels about the nine obstacles on the path of self-progression and realization. He begins with three physical disabilities: body ailments like disease, laziness or languor, and sloth and sluggishness. The mental obstacles include doubt or indecision, carelessness and sensory gratifications. Intellectual impediments arise from the philosophy of illusion or living in the world of illusion; failure to hold on to what is undertaken; and inability to maintain the progress achieved. Besides these nine obstacles, Patanjali notes that labored breathing disturbs the body; tremor of the body shakes the cellular body; despair makes the mind weak and fickle; and sorrow affects the intellectual caliber. Thus, these four accompanying distractions further scatter the consciousness, which is already in a disturbed state.

These afflictions and obstacles are nothing but imperfections in the health of the body and in the state of the mind. Hence, the science of Yoga begins with a philosophy of sorrow, aims at the purification of the body and mind, and ends in emancipating practitioners by releasing them from physical, mental, moral, or spiritual pains. Patanjali sums up the effect of Yoga in one Sutra. He says, "by regular and devoted practice of the eight components of Yoga, the impurities of the yoga practitioner's body, mind, and intelligence are consumed, the causes of afflictions removed, and the crown of spiritual light and wisdom is bestowed" (Sutra II. 28, p. 132 in Iyengar, 1993).

THE EIGHT COMPONENTS OF YOGA

Yama and Niyama

Yama is self-restraint, or the "don'ts" of life, whereas *niyama* is the fixed practices, or the "do's" of life. These form the framework of rules on which the individual and society are based. They are the core of every culture and the foundation of every society. The yama is of five parts: nonviolence, truthfulness, freedom from avarice, control of sensual pleasures, and freedom from possessions beyond one's needs. Yama helps to restrain the organs of action. The rules of yama are clearly laid out for us, to live in the midst of society while remaining a yoga practitioner. They are conducive to social harmony and integration.

As yama is a universal social practice, niyama evolves from the individual practices necessary to build up the *sadhaka's* (yoga practitioner's) own character. They are cleanliness, contentment, religious fervor or arduous practice, self-study, and surrender of the self to the Lord. These five observances not only are in accord with the five sheaths of man—the anatomical, physiological, emotional, intellectual, and spiritual—but also are useful in culturing the senses of perception.

There cannot be freedom without discipline. Without morality and discipline, spiritual life is an impossibility. Mastery of Yoga would be unrealizable without the observance of the ethical principles of yama and niyama.

Asana

Asanas (yoga postures), the third limb of Yoga, are basic in strengthening and cleansing the body and purging the impurities of the mind. I emphasize perfection in asanas because the body is the means through which we perceive and act, and therefore, a healthy and strong body is an incomparable asset in Yogic *sadhana* (path of Yoga).

Asanas strengthen and purify each and every limb, each and every fiber, each and every cell of the body. As such, the range of asanas is infinite. Traditional books mention that there are as many asanas as living species.

Asanas have a great depth and are a science and art in themselves. In asana, we proceed from the external to the internal, from the gross to the subtle, from the skin to the Soul, from the known to the unknown. I define asana as firmness in the body, steadiness in intelligence, and benevolence in consciousness. Whatever asana one performs, it should be done with a feeling of firmness and endurance in the body, goodwill in the intelligence of the head (consciousness), and awareness and delight in the intelligence of the heart (conscience). This is how each asana has to be understood and done, with a sense of nourishment and illumination. Infinite poise and balance are instilled in the asanas, in which the body, mind, and Soul become one.

Pranayama

Pranayama, the fourth constituent of Yoga, deals with the control of prana and energy, grossly translated as breath. Prana is a self-energizing force that permeates each individual as well as the universe at all levels.

It acts as physical energy, mental energy, intellectual energy, sensual energy, spiritual energy, and cosmic energy. All that vibrates in the universe is prana. It is the wealth of life. This self-energizing force is the principle of life and of consciousness. As the atmosphere carries fine ingredients of life's elixir, or the life force (prana), Yogis discovered the method of pranayama so that profound energy is earned, stored, and distributed, continuously providing needed energy to the body, mind, and spirit.

Prana (energy) and *citta* (consciousness) are in constant contact with each other. They are like twin brothers. Mind is mercurial and moves with infinite speed. But the breath moves slower, and hence it is easier to control. It is said, "as the breath moves so the mind moves, and as the breath is stilled so the mind is stilled."

Pranayama (yoga breathing practice) cannot be done with force. It needs a very delicate, subtle adjustment of the cells of the lungs, quietness of the brain cells, and alertness in attention and observation. Hence, it has to be learned under a competent teacher. Patanjali expressly advises the sadhaka to do pranayama only after attaining proficiency in asanas. For the first time, he shows a distinct step in the ascent on the ladder of Yoga.

Patanjali sums up the effects of pranayama, saying that it removes the veil covering the light of knowledge and heralds the dawn of wisdom. By its practice, illusion, ignorance, desire, and delusion, which obscure the intelligence, are destroyed, and the inner light of wisdom is allowed to shine. As the breeze disperses the clouds that cover the sun, so pranayama wafts away the clouds that hide the light of intelligence. Thus, pranayama becomes the gateway to *dharana* (concentration) and *dhyana* (meditation).

Pratyahara

Pratyahara (withdrawal of the senses), the fifth limb, begins with the inner quest and acts as a foundation in the path of renunciation. From here begins the return journey toward the seer or the Soul. Memory and mind are so much interwoven that it is hard to distinguish between them. In one's life, memory impels the mind to seek sensual pleasures.

Pratyahara helps the senses of perception and memory to rest quietly, each in its place, and to cease importuning the mind for their gratifications. They lose the taste and flavors of their respective objects. The mind, up until now, acted as a bridge between the senses and the seer, but now draws back from the contact senses and turns inward toward the seer to explore spiritual wealth. Pratyahara, in fact, is an effect of pranayama. The practitioner must focus attention on the one, which is ever fresh, changeless, and always in a state of bliss.

Dharana, Dhyana, and Samadhi

Dharana, dhyana, and *samadhi* are the other three limbs of Yoga. These three are so close to each other, that Patanjali had to coin a special term, *samyama,* meaning integration, to bring out that these three limbs of Yoga are without division. Dharana is confinement of citta's (consciousness's) attention to an object or region outside or inside the body. Dhyana, or meditation, is the uninterrupted flow of attention, and samadhi is total absorption in the object of meditation. Asanas and pranayamas can be explained, taught, shown, and corrected, whereas yama and niyama are explained by stories of great men as ideal examples to build up character. These last three stages of Yoga are experiencing states. They cannot be presented with explanations.

Meditation is the art of bringing complex mind to a state of simplicity, without arrogance, but with innocence. One who is free from doubt and confusion and has intuitive, instant clarity has reached the pinnacle of meditation.

Today, there is a craze for meditation and instant enlightenment. Meditation, being part of Yoga, cannot be separated from the parent body, from Yoga. However, dharana, dhyana, and samadhi are the effects or fruits of diligent practice. To bypass the other limbs and enter directly into these practices would be not only dangerous but also an abuse of Yoga. We have to build up that strength and vigor to face the light of the Divine when divinity graces its light upon us.

RENUNCIATION

Patanjali says that practice and detachment are the means to restrain the fluctuations and modifications of the mind. Practice is knowledge with action. It is a systematic, repeated performance involving a certain methodology in order to accomplish skill and proficiency. It is helpful in building up confidence and refinement in culturing the consciousness, whereas renunciation is cultivation of freedom from worldly desires and appetites. Renunciation is knowledge with devotion to God. Renunciation is the act of discharging that which obstructs the mind and the spiritual path. As a bird cannot fly with one wing, so also, a Yogi cannot ascend to spiritual height without proper disposition for practice and renunciation. Practice will be only sensual without discriminative powers.

Yama begins with nonviolence and ends with nonpossession. Niyama starts with cleanliness and culminates in the surrender of the ego. In asana, one learns to transcend the dualities, while in pranayama one lifts the veil that clouds the light of knowledge and takes one's consciousness nearer to the Soul.

Practice of pratyahara brings supreme control over the senses and mind. Without the mind being withdrawn from sensual objects, dharana and dhyana are not easy to practice or assimilate. Samadhi is a desireless state, a supreme state of renunciation.

Patanjali begins Yoga with the philosophy of sorrow and ends with emancipation. He recognizes the importance of the aims of individuals, namely, science of duty, purpose of life and wealth, desire and passion, and emancipation. The philosophy of Yoga is not meant only for celibates or renunciates. *Brahmacharya*, or continence, is not negation or forced austerity and prohibition. All aims of the individual are meant for the seer to experience the pleasures of the world, or for reaching emancipation with right perception. Married life is also one of the ways of moving from human love to divine love or union with the supreme Soul. Thus, Yoga acts as an instrument to develop purity in thought, word, and deed.

CONCLUSION

Scientists have begun to accept the moral codes of Yoga as essential for health and happiness. They are also clear in their thinking that *psyche* (brain) and *soma* (body) are interrelated, and it may not be too far for them to establish a psychospiritual understanding of human life. The World Health Organization (WHO) proclaims that the twenty-first century will be filled with physical health and mental well-being. I don't think there is another alternative to Yoga that can fulfill the ambitions of the WHO governments all over the world, governments that are spending millions for research on diseases and drugs to make unhealthy people healthy. But alas! No government has yet awakened to the need to keep *healthy* people healthy. Yoga is for all. To limit Yoga to the boundaries of one nation is the denial of Universal Consciousness. Human feelings, emotions, joys, and sorrows are the same the world over.

Yoga is a science, for it has a technique based on well-tried principles. It is a science that shows how to commune with the body, the mind, and the Soul. It thus establishes a highly intelligent communication, or, rather a perfect communion between the body and the mind, and the mind and the Soul. It thereby brings thorough understanding of one's nature, so that one lives a profoundly positive life. Such an individual is at peace with the self and with all people.

NOTE

1. From a letter to the editor of this book, Jennifer Chesworth, September 1994.
2. *Light on the Yoga Sutras of Patanjali*, B. K. S. Iyengar, 1993. New York: Aquarian Press, an imprint of HarperCollins. This unique edition contains a new translation of the Sutras and a commentary by B. K. S. Iyengar.

PART II

Policy Issues in Health and Health Ecology

11 Risk, Science, and Democracy

WILLIAM D. RUCKLESHAUS

In the study of history, nothing is more fascinating than the emergence of those ideas that periodically galvanize humankind into urgent action. Such ideas leap onto the center stage of public awareness, stay for a time, and then effectively vanish—either discarded, like witchcraft and the divine rights of kings, or absorbed into the public consciousness to become part of the status quo. The most interesting moments in this process, of course, are those when the idea is on stage, when it engages the public in passionate debate, when people struggle to fit the idea into the existing order, and when, through their efforts, people inevitably change both the existing order and the character of the idea.

Environmentalism has been an idea "on stage" in this sense for some thirty years. Born in its modern form in the writings of such people as Rachel Carson, Rene Dubos, and Barry Commoner, environmentalism entered the world of action with startling speed. In the United States, at all levels of government, dozens of important environmental laws were passed in a single decade. Government agencies were reorganized to administer the new legislation; at the federal level, this included the establishment of the Environmental Protection Agency (EPA) in December 1970. Hundreds of regulations were issued, all ensuring that the tenets of environmentalism would intrude into nearly every aspect of life.

AUTHOR'S NOTE: Reprinted with permission from William D. Ruckleshaus, "Risk, Science, and Democracy," *Issues in Science and Technology*, Vol. 1, no. 2 (Spring 1985), pp. 19-38.

Environmentalism has changed society, but over the same period, environmentalism itself has changed as well. During the past two decades, there has been a shift in public emphasis from visible and demonstrable problems, such as smog from automobiles and raw sewage, to potential and largely invisible problems, such as the effects of low concentrations of toxic pollutants on human health. This shift is notable for two reasons. First, it has changed the way in which science is applied to practical questions of public health protection and environmental regulation. Second, it has raised difficult questions as to how to manage chronic risks within the context of free and democratic institutions. People are afraid of these environmental risks, and fearful people all too often trade freedom for the promise of security.

THE SCIENCE OF RISK

In science, the majority does not rule, as the history of science amply demonstrates. Everybody but Semmelweiss was wrong on childbed fever. Everybody but Wegener was wrong on continental drift. Scientists outside the consensus, not averse to voicing their objections in public, may be cranks or they may be right. Public officials cannot make this distinction; only the slow mills of science can grind out the truth.

Public officials, however, do not have that kind of time. From its earliest days, the EPA was often compelled to *act under conditions of substantial scientific uncertainty.* The full implications of this problem were masked at the beginning because the kind of pollution we were trying to control was so blatant. Although scientists were often in the forefront of the early struggles against pollution, most people did not need a scientific panel to tell them that air is not supposed to be brown, that streams are not supposed to ignite and stink, that beaches are not supposed to be covered with raw sewage. Many of the grosser sorts of pollution are now under control in the United States. But the level of controversy about environmental protection has not diminished.

The risks of effects from typical environmental exposures to toxic substances—unlike the touchable, visible, and malodorous pollution that stimulated the initial environmental revolution—are largely constructs or projections based on scientific findings. We would know nothing at all about chronic risk attributable to most toxic substances if scientists had not detected and evaluated them. Our response to such risks, therefore, must be based on a set of scientific findings. Science, however, is hardly ever unambiguous or unanimous, especially when the data on which definitive science must be founded scarcely exist. The toxic effects on health of many of the chemicals the EPA considers for regulation fall into this class.

Risk assessment is the device that government agencies such as the EPA have adopted to quantify the degree of hazard that might result from human activities—for example, the risks to human health and the environment from industrial chemicals. Essentially, it is a kind of pretense; to avoid the paralysis of protective action that would result from waiting for "definitive" data, we assume that we have greater knowledge than scientists actually possess and make decisions based on those assumptions.

Of course, not all risk assessment is on the controversial outer edge of science. We have been looking at the phenomenon of toxic risk from environmental levels of chemicals for a number of years, and as evidence has accumulated for certain chemicals, controversy has diminished and consensus among scientists has become easier to obtain. For other substances—and these are the ones that naturally figure most prominently in public debate—the data remain ambiguous. In such cases, risk assessment is something of an intellectual orphan. Scientists are uncomfortable with it when the method must use scientific information in a way that is outside the normal constraints of science. They are encroaching on political judgments, and they know it. As Alvin Weinberg (1990) has written,

> Attempts to deal with social problems through the procedures of science hang on the answers to questions that can be asked of science and yet cannot be answered by science. I propose the term *trans-scientific* for these questions. . . . Scientists have no monopoly on wisdom where this kind of trans-science is involved; they shall have to accommodate the will of the public and its representatives.

However, the representatives of the public, in this instance in protective agencies, have their problems with risk assessment as well. The very act of quantifying risk tends to reify dreaded outcomes in the public mind and may make it more difficult to gain public acceptance for policy decisions or may push those decisions in unwise directions. It is hard to describe, say, one cancer case in 70 years among a population of a million as an "acceptable risk" when such a description may too easily summon up for any individual the image of some close relative on his or her deathbed. Also, the use of risk assessment as a policy basis inevitably provokes endless arguments about the validity of the estimates, which can seriously disrupt the regulatory timetables such officials must live by.

Despite this uneasiness, there appears to be no substitute for risk assessment, in that some sort of risk finding is what tells us there is any basis for regulatory action in the first place. The alternative to performing risk assessment is to adopt a policy of either reducing all *potentially* toxic emissions to the greatest degree technology allows, or banning all substances for which there is any evidence of harmful effect, a policy that no technological society could long survive. Beyond that, risk assessment is an irreplaceable tool for setting priorities among the tens of thousands of substances that could be subjects of control actions—substances that vary enormously in their apparent potential for causing disease. We must, therefore, use and improve risk assessment with full recognition of its current shortcomings.

This accommodation would be much easier from a public policy viewpoint were it possible to establish for all pollutants the environmental levels that present zero risk. This is prevented, however, by an important limitation of the current technique: the difficulty of establishing definitive no-effect levels for exposure to most carcinogens. Consequently, whenever there is any exposure to such substances, there is a calculable risk of disease. The environmentalist ethos, which is reflected in many of the environmental laws in the United States, and which requires that zero-risk levels of pollutant exposure be established, is thus shown to be an impossible goal for an industrial society, as long as we retain the no-threshold model for carcinogenesis.

OPPOSING VIEWPOINTS

This situation has given rise to two conflicting viewpoints on protection. The first, usually proffered by the *regulated* community, argues that regulation ought not to be based on a set of unprovable assumptions, but only on connections between pollutants and health effects that can be demonstrated under the canons of science in the strict sense. This community points out that for the vast majority of chemical species, we have no evidence at all that suggests effects on human health from exposures at environmental levels. Because many important risk assessments are based on assumptions that are scientifically untestable, the method is too susceptible to manipulation for political ends and, the regulated community contends, it has been so manipulated by environmentalists.

The second viewpoint, which has been adopted by some environmentalists, counters that waiting for firm evidence of human health effects amounts to using people as guinea pigs, and that is morally unacceptable. It proposes that far from overestimating the risks from toxic substances, conventional risk assessments underestimate them, for there may be effects from chemicals in combination that are greater than would be expected from the sum effects of all chemicals acting independently. Although approving of risk assessment as a priority-setting tool, this viewpoint rejects the idea that we can use risk assessment to distinguish between significant and insignificant risks. Any identifiable risk ought to be eliminated insofar as available technology can do so.

Both of these opposing viewpoints reflect the fear that risk assessment may be imbued with values repugnant to one or more of the parties involved. Some people in the regulated community believe that the structure of risk assessment inherently exaggerates risk, whereas many environmentalists believe it will not capture all the risks that may actually exist. This disagreement is not resolvable in the short run through recourse to science. Risk assessment is necessarily dependent on choices made from among a host of assumptions, and these choices will inevitably be affected by the values of the choosers, whether they be scientists, civil servants, or politicians.

This problem can be substantially alleviated by the establishment of formal public rules guiding the necessary inferences and assumptions. These rules should be based on the best available information concerning the underlying scientific mechanism. Adoption of such guidelines reduces the possibility that an EPA administrator, for example, may manipulate the findings of some risk assessment so as to avoid making the difficult, and perhaps politically unpopular, choices involved in a risk-management decision. Both industry and environmentalists fear this manipulation—from different brands of administrators, needless to say. Although we cannot remove values from risk assessment, we can and should keep those values from shifting arbitrarily with the political winds.

IS IT WORTH IT?

That this question must be asked, and asked carefully, is a token of how the main force of the environmental idea has been modified by the recent focus on toxic risk to human health. In truth, this question should have always been asked, but because the early goals of environmentalism in the United States were so obviously good, the requirement to ask "Is it worth it?" was not firmly built into all environmental laws. Who would dare to question the worth of Lake Erie? Environmentalism in the United States at its inception was a grand vision, one that nearly all Americans willingly shared. Somehow that vision of the essential unity of nature and of the need to bring industrial society into harmony with it has been lost among the parts per billion, and with it, we have lost the capacity to reach social consensus on environmental policy.

Why has this happened? I believe it is because environmentalism, like many another social movement, is suffering from the excesses of its own youthful vigor. In the United States, early legislation made promises that could not reasonably be kept; expectations were raised that were bound to be unfulfilled. The Clean Air Act, for example, promised absolute protection from airborne carcinogens, but we cannot keep that promise. The American people were also promised, under the clean air and water laws, that the air would be pure and that water pollution would be eliminated by a specific date; we have not kept those promises. Few things are more corrupting to a free society than grand promises unfulfilled.

Rational thinking requires a kind of democratic citizenship that is willing to dig deeper than the glib headlines and the usual invitations to panic. It also requires much more from a regulatory agency providing the facts; the agency must be willing to explain and be able to communicate, and most of all, it must admit the uncertainties buried in its calculations. Only then can the appropriate balancing decisions take place.

RISK IN THE LOCAL CONTEXT

Some years ago, René Dubos (1968) said that the way to cope with such massive problems as pollution control was to "think globally and act locally." It is still good advice, and may serve as a general prescription for successful management of technological risk in a democratic society. Global thinking in the present case means dealing explicitly with the central questions of risk management: how to reconcile technological systems with social values; how to develop consensus about potentially dangerous technologies; and how to establish and maintain trust in our protective institutions. We do not yet know how to deal very well with any of these questions.

That is why local action—a diversity of local actions—is necessary. The most efficient way for our society to learn how to cope with risk is to enable hundreds or thousands of locally based risk management endeavors to take place. Local risk-taking preferences could then be expressed, under broad limits set by higher levels of government. This will inevitably change public perceptions of risk, for in such perceptions familiarity breeds, not contempt, but the ability to discriminate between the significant and insignificant, between trivial and important risks. Fear is, after all, what has tended to paralyze public policy on these issues. As people begin to assess and manage risks at the local level, they will be preparing themselves to cope as citizens of a free, democratic society moving into a future that will be dominated by barely imaginable technologies and fraught with unfamiliar risks.

REFERENCES

Dubos, R. (1968). *So human an animal*. New York: Scribners.

Weinberg, A. (1990). In T. Glickman & M. Gough (Eds.), *Reading in Risk*. Washington, DC: Resources for the Future.

12 The Politics of Cancer

ROBERT N. PROCTOR

More than a thousand people die of cancer every day in the United States. For every American alive today, one in three will contract the disease; one in five will die from it. Cancer is the plague of the twentieth century, second only to heart disease as a cause of death in most industrial nations. Although most other diseases are on the decline, cancer is on the rise. The trend has been building for some time: Roswell Park (1899), a New York physician, noted as early as 1899 that cancer was "now the only disease which is steadily upon the increase" (p. 385). That year, cancer claimed about 30,000 U.S. lives. In 1996, cancer was projected to kill nearly twenty times that many: 555,000, according to American Cancer Society projections (American Cancer Society, 1996). If present trends continue, cancer will become the world's leading cause of death sometime in the twenty-first century. It is already the number one cause of death in Japan.

The tragedy is magnified by the fact that the causes of cancer are largely known—and have been known for quite some time. Cancer is caused by bad habits, bad working conditions, bad government, and bad luck, the latter including such things as the luck of the genetic draw and the culture into which one is born.[1]

Geographical and occupational differences give us clues as to what causes cancer. Cancer of the mouth is common among the peoples of India and southeast Asia, who chew betel nuts and tobacco leaves. Asbestos workers suffer cancer of the lungs and gut; dye workers suffer cancers of the bladder and stomach. Cervical cancer is rare in nuns but quite common in prostitutes. Bowel cancer is rare in countries where meat is not a regular part of the diet and where large amounts of fiber are consumed. Mormons, whose religious beliefs forbid them to smoke or to drink alcohol, coffee, or tea, die of cancer 20 percent less often than do non-Mormons. The Japanese vulnerability to stomach cancer—that nation's leading cancer killer—probably derives from their consumption of large amounts of pickled, burned, and high-salt foods cooked with soybean pastes and sauces. Liver cancer is especially common in Africa and Guam, because the food in those places is often contaminated with aflatoxin, a potent fungal toxin. In the United States, African Americans suffer significantly higher rates of death from nearly every form of cancer than do Whites (skin cancer being the only notable exception), although studies have shown that it is poverty rather than race that is the root cause of the difference. First-world poverty is surely one of the most potent carcinogens.

Cancer, in other words, is not a constant of the human condition but a product of the substances to which we are exposed at home or at work, the lifestyles we lead. Cancer is a historical disease in at least two separate senses: *Theories* of what causes cancer change over time, but so do the *causes* at work in carcinogenesis.

Theories of what causes cancer have included virtually every known vice and every known virtue. A short list would include humoral imbalances, hereditary predispositions, sunshine, obesity, syphilis, female sex hormones, radiation, tomatoes, tarred roads, grief and anxiety, arsenic, affluence, poverty, sexual abstinence, sexual promiscuity, and water derived from streams in which trout are abundant.

But cancer is also historical in the sense that what actually causes cancer changes over time. Pipe smoking was first recognized as a cause of lip cancer in 1761, two centuries after Raleigh's transatlantic transport of tobacco. Percivall Pott, an English physician, described soot-induced scrotal cancer among London's chimney sweeps in 1775—and there is reason to suspect that the shift from wood to coal as the primary fuel for English cooking and heating was at least partly to blame. In 1900, women died of cancer far more often than men; today, it is men who die more often then women, and tobacco is the primary cause of this reversal in fortunes. Two-pack-a-day smokers increase their risk of lung cancer by about twenty times. The World Health Organization estimates that about 3 million people are killed by cigarettes every year worldwide; that number is expected to grow to about 10 million per year in the early decades of the next century (Parkin et al., 1988). In short, who gets cancer, where, and how is a cultural artifact.

Such knowledge as we have of causes, however, has done surprisingly little to aid us in our search for solutions. Notwithstanding repeated and glowing pronouncements from the American Cancer Society, cancer treatment has made little progress since Richard Nixon declared war on the disease in 1971. Five-year survival rates for the majority of cancers (lung, colon, breast, and stomach, for example) remain essentially where they were twenty years ago—despite more than $30 billion spent on research by the National Cancer Institute. A 1993 study released by the institute showed that although people diagnosed with cancer do generally live longer (53 percent now live five years or more, compared with 49 percent in the mid-1970s), part of this meager improvement is due to statistical sleight of hand; people who used to die four years after diagnosis may now die after five, their "improvement" due to the discovery of their cancer a year earlier than used to be the case (Miller et al., 1993).

Even where survival rates really have improved, this may or may not have to do with the treatment patients receive. Chemotherapy has dramatically increased the life expectancy of children diagnosed with leukemia, and Hodgkin's disease and testicular cancer are now quite treatable. Malignant melanoma is nearly 100 percent curable if detected early, and many lymphomas respond well to chemotherapy. But the outlook is not so sanguine for the really big killers. About 95 percent of all lung cancers still prove fatal, regardless of what form of treatment one chooses. The *New England Journal of Medicine* in 1984 reported that people with colon cancer—America's second-largest cancer killer (after lung cancer)—who received chemotherapy alongside surgical removal of tumors did not live any longer than people who received no chemotherapy. The study also found that chemotherapy actually increased the risk of leukemia. Similar doubts have been raised concerning surgery and radiation—the other two legs of the therapeutic triad (also known as poison, slash, and burn). Even X-ray mammography turns out to be more and less than advertised. For women under the age of forty, for example, there are probably as many tumors caused by the procedure as are detected and cured as a result of it. The X-ray levels used in standard mammography have declined in recent years, but criticisms are still raised that too many younger women, and not enough older women, are being screened (Gastrointestinal Tumor Study Group, 1984).

In consequence of these gloomy findings, it has become hard to deny that the war against cancer is being lost. This was the conclusion of an article published in the 1986 *New England Journal of Medicine* by John

Bailar and Elaine Smith. Former Stanford University president Donald Kennedy expressed a somewhat stronger view when he called America's cancer campaign "a medical Vietnam." James Watson, codiscoverer of the DNA double-helix and one of the nation's most widely respected scientists, simply called it "a bunch of shit" (Kennedy & Watson quoted in Chowka, 1978).

What is going on here? How can one of the largest medical efforts in history have proved so futile? Why, if cancer is so obviously a product of such things as smoking, radon, and the "industrial way of life," has so little been done to solve the problem at its roots? Is it really the case that, as Samuel Epstein (1979) suggested fifteen years ago in his *The Politics of Cancer*, "While much is known about the science of cancer, its prevention depends largely, if not exclusively, on political action?" (p. 511).

SEAS OF CONTROVERSY

In regard to what is known and unknown about cancer, there is controversy virtually everywhere one looks: over the role of lifestyle and occupation in the genesis of cancer; over the role of stress, personality factors, and "natural carcinogens" in things like beer, charcoal, and bruised broccoli. No one really knows how serious is the hazard posed by radon gas seeping into basements or by electromagnetic fields from high-voltage wires and household appliances. Do cellular phones cause brain cancer? What about the cosmic rays absorbed while flying during sunspot activity, when the radiation one receives in an hour can exceed that allowed for nuclear workers in a year? How bad is it to eat Brazil nuts, the most radioactive natural food, or to dust a baby's bottom with talcum powder, which naturally contains asbestos?

I say no one knows, but it would be more precise to say that in most such matters, there are islands of agreement separated by deep seas of controversy. Evidence accumulates that chlorinated water causes bladder cancer, but the Chlorine Institute, a trade association, disputes that evidence (Anderson, 1993; Morris et al., 1992). Hair colorings are suspected of causing non-Hodgkin's lymphoma, but that too is disputed. Bruce Ames (1983) of Berkeley has generated endless controversy with his contention that peanut butter and barbecued meats contain potent carcinogens and that drinking a single glass of wine is thousands of times more hazardous than drinking a glass of pesticide-contaminated water (cf. Bollier, 1988). Doubts have been raised about whether hazards of dioxin have been exaggerated, whether all or only one kind of asbestos (amphibole) is dangerous, whether industrial life is as perilous as we are often led to believe.

Tempers run high in such debates, because much is at stake. Environmental groups depend to a certain extent on public fears to solicit funds, and manufacturers stand to gain or to lose from whether and to what extent a given chlorinated or halogenated hydrocarbon is judged a public health hazard. Cancer research itself is a very big business, and the research establishment has vested interests in particular kinds of approaches rather than others.

The interests at stake, in other words, are complex and sometimes shifting. Even "industrial interests" are not what they used to be. Billion-dollar industries have sprung up to "abate" or "remediate" environmental hazards such as asbestos, lead, and radon, and much of the twenty-first century will probably be devoted to cleaning up the industry of the twentieth. In 1988, for example, the Department of Energy estimated the cost of cleaning up the nation's twenty-eight nuclear bomb plants and testing facilities at between $40 billion and $110 billion (*New York Times,* July 2, 1988). The General Accounting Office reported shortly thereafter that the cost could actually be as high as $175 billion (*New York Times,* July 14, 1988). The commercialization of environmental troubles has led to unprecedented stakes in the exaggeration or diminution of environmental hazards, the net result being that experts commonly disagree about what is a hazard and what is a risk. Strange as it may seem, there is not even a well-defined consensus concerning whether overall cancer rates are on the rise. Environmentalists such as Devra Lee Davis argue that brain and several other cancers are rapidly increasing; Richard Doll and other "cancer conservatives" claim that the increases can be explained by reference to improved diagnostics and access to medical care.

What is strange to a historian is that many of these same debates have been going on for more than a century. As early as 1843, Stanislas Tanchou, physician to the king in Paris, presented statistics to prove that cancer was on the rise. Cancer for Tanchou and his followers was a "disease of civilization": more common in towns than in the countryside, in Europe than in Africa, among domesticated than among wild animals, and so forth. Medical missionaries and frontier doctors for the rest of the century tried to prove that cancer was absent or rare among the Athapaskans of Canada, the Inuit of the Arctic, the Hunza of the Himalayas, and other purported primitives. Skeptics charged the investigators with having ignored the fact that societies such as these may simply not have had the medical services required to evidence death by cancer.

Lurking behind much of the present discussion is a similar question of whether environmental degradation is really as unhealthy as environmentalists have made it out to be. Especially since the election of President Ronald Reagan in 1980, we have heard that the risks posed by toxic contaminants have been exaggerated; that the widely publicized "alar scare" of 1989, for example, was hysterical media hype fostered by power-hungry environmentalists; and that fear of chemicals may do more harm than the agents feared. We have witnessed the medicalization of environmental protest, so that the fear of living near an environmental hazard is now labeled a mental illness, amid growing talk of things like fiber phobia, fumaphobia, radiophobia, chemophobia, nosophobia, riskophobia, and so forth.

GENERAL PRINCIPLES

Let me stand back from particular controversies for a moment and say something about methodology. The central questions of what I like to call "political philosophy of science" include the following:

1. *Why do we know what we know, and why don't we know what we don't know?* There is a great deal of talk about the "culture of science," but where is there discussion of the "cultivation of ignorance"? If the politics of science consists (among other things) of the structure of research priorities, then it is important to understand what gets studied and why, but also what does *not* get studied and why not. One has, in other words, to study the "social construction of ignorance." The persistence of controversy is often not a natural consequence of imperfect knowledge but a political consequence of conflicting interests and structural apathies. Controversy is often engineered; ignorance and uncertainty are manufactured, maintained, and disseminated.

2. *Who gains from knowledge (or ignorance!) of a particular sort and who loses?* Scientists and science mongers often speak royally about how "we" know this or that—but who is that *we,* and why does it know what it knows? What, for example, is the connection—if any—between the fact that 90 percent of cancer researchers are males and that men predominate as subjects in clinical trials for cancer drugs? (Rosser, 1994). Why are the cancers that affect men better understood than cancers that affect women?[2] Who does science, and who gets science

done to them? What or whom is knowledge for, and what or whom is it against?

3. *How might knowledge be different, and how should knowledge be different?* What are the virtues of looking at ultimate rather than proximate causes, for example, or of seeking prevention rather than cure? What are the social responsibilities of the cancer theorist or, for that matter, the social science theorist?

Science has a face, a house, and a price: One has to ask who is doing science, in what institutional context, and at what cost. Understanding such things can give us insight into why scientific tools are sharp for certain kinds of problems and dull for others—it might also help us to see why the war against cancer is going so badly.

How does one put such ideas into practice? Let me give two examples: the life and times of Wilhelm C. Hueper and the story of the trade associations. The first illustrates the power of the state to intervene in this area; the second, the power of economic agents to rule you, fool you, and make you rest assured.

Hueper's suppression by the Atomic Energy Commission (AEC) in the 1950s is surely one of the most dramatic and consequential examples of U.S. state-sponsored censorship. Hueper was head of the Environmental Cancer Section of the National Cancer Institute from 1948 to 1964, and was celebrated by Rachel Carson in *Silent Spring* as "the father of environmental carcinogenesis." In 1948, he had begun a project to document lung cancers among the uranium miners of the Colorado plateau, but his efforts were stymied by the AEC's director of biology and medicine, who ordered him to delete all references to uranium mining at a scientific meeting he planned to attend. Hueper protested the order and was thereupon barred from all epidemiological work on occupational cancer, ironically, in the same year that the National Institutes of Health's chief of research—Hueper's own boss—was trumpeting the freedom of science. Hueper later complained that censorship of his other studies had delayed measures to remedy the situation, leaving countless men to die who may have been saved (for more on this man, see Proctor, 1995, pp. 36-48).

The same was true, interestingly, in other countries, such as East Germany and Czechoslovakia, which had their own Huepers and many more victims kept in the dark. I traveled to Czechoslovakia in the summer of 1992 to examine archives pertaining to the 1879 discovery of the so-called *Schneeberger Krankheit* (uranium mine-induced lung cancer); what I found was that more people have died from the disease since the 1950s than in the previous five hundred years of the mine's operation. The famous Joachimsthal mines were reopened by Soviet occupation authorities soon after the Second World War, following a secret agreement on November 23, 1945, that granted the Soviets exclusive rights to all uranium produced in the country. Vladimir Rericha, the chief epidemiologist at the Czechoslovakian Health Institute of the Uranium Industry, told me that he and his colleagues had shown that Czech uranium miners were dying from lung cancer at about five times the rate of coal miners. Rericha tried to publish his findings in 1966 but was barred from doing so by the State Security Police. Czech security authorities were purportedly afraid that uranium health statistics could be used to calculate uranium production levels and the quality of uranium being mined. The cynicism of such a ban was made apparent in 1970, when the administrative chief of all Czech uranium mining—Karel Bocek—defected to West Germany. Rericha requested and was again refused permission to publish; one can only conclude that Czech authorities feared that revelation of the sacrifice of its miners for Soviet atomic power might not sit well with the Czech populace (Proctor, 1993).

Rericha provided me with details on the number of miners and their lung cancer rates, but there was a part of the story that even he didn't know about. One of his colleagues at the Health Institute led me to papers from the newly opened state security archives describing conditions at seventeen "uranium mine concentration camps" established in the late 1940s and early 1950s to provide mine workers. Thousands of political prisoners labored in these camps: 64 in 1946 (all Germans, presumably Nazis); 5,500 in 1950; culminating in 11,816 in 1953. Prisoners worked the hottest ores.

The Cold War quest for national security claimed lives on both sides of the Iron Curtain; state authorities on both sides engineered cancer clusters and then silenced efforts to expose or ameliorate those clusters.

"DOUBT IS OUR PRODUCT"

There are forty thousand trade associations in the United States, the primary purpose of which is to do in aggregate what a single firm is often unable or unwilling to do—take the heat, respond to the press, coordinate product safety and legal research, and so forth. Many such groups have been formed in response to specific regulatory proposals: when the National Academy of Sciences published a review of evidence linking breast and colon cancer to the consumption of meat, the American Meat Institute organized a coalition of dairy, poultry, and livestock associations to discredit the charges (Proctor, 1995, pp. 101-132). When the *New England Journal of Medicine* published evidence that caffeine causes pancreatic cancer (MacMahon et al., 1981), the National Coffee Association (1987) responded with a position paper refuting the charges. The Calorie Control Council kept saccharine on the market after it was shown to cause cancer in rats. The Chlorine Institute has helped to rescue the reputation of dioxin; and the American Council on Science and Health even manages to claim that a little bit of dioxin is good for you.

The dollars behind these "Hertz rent-a-scientists"—as *Time* magazine has christened them—are often substantial.[3] The Council for Tobacco Research (1995) is one of the largest private supporters of medical research in the world, having spent $240 million for this purpose since the 1950s, resulting in the publication of more than three thousand scientific articles. The American Industrial Health Council is a leading advocate of "go-slow" policies in the area of environmental regulation—as is the Synthetic Organic Chemicals Manufacturers Association, a consortium of twenty-one associations ranging from the Silicones Health Council to the Methyl Tertiary Butyl Ether Task Force. All use science as a form of public relations; all prove the verity of Gibson's Law—I refer of course to the principle that "for every Ph.D. there's an equal and opposite Ph.D."

Trade associations such as these make it their business to exploit, disseminate, and, if need be, produce uncertainty in the area of environmental carcinogenesis. This has important consequences for public perceptions of science. The production and management of uncertainty has facilitated what one might call the "MacNeil-Lehrerization of science": the media display of equal and opposing views on apparently settled questions, generating the sense that endlessly more research is needed to resolve guilt or innocence in questions of carcinogenesis.

Bias in such cases, however, is more subtle than is commonly imagined. The Tobacco Institute can support "good" medical research, but the hoped-for effect may be goodwill toward the industry. A chemical manufacturer may promote research into the hazards of a hydrocarbon, but the hoped-for effect may be to insinuate ambiguity and therefore delay regulation. A lead-zinc trade association may call for more study of the effects of lead on intelligence, but the main goal may be to raise doubts about evidence of a health risk.

Bias in such efforts does not necessarily mean that science is bogus; support even of "good science" may assist an industry in deflecting attention from the hazards of a product—as when the Council for Tobacco Research (1995) promotes genetics research. I call this the smoke-screen effect—the effort to jam the scientific airwaves with true but trivial work, the net effect of which is to distract from what is going on underneath. Bias in such cases lies typically not in the falsification of research but rather in the diversion of attention from one problem to another—from causes onto mechanisms, for example, or from questions of public health onto questions of free speech. Bias also emerges, however, from the fetishization of certain of the self-avowed idols of conventional science. Science requires empirical verification, but the rabid distrust of a well-founded hypothetical can be used to dismiss a plausible point (as when animal evidence of carcinogenicity is dismissed by industry-financed skeptics). Science seeks to reduce uncertainty—but the demand that regulators hold back until all uncertainty is eliminated can be used as an excuse to do nothing.

The manufacturer and distribution of uncertainty is, I would suggest, an insufficiently recognized social function of science. (As one tobacco company puts it: "Doubt is our product.") Philosophers have not yet focused on science as an instrument of public relations, perhaps because the story to be told is not a very cheerful one. More attention needs to be paid to the ideological uses of science—how light is used to cast confusing shadows.

THE SOCIAL CONSTRUCTION OF IGNORANCE

Ignorance is surely one of the most prominent features of knowledge about cancer in the late twentieth century. Some of that ignorance is not just a natural consequence of the ever shifting boundary between the known and the unknown but a political consequence of decisions concerning how to approach (or neglect) what could and should be done to eliminate the disease. Ignorance is politically constructed by outright censorship (admittedly rare), by failures to fund, by the absence or impotence of interested parties, and by efforts to "jam the scientific airwaves with noise" (Marshall, 1987). Science, public policy, and public opinion are all affected.

I do not want to leave the impression that there are not inherent features of the cancer problem that make it difficult to obtain solid knowledge. Unambiguous knowledge of genetic susceptibility may have to wait for new techniques of DNA analysis, and improvements in therapy may well have to await dissection of the protein products of cancer genes. Epidemiologists face methodological obstacles that often reduce to such practical questions as, How large can I afford to make my study? Many nickel-and-dime carcinogens conferring, say, a 5 percent or 10 percent increased likelihood of disease are epidemiologically invisible, because the number of people one would have to study to obtain statistically significant results would be too large to be feasible. Animal studies and bacterial bioassays are invoked to solve this problem, though these, too, are not without flaws.

My concern is that inadequate attention has been given to how one should look and act to discover causes and organize prevention. The concept of causation is part of the problem; much of the politics of cancer research lies in how far down in the chain of causation one is willing and able to look. Does one stop (or start) with genetics, or immunology, or epidemiology? When is a nation's health or environmental policy (or the absence thereof) the cause of cancer? Can cancer be caused by elections, or recessions, or ad-induced habits and fashions? Was Ronald Reagan a carcinogen? The question of where the "real cause" lies is politicized, with the moralistic left favoring attention to ultimate (or social) causes and the stonewalling right favoring attention to more proximate causes or mechanisms. The emphasis on immediate mechanisms is attractive for those who believe that the large is to be explained by the small but never vice versa; the search for underlying causes exclusively in terms of biological mechanisms—flaws in the somatic genome, the molecular biochemistry of initiators and promoters, the activity of oncogenes, and the like—effaces the diversity of social causes that "ultimately" produce the real-world variety of cancers in the first place.

A related kind of shortsightedness can be found in the effort to rest analysis after classifying a given percentage of cancers as due to "lifestyle factors." About 30 percent of all cancer, for example, is said to be due to smoking, but what is smoking due to? The poor smoke more than the rich, and high school dropouts are much more likely to smoke than high school seniors. Why not say that poverty or faulty education is the primary cause of lung cancer? Why not say that cancer is caused by cigarette advertising, tobacco subsidizing, fear of fat, or youthful illusions of immortality? (See Brandt, 1990; Ernster, 1993; Wynder, 1993.)

Cancers are misfits in the world that epidemiologists want to attribute neatly to lifestyle, occupation, genetics, and infection. The search for percentages to be accorded each of these "factors" belies the extent to which occupation is shaped by culture, culture by skills and technologies, technologies by lifestyles, lifestyles by infectious possibilities, infectious agents by economic structures, and so on. Dietary cancers are usually classed as lifestyle cancers, but how much can one blame the changes in eating habits that have followed the triumph of transport-based petrochemical agribusiness? Fat consumption, linked to colon cancer, usually registers as diet (= lifestyle)—but what does one make of the fact that people in low-earning jobs are more likely to eat fatty, high-salt, carcinogenic foods (Polednak, 1989)? The Bilharzia bladder cancers of the Nile Valley and Brazil usually figure in the "infection" columns of causal tables, but what does one do with the fact that the 200 million people exposed to the parasite suffer mainly because they bathe and wash in sewage-contaminated water?

How, in other words, in a discourse dominated by concepts of genetics, germs, lifestyle, and occupation, does one come to grips with cancers caused by chronic poverty, medical neglect, environmental injustice, media-induced fashions, or industrial malfeasance? If poverty is what distinguishes African American cancer rates from European American rates, why does the National Cancer Institute classify by race rather than by income? If physical exercise is one way to prevent breast cancer, why not pin at least some of the deaths on the failure to provide support for female athletics? Looking to the future: If the U.S. Army's $210 million strategic breast initiative suddenly comes up with a miraculous cure or even moderately successful treatment, how should one regard the historical neglect of the malady that, for most of human history, has been one of the most deadly forms of cancer?

I don't intend all this to be depressing, although I must confess that I do appreciate what Wilhelm Hueper meant when he characterized his method as "one piece of dirt leading to another." The story of cancer is not a very upbeat one, and the stables of the research establishment are not exactly clean. We need to focus on the seamy sides of science and not just its polished carapace. We are rightfully suspicious of fairy tales that recite the triumph of medical research over popular superstition, but I don't take this as grounds for pessimism. There are good reasons to believe that critically informed public health measures could greatly lessen our cancer load, and this is reason, I believe, for optimistic activism.

Optimistic activism, however, requires a solid understanding of the politics of science: how priorities are shaped by power formations, ideological gaps, interests and disinterests, government and industrial support (or lack thereof), disciplinary dogmas, and professional and institutional parochialisms. Recent debates over what causes cancer bring these concerns into focus, because the terrain is among the most highly contested in all of modern science. My hope is that by examining how and why such questions have become the objects of controversy, we may learn more about how politics shapes science—and perhaps even more about what really causes cancer and what to do about it.

NOTES

1. Old age is, of course, a major cause of cancer, which is why death rates are generally presented as age-adjusted figures. Florida, for example, has a much higher annual cancer death rate than Alaska (250/100,000 vs. 80/100,000) due to the fact that Floridians are, on average, significantly older than Alaskans. Adjusting for age, one finds that Floridians actually have a slightly lower cancer mortality rate than Alaskans (163/100,000 compared to 184/100,000). See the American Cancer Society, 1992, p. 7.

2. Early childbirth is known to lessen one's risk of breast cancer, and late or no childbirth at all seems to heighten the risk. (Nuns have long been known to have very high rates.) Hormonal fluctuations are commonly invoked to explain the disease, but surely there is something wrong with the explanation offered by some that the disease is due to women's "incessant ovulation." We are similarly dissatisfied with reassurances that Long Island's high breast cancer rate can be explained by the high proportion of Jews living on the island; Jewish women may have high breast cancer rates, but why, the question then becomes, is that the case?

3. The American Hospital Association, for example, based on Lake Shore Drive in Chicago, has a staff of 884 and an annual budget of $79 million. Washington, D.C. is the headquarters of some 1,700 trade associations, making trade association business, after tourism, the second-ranking private industry in the nation's capital. See Hirsch, 1993.

REFERENCES

American Cancer Society. (1992). *Cancer facts and figures—1992.* New York: ACS.

American Cancer Society. (1996). *Cancer facts and figures—1996.* New York: ACS.

Ames, B. N. (1983). Dietary carcinogens and anticarcinogens. *Science, 221,* 1256-1264.

Anderson, E. V. (1993, May 10). Chlorine producers fight back against call for chemical's phaseout. *Chemical & Engineering News,* pp. 11-12.

Bailar, J. C., III, & Smith, E. M. (1986). Progress against cancer? *New England Journal of Medicine, 314,* 1226-1232.

Bollier, D. (1988, September/October). Leading scientist laughs at DDT, worries about peanut butter, believe it or not! *Public Citizen,* pp. 12-20.

Brandt, A. M. (1990, Fall). The cigarette, risk, and American culture. *Daedalus,* pp. 155-176.

Carson, R. (1962). *Silent spring.* Boston: Houghton Mifflin.

Chowka, P. B. (1978, January). The National Cancer Institute and the fifty-year coverup. *East West,* p. 23.

Council for Tobacco Research. (1995). *Report of the Council for Tobacco Research: U.S.A., Inc., 1995.* New York: Author.

Epstein, S. S. (1979). *The politics of cancer.* New York: Anchor.

Ernster, V. L. (1993). Women and smoking. *American Journal of Public Health, 83,* 1202-1203.
Gastrointestinal Tumor Study Group. (1984). Adjuvant therapy of colon cancer: Results of a prospectively randomized trial. *New England Journal of Medicine, 310,* 737-743.
Hirsch, V. R. (1993). Industry performance and public opinion. In N. F. Estrin (Ed.), *The cosmetic industry: Scientific and regulatory foundations.* New York: Dekker.
MacMahon, B., et al. (1981). Coffee and cancer of the pancreas. *New England Journal of Medicine, 304,* 630-633.
Marshall, E. (1987). Tobacco science wars. *Science, 236,* 250-251.
Miller, B. A., et al. (1993). *SEER cancer statistics review, 1973-1990.* Bethesda, MD: National Cancer Institute.
Morris, R. D., et al. (1992). Chlorination, chlorination by-products, and cancer: A meta-analysis. *American Journal of Public Health, 82,* 955-963.
National Coffee Association. (1987). *Coffee consumption and pancreatic cancer: A scientific update.* New York: Author.
Parkin, D. M., et al. (1988). Estimates of the worldwide frequency of sixteen major cancers in 1980. *International Journal of Cancer, 41,* 184-197.
Polednak, A. P. (1989). *Racial and ethnic differences in disease.* New York: Oxford University Press.
Proctor, R. N. (1993). The Oberrothenbach catastrophe. *Science, 260,* 1676-1677.
Proctor, R. N. (1995). *Cancer wars: How politics shapes what we know and don't know about cancer.* New York: Basic Books.
Rosser, S. V. (1994). *Women's health—Missing from U. S. medicine.* Bloomington: Indiana University Press.
Wynder, E. L. (1993). Toward a smoke-free society: Opportunities and obstacles. *American Journal of Public Health, 83,* 1204-1205.

13 Radiation: The Ghost in the Biosphere

JUDITH H. JOHNSRUD

Irradiation of biological organisms occurs when unstable matter decays, releasing its radiant energy, which in turn comes into contact with a living being. That radiation, striking or passing through a cell or through a cell nucleus, may disrupt any atom or molecule with which it comes in contact. It may have no effect, or it may cause cellular death or a mutation that alters the structure or function of the cell's constituents, subsequent cell reproduction, or the organism as a whole.[1] Ionizing radiation received from cosmic and terrestrial sources is thus an agent of genetic change. It is one of the means by which we humans and all other fauna and flora have evolved slowly over time, at naturally occurring radiation exposure levels that are relatively constant worldwide and have remained so for thousands of years.

"Ghost in the biosphere" aptly characterizes ionizing radiation: We are bombarded continuously by that which human beings cannot detect with our ordinary senses. We cannot see, smell, taste, or feel it. It is present in the atmosphere, in water, soil, bedrock, and in plants and animals. Radiation exists, and, in itself, it is neither a positive nor a negative entity.

The nature and extent of the detrimental health effects that may result from exposures to ionizing radiation, from either naturally occurring or man-made sources, is a subject of substantial controversy in medical and other scientific circles. The significance of the disagreement to

members of the public lies in the experimental nature of permitting increased doses to the population as a whole from nuclear energy facilities and activity beyond the exposures we receive from natural background radiation. The ethical dictum that guides the medical profession is pertinent: *primum non nocere;* first, do no harm. This commentary is based on the conservative public health principle that, absent certainty of safety, an excess of caution is prudent when an entire population, present and future, is at risk.

THE HAZARD OF IONIZING RADIATION TO HUMAN HEALTH

Undetected, gamma and X rays pass through our bodies, sometimes harmlessly and sometimes randomly causing injury. Charged alpha and beta particles may enter the body via ingestion and inhalation or through cuts and skin abrasions. Depending on their rates of decay ("half-life") and length of retention in the body, they can long remain, residing in the lungs and blood, or building into bone and tissue. These particles then undergo radioactive decay internally, causing their disruptions at the cellular or molecular level. Often, after an exposure, the resultant damage has a long latency period, with the lapse of many years or decades—or even generations for genetic effects—before any injury can be clinically observed. The intense irradiation by alpha particle decay internally is believed to be particularly dangerous; recent research indicates that a "delayed mutational effect" may be experienced in a cell that appears to reproduce normally for several cell generations before the harmful mutation can be detected (Kadhim et al., 1992; see also Nagasawa & Little, 1992).

In the introduction to his recent physician's guide to identification and medical management of radiation injuries, Donnell W. Boardman (1992) explained,

> The risks inherent in the manufacture, storage, and distribution, as well as use, of radioactive materials have been minimized. . . . Many ill-effects have been newly identified and are as yet poorly defined and understood. Diagnosis is difficult, partly because no two people will have the same dose or injury, partly because access to official records and pertinent scientific literature is restricted . . . [and] because specific radiobiologic effects cannot be reproduced in the laboratory.

Ionizing radiation targets only a part of any one of the billions of atoms in a single cell; its energy is dispersed unevenly among many atoms of any of the approximately 75 trillion cells in the human body. No two people, or even comparable DNA segments of any two cells, can receive the same dose of ionizing radiation.

Much molecular damage is done . . . before symptoms can be recognized. Few radiation recipients will have early definable symptoms, though some may exhibit vague symptomatology, including fatigue, joint and muscle pain, and gastro-intestinal discomfort. No two will have the same clinical picture.

EVOLUTION OF RADIATION PROTECTION

Historically, it had been known for centuries that miners in certain mountainous areas of eastern Europe experienced lung disease. The late nineteenth- and early twentieth-century research of Henri Becquerel and, later, Marie and Pierre Curie identified radioactive properties of uranium, radium, and other unstable elements. But the development of the first internationally accepted radiation protection standards for workers and the public did not come about until 1925. As more information about the carcinogenic qualities of ionizing radiation has become available over the last seventy years, radiation exposure limits have become progressively more restrictive (U.S. Department of Energy, 1995).

At first, health physicists who recommended the public exposure limits had assumed that there would be relatively few domestic nuclear facilities and that only nuclear industry workers and a small portion of the total population would therefore receive appreciable doses. It was, however, understood from the outset that those members of the public who did receive exposures from the permissible routine releases would be at some increased risk of radiation-induced diseases or life-shortening effects. In determining acceptable radiation exposure limits, these scientists made a judgment that the overall benefits to society from the commercial uses of atomic energy would outweigh the risks and injuries incurred by the individuals exposed.

A second assumption of the standard setters in the earlier period was that there is some safe threshold of exposure, below which no harm would occur. Despite the knowledge among geneticists, such as Herman Muller, of adverse mutational effects, there was a lack of statistically significant observations of negative health effects at low doses in human beings. This lack, combined with some evidence of cell repair mechanisms, led to the conclusion that human beings would not experience important damaging impacts from low-level radiation exposures.

It was only in 1990 that the National Academy of Sciences Committee on the Biological Effects of Ionizing Radiations (BEIR Committee) addressed biomedical studies of the alterations of genes and chromosomes resulting from low doses and low dose rates. This committee, which had earlier supported the assumption of a safe threshold of exposure, reached the conclusion that the frequency of such effects as cancer induction and heredity genetic effects increases with low-level radiation as a linear, non-threshold function of the dose, in spite of evidence that molecular lesions which give rise to somatic and genetic damage can be repaired to a considerable degree.

In short, the Academy's National Research Council BEIR Committee now agrees that there is no safe radiation dose. It had long been recognized that some number of spontaneous cancers (variously estimated at about 20,000 per year) were attributable to naturally occurring background radiation exposures (Morgan, personal communication, c. 1976-1978). But this statement by the conservative BEIR Committee was a marked departure from its prior positions that small, incremental doses were essentially harmless.

Why had it taken so many decades for the deleterious consequences of radiation exposures to be recognized? The explanation lies, at least in part, in the intricate relationships of the development of nuclear technologies in secrecy in wartime, the use of atomic bombs by the United States, the federal government's desire to establish constructive commercial uses of the atom for peaceful purposes, the electric utility industry's wish to allay public reservations about nuclear safety, and the continuing context of military weaponry and secrecy throughout the years of the Cold War. The Energy Department only revealed its role and that of its predecessor, the Atomic Energy Commission, in human radiation experimentation in 1993-1994, as part of the agency's effort to regain public confidence.

The delay in recognition of the variety and extent of radiation effects can also be explained by the length of time and the size of a study population that are required to obtain reliable data on latent injuries in a civilian population. Our society does not keep national data banks of health-related information. Our population is mobile; it is difficult to trace people who have received radiation doses in years past or to determine their exposures —especially low-level doses—from sources in the environment. Robust epidemiological data were rare, even if there had been a will on the part of governmental agencies to detect the full range of negative health effects.

U.S. radiation protection standards have, in the past, been based largely on the data obtained from post-World War II studies of Japanese who survived the 1945 U.S. atomic bombings of Hiroshima and Nagasaki. Some scholars have noted that the study subjects were an anomalous population, composed of those who are known as "healthy survivors"—that is, the people who were still alive, despite deprivations of food, shelter, and medical care, by the end of the decade, when the Atomic Bomb Casualty Commission (ABCC) began its observations (Stewart, personal communication, 1982). The initial dose estimates were uncertain. Cancers, leukemia, and genetic malformations were the principal consequences for which the ABCC scientists were looking in the decades that followed.

Research in the 1980s by a successor scientific organization—the Radiation Effects Research Foundation, sponsored jointly by the United States and Japan—undertook dose reconstructions of the Japanese survivors. These researchers concluded that the cancer effects per unit of dose received were in fact higher than the earlier data had indicated (Preston & Pierce, 1987, 1988; Preston et al., 1987; Radiation Effects Research Foundation, 1987, 1988).

During the 1980s, both international bodies that recommend regulations and the responsible federal agencies in the United States reviewed the emerging scientific literature on radiation impacts. A long enough time had passed that latency periods had expired for the appearance of leukemia (typically less than a decade) and solid tumors (two or more decades). Once again, authorities found that exposure limits were too lax to provide sufficient protection of public health and safety. The previous decade had seen rapid expansion of the nuclear power industry, especially in the United States and Europe. By the mid-1970s, American utilities expected nearly 200 large nuclear power reactors in operation by the year 2000, although only about 115 reactors were eventually built. The proportion of the population receiving occupational radiation doses had grown, as had the exposures from multiple sources for the general public. The March 1979 Three Mile Island, Unit 2, (TMI) accident provided a sobering realization among members of the nuclear industry and its regulators that large amounts of radioactivity might be disseminated broadly into the planetary environment in consequence of accidents more severe than anticipated by the regulators.

The level of naturally occurring background radiation—between 100 and 200 millirem (a measure of dose received)—was being augmented by the total of allowed emissions from each licensed facility and also by accidental releases, plus the doses received from medical practices. In the aftermath of the TMI accident, the nuclear industry noted that yet another source of exposure had been overlooked: accumulations of radioactive radon gas in poorly ventilated buildings. In the 1980s, the national and international commissions that recommend standards estimated that, if radon was included, the average dose to the public had risen to between 300 and 400 millirem per year, and it adopted an annual average dose of 360 millirem. Independent anecdotal monitoring, however, indicates that few outdoor locales register even half that amount.[2]

To meet the need to apply more restrictive standards in this burgeoning technology, the International Commission on Radiological Protection recommended tightening dose limits from routine emissions. In 1994, after more than a dozen years of review, the U.S. Nuclear Regulatory Commission (NRC) implemented revised regulations that appeared to set more stringent exposure standards for the public by reducing the maximum permissible individual dose from 500 millirem to 100 millirem per year (but permitting licensees to request exceptions that allowed the older dose limit). However, the method of calculating the dose was changed as well, substituting for specific dose limits to the critical organs an approach that used weighting factors to account for organ doses in estimating an annual total effective dose equivalent to an individual member of the public (U.S. Code of Federal Regulations, Title 10, Part 20).

THE ROLE OF LAW AND REGULATION

It is important to understand that licensed producers and users of radioactive materials are self-reporting to the regulatory agency. The data they submit on radiation releases into the environment from an operating facility are applied in dispersion models to calculate doses received by individuals. The U.S. Environmental Protection Agency (EPA) sets environmental standards for exposures to the public from licensed facilities; the NRC implements those standards or, in certain circumstances, its own standards under a Memorandum of Understanding with EPA. The NRC does not monitor real doses to real people.

As for irradiation from nuclear weapons production and testing facilities operated by the U.S. Department of Energy (DOE) under the guise of national security, that agency has not in the past been subject to EPA and NRC radiation protection standards. Radiological contamination of weapons-production facilities has been severe; the costs and difficulty of decommissioning and decontaminating those sites are only beginning to be comprehended. In 1991, the EPA reported to Congress that more than forty-five thousand sites in the United States were either radiologically contaminated or potentially contaminated. Although some of those sites may be readily cleaned up and released for unrestricted use, the NRC, in its 1994 Staff Draft Criteria for Decommissioning, stated that there may be "a few tens of sites" where the radioactive contamination is so pervasive that public health and safety will be best protected by permanent on-site stabilization and disposal, "despite the failure to meet the 100 millirem per year cap" on doses to an average member of the critical group of people who are most likely to receive exposure at the site in the future, after it has been released for restricted use.

Moreover, the standards for present and future exposures to members of the public from radioactive waste storage and disposal facilities may be subject to relaxation, either by changes in agency definitions and regulations, by economic factors, or by congressional action. The allowable exposure limits for waste disposal sites are of particular significance, because the proposed disposal technologies will not permit easy recovery in the event of repository failure. Although a congressman once observed that "radioactive waste is our grandchildren's problem; let them worry about it," an axiom of nuclear waste management has long been that the generation that produces the waste should be responsible for its disposal.

Nonetheless, the DOE and the states have struggled unsuccessfully for decades to site, build, license, and operate new disposal facilities for both high- and low-level wastes. Waste generators resist paying the full costs for reliable long-term containment of radioactive wastes in isolation. The technologies that have been devised for sequestration in the fifty years of the Atomic Age are, quite obviously, still experimental, relative to the duration of the hazardous life of some of the wastes, which extends into the hundreds of thousands of years or longer. As more and more wastes accumulate from the operation of more than one hundred reactors, plus nuclear weapons wastes, the costs of isolation continue to escalate.

In consequence of the escalating costs of waste management and disposal—even if one imagines that it is possible to "dispose" of anything—the nuclear industry has turned to the deregulation of some nuclear wastes. Since the late 1970s, the NRC has attempted repeatedly to declare some radioactive wastes to be *de minimis* (trivial) in hazard and hence capable of being categorized as "Below Regulatory Concern." Under policies developed in 1986 and 1990, the NRC had planned to release low-activity wastes into the biosphere without restriction or labels, to be "disposed" of in municipal landfills, the liquids dumped into sewers, and radioactive materials recycled into consumer products (NRC Final Policy Statement, *Federal Register*, July 1990). For each "justified practice," an individual in the public would have been permitted to receive an annual dose up to 10 millirem, an additional 10 percent above natural background levels. There appeared to be no limit to the number of such justified practices that the NRC might approve. This potentially massive deregulation of low-level radioactive waste was halted by a provision of the 1992 National Energy Policy Act, but current low-level waste "minimization" practices allow incineration, with some release into the atmosphere and a concentration of activity in the ash.

The United Nations Scientific Committee on the Effects of Atomic Radiation (UNSCEAR) published two massive reports in 1993 that summarized the current state of knowledge concerning low-dose and chronic low-dose radiation impacts. Although this committee continues to support the efficacy of cellular repair and organic adaptive response mechanisms in lessening the negative effects of irradiation, UNSCEAR, too, concludes that low-dose radiation is associated with initiation of fatal cancers, leukemia, and genetic damage—and also with noncancer illnesses and dysfunction of the immune system.

THE DARK SHADOW OF CHERNOBYL: CHRONIC LOW-DOSE EFFECTS FROM RESIDUAL RADIATION

The catastrophic explosion in April 1986 of the Chernobyl Block 4 reactor, located on the Ukrainian-Belarussian border, spewed out more than 100 million curies of radioactive gases and particulates, contaminating much of Europe and vast areas of the then-Soviet Union with long-lived radioisotopes. In the following years, government authorities in Moscow dismissed the complaints of illnesses among the children in Ukraine and Belarussia as "radiophobia" or "radiation hysteria," and prohibited physicians from linking radiation with the sicknesses they were treating (A. Guskova, Ministry of Health, Moscow, personal communication, 1989, 1991; Yevgeny Velikov, Deputy Director of the Kurchatov Institute for Nuclear Physics, Moscow, personal communication, 1991).

Nearly a decade after the disaster, Belarussian and Ukrainian health officials report that some 125,000 deaths are believed to have resulted from Chernobyl. Moreover, radiation biologists find that residual radioactivity, deposited unevenly over extensive regions, has spread, entering the soil, water supplies, and the food chain. Slightly contaminated foodstuffs are shipped throughout the former Soviet Union, consumed by people far from Chernobyl. Day after day, from slightly contaminated food and water and from radioactive dust particles, individuals receive repeated low-dose exposures via ingestion and inhalation pathways, a ghostly presence in the lives of many and a source of anxiety about the future well-being of these radiation recipients.

Doctors and radiobiologists, now free to speak out since the dissolution of the Soviet Union, assert that the health consequence of chronic low-dose radiation exposures, especially for rapidly growing young children, is damage to the immune system. Immunological dysfunction, they find, in turn increases susceptibility to infections and many other diseases. Even from the normal diseases of childhood, children are sicker, stay sick longer, and experience frequent recurrences. They suffer from increased allergies, asthma, diabetes, and disorders of respiratory, gastrointestinal, and endocrine systems.

Teachers and sports instructors report that their students exhibit chronic fatigue, lack of stamina, a marked inability to concentrate and learn, and consequent stress-related sociopathic behaviors. Overall, the physicians have identified the medical condition known as "failure to thrive." These noncancer effects are observed in addition to the leukemias and rare childhood thyroid cancers that already have increased many times within the first few years since the accident (E. Burlakova et al., Soviet Academy of Sciences, personal communication, 1991).

In April 1991, leading radiobiologists in the Soviet Academy of Sciences declared flatly that "the Hiroshima model of dose-response does not apply to the situation of Chernobyl." At Hiroshima, the bomb had been a single above-ground blast; the plume had moved off over the ocean. At Chernobyl, there was the initial powerful explosion and the stratospheric rise of the plume and fallout; but, also, the reactor burned for nearly two weeks, producing intense near-ground radiation that caused heavy contamination.

It is, however, the lingering residual radioactive contamination that gives rise now to the protracted low-level radiation exposures, the chronic doses that damage in subtle and indirect ways. "The Chernobyl model of dose-response is very different. We are rewriting classical radiation biology," said Dr. Elena Burlakova, chairperson in 1991 of the Soviet Academy of Sciences Scientific Council on Problems of Radiation Biology (personal communication, 1991). She dismissed the former government's claim that these illnesses are "merely due to stress." As for the laboratory dogs that are given radiation doses comparable to those received by the children, she said, "The dogs don't suffer from radiation hysteria. They get sick, just like the children."

In the long run, it is that ghostly shade over the environment, everywhere increasing "radiation loading" throughout the biosphere, that may eventually pose the most injurious threat to human health, undermining well-being of children. Quite apart from personal suffering, the health care costs and losses of economic productivity that may result from higher radiation levels have not been calculated. The electorate has not been offered a choice. Chernobyl should stand as a warning for the future, of the thickening of the radiation environment all around us, as more and more emissions are allowed to enter air and water, as more and more waste accumulates, as accidents happen.

ISOLATING THE RADIOACTIVE GHOST FROM THE BIOSPHERE

As the world enters the second half-century of the Atomic Age that began with the splitting of the atom and approaches a new millennium, nuclear nations have generated thousands of tons and millions of cubic meters of radioactive wastes. Nuclear weapons production and the commercial use of nuclear energy to generate electricity account for the majority of these wastes, some of which are intensely radioactive and possess very long hazardous lives. In the absence of proven capability to ensure permanent isolation of wastes, the continuing reliance on nuclear power in many countries, plus the numerous industrial, medical, and research uses of the atom, contribute to the total accumulating quantities and long-term biological dangers of nuclear wastes.

Furthermore, the operations of nuclear facilities of all types continue to allow both sanctioned "permissible" routine emissions and occasional accidental releases into the biosphere. There, even as the various radioactive isotopes are decaying at their differential rates, dispersing and diluting, they are also accumulating and reconcentrating in the food chain. They affect the quality of the environment and, ultimately, the health and safety of human beings, whether they are near the source or far away from the point and time of origin of the releases. It is, therefore, virtually impossible for a radiation recipient to be able to trace the causation of an illness, a cancer, leukemia, or birth defect, to the original source.

The ghostly presence of radiation in the environment will not go away. It cannot be "treated" and neutralized; it will remain with us for many generations, slowly decaying at given physical rates, releasing its energy, causing random biological injury. But the option exists to curtail the production of ever more radioactive materials and wastes. We already possess technologies to replace most uses of the atom. Extension of the Non-Proliferation Treaty and the continued dismantling of nuclear weapons, although the latter creates serious unresolved problems of preventing diversion of fissile materials and of plutonium disposition, are positive steps toward a less dangerous "denuclearized" future. An end to production of additional quantities of radioactive waste would "bound the problem," allowing us to know how much and what kinds of nuclear materials and wastes must be sequestered for the hundreds and thousands of years of their hazardous lives. We can then undertake to minimize the biological damage that may result from wastes already generated.

It seems reasonable that a first step should be to change our nation's nuclear energy policy. It is a relic from the now-failed hope of the peaceful atom, enshrined in an outmoded statute. The introductory declaration that opens the 1954 Atomic Energy Act, the governing law, states,

> Atomic energy is capable of application for peaceful as well as military purposes. It is therefore declared to be the policy of the United States that—
>
> a. the development, use, and control of atomic energy shall be directed so as to make the maximum contribution to the general welfare, subject at all times to the paramount objective of making the maximum contribution to the common defense and security; and
>
> b. the development, use, and control of atomic energy shall be directed so as to promote world peace, improve the general welfare, increase the standard of living, and strengthen free competition in private enterprise.

Missing from this policy, nearly half a century old, is any specific statement that the true paramount U.S. objective, with respect to ionizing radiation, is to protect the health and safety of the American people and the quality of the environment. A political will to make that transition to a policy based on prevention of radiation damage is essential if the slow but inexorable spread of ever more radiation into the biosystem is to be halted, and if the thickening of the radiation environment around us is ever to be reversed.

No one set of actions will end the nation's commitment to the uses of nuclear energy. Nuclear technologies have embedded themselves deeply in the economy of our nation and many other countries. Not all atomic uses would, or doubtless should, be ended. Some uses of the atom would be easy to replace; some would not. Alternative and innovative technologies, however, are already starting to reduce reliance on nuclear materials and nuclear-generated electricity. The half-century focus on nuclear armaments has shifted to their disposition. Economic realities associated with operations, maintenance, equipment replacement, and, above all, nuclear waste isolation are being taken very seriously, with an increasing demand for full cost accounting of the entire system of nuclear energy production and utilization; we begin to internalize the externalities.

Many people have come to believe that a political will to denuclearize can bring about a safer, less expensive national energy and security future, as the Union of South Africa has done and the Ukraine proposes to do. The United States can do so, too, if it so chooses. The radioactive ghost will not vanish altogether, but it can be brought under watchful control. High priority must be given to seeking better means of nuclear guardianship that will ensure equal opportunity for future peoples to be able to maintain control over the nuclear waste produced during our time on Earth. Surely it is prudent to try.

NOTES

1. I am indebted particularly to the late Donnell W. Boardman, M.D., founder and president emeritus, Center for Atomic Radiation Studies, Cambridge, Massachusetts, for his insights into low-dose and noncancer effects of exposures to ionizing radiation, and to John W. Gofman, Ph.D., M.D., and Alice M. Stewart, M.D., for patient tutelage in the health effects of ionizing radiation.

2. The author has engaged in informal monitoring since 1989; except at high elevations or in areas of high uranium or thorium bedrock, the average figure observed in most of the United States is closer to 120-150 millirem per year dose level. Citizen groups near nuclear facilities have begun to develop independent radiation monitoring capability.

REFERENCES

Atomic Energy Act of 1954, 42 USC sec. 2011, in U.S. Nuclear Regulatory Commission, Office of the General Counsel, Nuclear Regulatory Legislation, 102d Congress, NUREG-0980, Vol. 1, No. 2, 1993.

Boardman, D. W. (1992). *Radiation impact: Atoms to zygotes: Low level radiation in the nuclear age*. Cambridge, MA: Center for Atomic Radiation Studies.

Kadhim, M. A., et al. (1992). Transmission of chromosomal instability after plutonium alpha-particle irradiation. *Nature, 355,* 738-740.

Nagasawa, H., & Little, J. B. (1992). Induction of sister chromatid exchanges by extremely low doses of alpha-particles. *Cancer Research, 52,* 6394-6396.

National Academy of Sciences, National Research Council, Committee on the Biological Effects of Ionizing Radiations (BEIR Committee). (1990). *Health effects of exposure to low levels of ionizing radiation*. Washington, DC: National Academy Press.

Preston, D. L., Kato, H., et al. (1987). Cancer mortality among A-bomb survivors in Hiroshima and Nagasaki, 1950-1982. *Radiation Research, 114,* 437-466.

Preston, D. L., & Pierce, D. A. The effect of changes in dosimetry on cancer mortality risk estimates in the atomic bomb survivors," RERF Technical Report TR-9-87, Hiroshima, Japan, 1987; Radiation Research, 1988.

Radiation Effects Research Foundation. (1987). U.S.-Japan joint reassessment of atomic bomb radiation dosimetry in Hiroshima and Nagasaki: Volume 1.

Radiation Effects Research Foundation. (1988). U.S.-Japan joint reassessment of atomic bomb radiation dosimetry in Hiroshima and Nagasaki: Volume 2.

Stewart, A. M. (1982). Delayed effects of A-bomb radiation: A review of recent mortality rates and risk estimates for five-year survivors. *Journal of Epidemiology and Community Health, 36,* 80-86.

United Nations Scientific Committee on the Effects of Atomic Radiation (UNSCEAR). (1993). *Sources and effects of ionizing radiations* (UN Pub. Sales No. E.94.IX.2). New York: Author.

United Nations Scientific Committee on the Effects of Atomic Radiation (UNSCEAR). (1994). *Sources and effects of ionizing radiations* (UN Pub. Sales No. E.94.IX.11). New York: Author.

U.S. Department of Energy, Office of Environmental Management. (1995). *Closing the circle on the splitting of the atom*. Washington, DC: Author.

14 A Molecular Basis for Development

An Environmental Policy for the 1990s

DAVID MORRIS

The environmental threat facing us is growing, but so is our capacity to face that threat. We have tools available to us today that did not even exist a decade ago. Ideas that were then restricted to academia have been put into practice on a commercial scale. Technologies that can form the basis for an ecological economy existed then only in the laboratory or, at best, in pilot plants. They are now commercially available. Industries that were just emerging eighteen years ago now form an important constituency for a green economy. And governments are now fashioning and enacting regulatory and fiscal incentives that are changing the economic underpinnings of the material foundation of industrialized economies.

It is a moment fraught with peril and opportunity. The puzzle pieces of renewal now exist. What is lacking is a coherent strategy that can excite the popular imagination and galvanize the political will to embrace solutions commensurate with the scale of the problem and of the opportunity.

AUTHOR'S NOTE: This chapter is excerpted from *A Molecular Basis for Development: An Environmental Policy for the 1990s* (1990), published by the Institute for Local Self-Reliance, Washington, D.C.

THE NEW ENVIRONMENTALISM

The environmental movement has had three distinct, although overlapping, historical phases. The first, and still the largest in terms of constituency and influence, was initiated in the early twentieth century. Its objective is wilderness preservation. Anglers, hikers, and hunters make up the bulk of its members, and the national park system is its most enduring legacy.

The second phase began in earnest in the 1960s with the publication of Rachel Carson's (1962) book, *Silent Spring*, and had its coming out party on Earth Day 1970. Its objective is to restrict chemicals directly harmful to animals or humans. The toxic reduction movement led to bans of DDT, PCBs, and leaded gasoline and the development of quantitative emission standards for dozens of other chemicals. The most important legacies of this era are the environmental impact statement and the development of statistical techniques to measure the impact of environmental degradation.

The third phase of the environmental movement began with the discovery of the ozone hole over the South Pole in the mid-1980s and was reinforced by the growing concern over global warming and acid rain. Its concerns go beyond the short-term dangers to life posed by toxic chemicals to the long-term dangers to life and world economies from chemicals toxic to nature as a system. In other words, it concerns itself with sustainability. Chlorofluorocarbons are nontoxic. Indeed, the inventor introduced freon at the 1930 American Cancer Society meeting by inhaling a lungfull and blowing out a candle, demonstrating the refrigerant's nontoxic and nonflammable nature. Nor is carbon dioxide toxic. It is a natural and necessary part of living systems. Even nitrogen and sulfur, the individual components of acid rain, are relatively nontoxic until they become dangerous acids when mixed with water. Then, like many anthropogenic chemical interactions, they undermine the equilibrium of natural systems.

The new environmentalism is global in its orientation and radical in its objectives. It provides the opportunity to develop strategies that address the weaknesses of previous environmental efforts. Wilderness preservationists, for example, traditionally focus their efforts on stopping destruction rather than redirecting development. This puts them at odds with those who worry about economic growth and jobs. The toxic reduction movement successfully organizes the grass roots by playing on fears. That can lead to the not-in-my-backyard syndrome, a philosophy which, like that of wilderness preservation, does not embrace

brace a new development paradigm. A focus on toxics can paralyze a citizenry unschooled in chemistry. Moreover, by targeting hundreds of discrete chemicals, it can win many battles while losing the war against pollution.

A MATERIALS POLICY

What is needed is a strategy that (a) cuts across the concerns of the various elements of the environmental movement; (b) is easily understood by the average citizen; and (c) bridges the concerns of worker and consumer, First World and Third World, urban dweller and farmer alike. What is needed is a policy that embraces a positive vision of the future: one that can be the basis for a new kind of economic development strategy. We need a comprehensive materials policy, that is, a focus on the molecular foundation of a green economy.

This policy must rest on a moral and an economic underpinning. The moral imperative has the following two components:

> Each nation is entitled only to its proportionate share of the Earth's resources.
>
> All nations must use materials on a sustainable basis, both in terms of the available reserves and the carrying capacity of air and water to absorb the pollution that comes with consuming those reserves.

To achieve the first objective requires a drastic reduction in the industrialized world's consumption of raw materials. To achieve the second requires not only a reduction but a shift from use of the most polluting of all massively used materials, fossil fuels, to the use of direct solar energy or stored solar energy in plant matter.

We need not rely on a moral imperative. The economic benefits of a materials policy can provide an equally persuasive justification. An ecological economy can lower operating costs and strengthen domestic, local, rural, and Third World economies. It can enhance national security while it strengthens economic security. And it can achieve these ends while making local and regional economies more self-reliant.

ADVANTAGES OF A MATERIALS POLICY

A materials policy is quantifiable. Therefore it allows us to measure our progress and establish quantitative goals. We can decide to save *x* amount of kilowatt hours or to reduce our per capita consumption of fossil fuels by *y* amount, and verify our performance with relative ease.

A materials policy can be implemented at all levels of government and enterprise. It need not wait on national and international actions. Recycling, energy efficiency, and the substitution of plant matter can be strongly encouraged by cities, counties, and states, as well as nations, at the same time that all work together to fashion global rules to further promote such efforts. Thus, the potential for wide participation and public education is great.

Such a policy offers a positive development vision, something to advocate as well as something to oppose. Its benefits accrue not only to the planet or the nation, but also to the region, and even to the household. Higher energy efficiency reduces the amount of money that leaves a region to pay for imported fuels. Increased recycling generates a pool of valuable scrap that can spur the development of regional industries. Increasing the demand for plant matter strengthens rural economies not only by raising the price of agricultural materials, but also by encouraging the location of processing and even product manufacturing facilities in these same communities. The use of direct solar energy potentially allows for even greater decentralization. A rooftop photovoltaic array, even at current efficiencies, could make the household virtually self-sufficient in electricity.

A comprehensive materials policy can integrate concerns about social justice and equity with environmental considerations. A radical drop in materials consumption by industrialized countries, one might argue, would harm Third World economies dependent on export of raw materials. However, even though the volume of materials trade might decline, the value of materials and therefore the overall revenue accruing to the Third World would increase. Moreover, technologies developed in industrialized countries that extract the maximum amount of useful work and value from renewable resources may be appropriate for Third World countries, allowing them to reduce dramatically the need for imported fuels and consequently, the need for hard currency. The need of Third World economies for hard currency to pay for imports has driven them to increase exports, often at the expense of the local and global environment. Increasing capacity to convert raw materials into products for domestic consumption in the developing world can raise the standard of living of the poorest, most rural segments of these countries.

A materials policy offers a benchmark against which to evaluate specific public policies, namely the extent to which we reduce materials consumption and substitute renewable resources for fossil fuels. Consider the environmental movement's changing response to the garbage crisis. When, in the late 1970s, it was discovered that leaking landfills polluted groundwater, national environmental groups supported incinerators as a viable alternative. In the mid-1980s, when incinerators themselves turned out to be serious polluters, the environmental community turned against them. The result was an understandable confusion and hostility from policymakers, who viewed environmentalists as negative not-in-my-backyarders.

Given a clearheaded materials policy, we would have argued against incinerators from the outset for the simple reason that incinerators destroy materials. Even if we could snap our fingers and have our wastes disappear into thin air, we would still be opposed to such a device because it encourages the consumption of raw materials and discourages recycling. Moreover, incinerators are usually sized to accommodate the majority of a community's garbage. Once in place, incinerators require major portions of the waste stream to operate economically and consequently tend to undermine efforts to achieve high levels of materials recovery.

Materials policy also clarifies the issue of degradable plastics. The environmental community at first supported such plastics, only to turn against them when it was discovered they were not truly degradable. A materials policy based on frugality would have opposed degradable plastics because, as with incineration, degradability encourages materials destruction. Materials recovery, not materials destruction, should be our goal.

Using a similar evaluation, we would oppose methanol derived from natural gas and favor ethanol derived from plant matter. Methanol is the fuel of choice by some environmentalists because natural gas is less polluting than gasoline, whereas ethanol is now made from energy-intensive, input-intensive corn crops. However, if fuels based on plant matter were to become our primary fuel supply, we would be relying not on corn, but on less input-intensive crops, such as sweet sorghum, woody grasses, and ultimately, single-celled algae. We would forestall the technological dynamic that would lead us in this direction if we were to move aggressively to a transport system based on natural gas.

INTERNATIONAL ORIENTATION

The environmental movement is formulating numerous regulations such as global greenhouse gas-emission standards, global forestry standards, sustainable fishery standards, and so on. These global conventions should have teeth in them. Violators should be viewed as international outlaws. The Montreal Protocol, which led to a phaseout of ozone-depleting chemicals, set an interesting precedent. The protocol allowed signatories to boycott products from nonsignatory nations. In other words, the world saw the threat to the biosphere as aggression and nations that continued to emit ozone-depleting chemicals as criminals subject to sanctions.

While global conventions related to environmental standards are being developed, so are global free-trade agreements. The latter may well undermine the former. Already the U.S.-Canadian free trade agreement undermines either country's ability to protect its environment rigorously. In Europe, Denmark has recently been ruled in violation of the European free-trade treaty because of its refillable bottle rule, and Germany's returnable container legislation is the subject of another complaint. In the proposed round of negotiations over the General Agreement on Tariffs and Trade (GATT), the United States proposes to eliminate the ability of countries and states to enact environmental standards more stringent than the global minimum standards.

The environmental movement should support global environmental standards while defending the right of individual nations and subnational units to exceed these standards and impose their more rigorous standards on imports.

FOCUS ON STATES AND CITIES

While national and international policies are important, much can be accomplished now on the state and local levels. States and cities have significant authority over materials use. They regulate and sometimes own electric and gas utilities, establish building codes, are responsible for collecting and disposing of garbage and sewage, manage forests, finance technical schools and state universities, and often possess significant economic development capabilities.

Focusing on state and local levels allows for more grassroots organizing, more public education, and more interaction with business, government, labor, and community groups than can be easily achieved on the national and international levels.

To concentrate on a state is to concentrate on a delimited territory. The goal is material self-reliance. Defining the goal territorially encourages comprehensive thinking, which simplifies the task. The focus on a state makes it easier to conceptualize a comprehensive strategy and to bring together the principal players.

This does not mean that operating on a state level will be easy. State agencies, after all, are fragmented along traditional lines in a way that undermines the ability of agency officials to think comprehensively. State departments of agriculture, for instance, are responsible for plant matter that grows in less than two years, whereas state forestry departments are responsible for biomass that matures over longer periods. Sewage authorities dispose of what could be excellent plant fertilizer. The sanitation department disposes of organic waste, an excellent complement to human waste for compost. The utility department regulates electric utilities, a potential consumer of biomass for fuels. The environmental department issues car emissions regulations that could spur the use of alternative fuels. And so forth.

DEVELOPING BAROMETERS OF SUCCESS

We need to know how well we are doing. When charities embark on fund-raising drives, they almost always post a large thermometer outside their buildings. The goal is clearly indicated, and the red mercury level marks how far along the community has progressed toward the goal.

We need barometers of success in moving toward an equitable and sustainable materials economy. One might measure the overall per capita raw materials used in a city/state/region. The goal would be 50 percent reduction in per capita raw materials consumption in twenty years. All recycling or energy efficiency efforts, for example, would be measured against progress toward this goal. A second barometer would measure a shift from fossil fuels to renewable fuels. The goal would be a 50 percent substitution of the latter for the former within twenty years.

With such barometers, we would no longer be satisfied when a city announces it has increased its recycling levels, or when a utility tells us it has saved electricity, or when automobile fuel efficiency standards have increased. For if recycling levels go up but garbage levels do likewise, if conservation improves but demand increases, if fuel efficiency rises but so does the number of miles traveled, then we are failing to move toward our goal. The twin barometers of our success would enable us to visualize our progress—or lack thereof.

CONCLUSION

Focusing on a molecular basis for a new economy offers a positive, workable, economically sound vision of the future. It spurs the development and refinement of technologies that are as appropriate for the Third World as for the industrialized world. It also combines a moral imperative with a hardheaded economic analysis. A comprehensive materials policy provides a strategy that can be the basis for concrete actions while also providing a vision of a just, equitable, and self-reliant future. By making every molecule count, we can create a new, sustainable economy.

REFERENCE

Carson, R. (1962). *Silent spring.* Boston: Houghton Mifflin.

15 Reproductive Technologies

The Necessity for Limits

JANICE RAYMOND

The necessity for limits has been a forceful tenet in environmental circles. Recycling, reusing, and reducing waste, with the emphasis on not generating problematic products to begin with, has been crucial to the present current of environmental activism. Would that the same commitment to prohibiting problematic drugs and technologies were prevalent in the reproductive realm.

As environmental engineer H. Patricia Hynes (1990) has noted, toxic reproductive chemicals are exempted from an environmental consciousness; as a wave of green lifestyle washes over industrial countries, making people conscious of not putting any unnecessary synthetic substances on and into their bodies, why are women being advised to use synthetic hormones? Furthermore, why is there an unmitigated increase in the number and kinds of drugs and technical fixes that are being prescribed for women—especially in the reproductive realm—at a time when the rest of the planet is being warned about the risk of chemicals and technical fixes? Can we be disturbed about chemically fed plants and animals and remain unconscious about chemically fed women, many of whom take scores of drugs from menstruation to menopause?

AUTHOR'S NOTE: This chapter is excerpted from *Women as Wombs*, by Janice Raymond, and is reprinted by permission of HarperCollins Publishers, Inc.

Are women being exempted from the natural world as more and more bodily processes become subject to the medicalization of technical progress? Surely, a genuine ecological consciousness should spot this glaring pollution of women. If environmentalists are quick to recognize the mechanizing of nature, why are they so slow to recognize the pathologizing of women's natural bodily processes? Why are synthetic and technical procedures being limited on plants and animals, yet being increased on women?

Environmentalism has increased consciousness of the limits of the ecosystem. The necessity for limits has also been raised in medical-ethical circles. Much of this debate was initiated with the publication of Daniel Callahan's (1989) book, *What Kind of Life? The Limits of Medical Progress,* in which he talks about medical and human priorities and the American unwillingness to set limits on medical interventions. The debate about the limits of medical interventions and innovations has also been raised in legislatures and health-financing contexts, as federal, state, and private health providers wrestle with decisions about how much and what kind of health care and techniques to cover. Yet, many state and federal bills seem bent on expanding, rather than limiting, coverage for costly, high-tech procedures such as technological reproduction.

THE POLITICS OF REPRODUCTION

In 1987, Massachusetts signed into law a bill that would require insurance companies to pay for the medical treatment of infertility. It covers all aspects of diagnosis and treatment of infertility, including superovulation, in vitro fertilization (IVF), and embryo transfer. Earlier, Maryland passed a law that extended coverage to IVF. And more recently, Hawaii and Texas have passed laws requiring coverage of infertility procedures.

On the federal level, Representative Pat Schroeder introduced a bill into Congress in 1990 covering many aspects of women's health and reproductive services. Launched in the midst of the antiabortion climate in the United States, especially in the aftermath of the 1989 Supreme Court decision on abortion, the purpose of H.R. 1161 was to offset this climate by promoting "greater equity in the delivery of health care services to American women through expanded research of women's health issues, improved access to health care services, and the development of disease prevention activities responsive to the needs of women" (U.S. Congress, H. R. 1161, 102d Cong., 1st Sess., 1-182).

Many parts of this legislation were excellent and much needed, such as research into contraception for men and improved barrier methods such as diaphragms and condoms. However, along with these laudatory provisions, this legislation required insurance programs for federal workers to cover "family building" expenses such as infertility treatments, "including procedures to achieve pregnancy and procedures to carry pregnancy to term" (H. R. 1161, Subtitle F, Federal Employee Building Act, § 252, at 11-13).

With Representative Olivia Snowe as cosponsor, Schroeder also built into this bill an appropriation request for $75 million to set up five federal centers to conduct research into birth control and fertility. This section, entitled "Contraceptive and Infertility Research Centers Act," provided for continued research "for the purpose of diagnosing and treating infertility." Schroeder said that this would cover IVF research as well as "clinical trials of new or improved drugs and devices for the diagnosis and treatment of infertility in both males and females" (H. R. 1161, Subtitle F, Contraceptive and Infertility Research Centers Act, § 151, at 7-10). Since no technologies or drugs are detailed in this section, it is difficult to know what specific research and technologies would be investigated. However, one thing is certain: Instead of recognizing the need to limit costly and experimental research and treatments that serve the few, this legislation promotes medical expansionism over reproduction and the lives and bodies of women.

The United States is not alone in this debate about insurance coverage of new reproductive technologies such as in vitro fertilization. Other countries have been more critical and controlling of high technologies. Australia has begun to survey the costs of burgeoning high technologies and drugs, and in 1988 the Australian Family Association called for ending Medicare benefits for in vitro fertilization. The secretary of the association, Michael Barr, pointed out that in that year each live birth by IVF cost $40,500 (Australian). Other governmental groups and individuals called for a review of the cost-efficiency of such procedures and blamed increased coverage of high-tech procedures for a "health care cost blow-out."

DESIRE OR NEED?

At a conference on biomedical ethics, ethicist Arthur Caplan (1987) noted that the usual measure employed by insurers to evaluate a treatment's efficacy is a 50 percent success rate over a five-year period, based on performance of all providers. In no country in the world does IVF technology fulfill this standard of efficacy. The question is, then, why should it be insured? Also, technologies such as IVF are promoted as cures for infertility when, in reality, they do nothing to treat infertility. They may provide some very few people with biological children, but they do not alleviate infertility.

Most important, in the reproductive context, certain desires have been transformed into needs. The desire for a child, for example, has been represented as a need of supposedly infertile couples. As science invents new needs for people, often for people who can pay and who are of the right race, sex, class, or sexual preference, the critical health needs of most people go unattended and uncovered by medical insurance.

Although usually framed in economic terms, the issue of limits is much more than economic cost containment. Progress cannot simply be equated with the unlimited development and application of more reproductive technologies. We must pay attention to the values and circumstances surrounding their use. For example, when surrogacy promotes a class of women who can be bought and sold as breeders, is it really progress that more supposedly infertile couples can have babies in this way? Progress for whom?

Reproduction is on the frontier of an endless technical and medical horizon, where we could simply spend more and more money, intervening in the bodily processes of more and more women, at great cost to women's health and well-being and at the expense of providing for the genuine needs of others. The increased medicalization and technologizing of reproduction is part of the debate over the limits of medical progress and the concomitant necessity for limiting what insurance can and cannot cover. We cannot continue to develop these technologies with total indifference to any kinds of limits and priorities.

WHO BENEFITS?

Because women are the primary "patients" in this realm of reproductive techniques, the critical question is, do these technologies benefit women as a social group—not just individual women? Furthermore, limits and priorities should be measured by what is happening in other areas of health care. Attention is currently being drawn to the crisis of AIDS women and babies; one out of eight women suffers from breast cancer; maternal morbidity and infant mortality rates are high. In industrial nations, these deaths often take place in the same hospitals where elite reproductive technologies are being developed and expanded for the select few who have access to them. For African Americans in the United States, the neonatal death rate is more than twice the national average, and for Native Americans, it is five times the national average.

The issue should not be increasing access to experimental, costly, and potentially debilitating technologies but rather implementing priorities that prevent maternal morbidity and infant mortality, as well as ensuring access to basic health needs such as nutrition, sanitation, prenatal care, and prevention of disease. Some will say that these reproductive technologies need not be pitted against access to basic health care. Yet, these technologies can only be defended in the interests of servicing the few, not the many others whose pressing needs go unmet because research money and expertise are siphoned off in quest of more profitable and high-tech fixes in reproduction.

The development of more reproductive drugs and technologies is not in keeping with an ecology of women's health. The marketing of medical progress through new reproductive technologies assures continued experimentation on women's bodies and a spiraling of the cycle in which women are encouraged to try every new, sickening, and debilitating technique or drug, hyped as the next miracle cure, to have a child. Progress ultimately is a moral, social, and political standard not measured by increased medical and technical innovation. When the fullness of this standard is ignored, and when science and technology separate themselves from this standard, progress is a form of social self-deception. The correction of this limited standard of progress cannot come from more reproductive technologies but from the progress that ensures welfare, not only of women as individuals, but of all women in all areas of the world.

REFERENCES

Callahan, D. (1989). *What kind of life? The limit of medical progress.* New York: Simon and Schuster.

Caplan, A. (1987, September 1). Calls IVF sage but questions efficacy rates. *Ob Gyn News,* p. 3.

Hynes, P. (1990). Reconstructuring Babylon: Women and Appropriate Technology. Keynote address given at Nordic Conference on Women, Environment, and Development, Norwegian Research Council for Science, the Secretariat for Women and Research, University of Oslo, Center for Research for Women, Oslo, Norway, November, 1990, p. 20.

16 Primary Health Care

Commitment to the Health of All

MARILYN MARDIROS

The Declaration of Alma Ata (WHO-UNICEF, 1978) delineates a dynamic paradigm, that of primary health care (PHC), through which the health needs of the world's population are addressed by placing emphasis on self-reliance, self-determination, and social justice in matters related to human health and well-being. Beginning with the formation of the World Health Organization (WHO) in 1947-1948, this chapter traces events from 1948 to 1978 leading to the Declaration of Alma Ata. An overview of the thrust of primary health care as an ideological shift from the biomedical model of health care is provided and includes consideration of the relevance of traditional forms of health care to contemporary health needs. The chapter ends with a discussion of the significance of ecological sustainability in health by fostering new partnerships between providers and consumers of health services through community involvement and control of relevant resources and services related to health.

BACKGROUND

In 1948, WHO was established as a specialized agency within the United Nations, responding to the need to consolidate activities in international health and address the health-related needs of the world's population. From its inception, WHO was mandated to unite activities within international health through cooperation, coordination, and information sharing among member states. Its goal was to work toward the well-being and security of all people through their attainment of the highest possible level of health; health was defined as a state of complete physical, mental, and social well-being and not merely the absence of disease or infirmity (WHO, 1986).

Increased emphasis on world economic development and interdependence occurred at the end of World War II, holding implications for health worldwide (Ebrahim & Ranken, 1988). Advances in technology and industrialization accelerated, rapidly reshaping the world. The roles of science and technology were reinforced as focal points within medicine and, by extension, within other health sciences. The biotechnological, scientific, empiricist model of health dominated the delivery of health care in Western industrialized nations to the exclusion of other perspectives. Notions of health and health care were, in actuality, sickness and sickness care, placing emphasis on the etiology of disease as defined by medical science. Many other factors affecting that etiology were of minimal or no interest as they were neither within the control of nor curable by medical science.

During the mid-twentieth century, nations in Latin America, Asia, and Africa that sought independence from colonial powers were left with a legacy of inappropriate health care establishments. Health services, imported from colonizing nations, were oriented to serve the colonial administrators, the military, and the nation's elite, with biomedically and institutionally oriented services situated in major urban centers, while poor and rural people remained essentially unserved. Also, xenophobic missionaries from Europe and North America facilitated the destruction of indigenous health care systems, leaving a fragile physical infrastructure dependent on outside help with no effective model of health care delivery to respond to the needs of the majority of people within a nation. The provision of health service had not met the needs of the majority and was never intended to be economically viable for developing nations. Instead, the impact of the imported model of service delivery contributed to dependency and promoted poorer health. As nations won their fight for independence, the expectations of economic self-sufficiency were turned into dependence and permanent debt (Mull, 1990).

Through the period from 1948 to 1977, it became evident that these factors mitigated against WHO's goals of achieving health for all. People continued to lack access to services where they could have their problems addressed appropriately (Mull, 1990). Imposed solutions from

Westernized nations and urban centers within developing nations did little to improve health of local rural populations. Unequal access to health care and the maldistribution of health professionals, who preferred to work in urban settings where there was access to prestigious, specialized, institutionally (hospital-) based services, often reliant on technology, contributed to the poor health of the majority of people. Health professionals, in particular physicians, were often educated overseas and were inappropriately trained to understand and respond to the needs of their own populations, holding to Western standards of medical care and medical education that focused on individual, not population, health. Contributing to poor health were government initiatives that put no priority on basic education, placing emphasis on military instead of social expenditure (Last, 1987).

Medicalization of health problems was perpetuated through the reliance on the biomedical/scientific/institutionally based approach to health care, with its inherent imposition of technological solutions to problems that are fundamentally social, political, and economic (Morley, Rohde, & Williams, 1983). For example, infant diarrhea is treated effectively with oral rehydration therapy (ORT). This potentially empowering and appropriate health technology, once provided free or for very low cost, can be made in most kitchens of the world as a cereal-based gruel. This effective solution that saves children's lives has become a multimillion-dollar industry and is tied to economic aid, forcing governments to charge for ORT to ensure profit for the multinational corporations that supply the electrolyte mixture in aluminum foil packages (Werner, 1994). The result is ongoing exploitation and disempowerment of the poor.

From the founding of WHO until the mid-1970s, it seemed apparent that science and technology were extending the longevity of many inhabitants of industrialized nations and improving their quality of life. Medical science was beneficial to nations holding economic and political power, whereas the majority of people worldwide remained underserved or not served at all by the advances of medicine. Those services that were provided were often not oriented toward the social, cultural, and economic circumstances of the populations they served. Hospitals continued to respond to injury and disease, with minimal attention paid to health promotion. The prevalent biomedical system, its practitioners, and structures have been unable to respond to the health-related needs of millions of people worldwide, mostly women and children, with the result being high levels of disability, endemic illness, and premature death (NCEPH, 1992). Modern (Western) medicine does not address poverty, the biggest cause of morbidity and mortality. Yet, it is the multiple causes of poverty, not the poverty itself, and the ill-health conditions created by poverty that must be addressed if people are to attain and maintain health (Werner, 1988).

During this same time, however, some nations, notably those where revolutions had been fought and won, such as Cuba and Nicaragua, were effectively responding to their people's health: lowering rates of disease; improving longevity and quality of life through an approach to health care that placed priority on the education of all citizens, in particular of women and girl children; and providing appropriate health services as shaped by people, not just professionals. In 1975, Dr. Carroll Behrhorst, a U.S. physician working in Chimaltenango, Guatemala, identified a list of priorities prerequisite to achieving health among the world's millions of rural poor. In order of priority, he lists social and economic injustice, land tenure, equitable agricultural production and marketing, population control, alleviation of malnutrition, health training, and finally, curative medicine (Behrhorst, 1975). It may be added that basic literacy and numeracy are prerequisite to social justice as these allow people to obtain knowledge about the factors that influence their lives.

PRIMARY HEALTH CARE

WHO and the United Nations International Children's Emergency Fund (UNICEF) jointly sponsored a conference in 1978 to develop strategies to respond to the existing gross inequalities in the health status of the world's population, particularly between developed and developing countries, but also within countries. This meeting, attended by 60 international organizations and 138 member nations, resulted in the Declaration of Alma Ata, 1978. Its objective was health for all by the year 2000 (HFA2000) through primary health care. Economic and social development, based on a New International Economic Order, were recognized as being of basic importance to the fullest attainment of health for all and the reduction of the gap in the health status between and within nations.

Health as defined by WHO in 1948 was reaffirmed in 1978. The Declaration of Alma Ata identifies health as a fundamental right of every person without distinction of race, religion, political belief, and economic, cultural, or social condition. The health of all people is held to be fundamental to the attainment of peace and security; another tenet is that individuals and their governments, through informed opinion and active participation, have a shared responsibility to work toward health. Health, a cultural construct, is viewed relativistically as a subjective state of well-being, influenced by the total environment within which people live, work, and play. As such, health is a resource to people and to their society, enabling them to lead economic and socially productive lives and to achieve conditions leading to physical, mental, and social well-being (WHO-UNICEF, 1978).

The Declaration of Alma Ata delineated the concept of primary health care as essential health care based on practical, scientifically sound, and socially acceptable methods and technologies made universally accessible to individuals and families in the community through their full participation, and at a cost that the community and the country can afford to maintain at every stage of their development in the spirit of self-reliance and self-determination (WHO-UNICEF, 1978). Primary health care is not in competition with the biotechnological medical model; it encompasses the medical model, its structures, and its practitioners as part of health and health care delivery. However, the goals of primary health care are much wider than those of conventional health care and range from that of health as a political and social right to that of health as an expression, or spinoff, of a quietly functioning informed community (Newell, 1975, p. 192).

Primary health care evolves from and reflects the economic conditions and sociocultural and political characteristics of a country and its communities. It is based on the application of the relevant results of social, biomedical, and health services research and public health experience, and it addresses the main health problems in the community (WHO-UNICEF, 1978). Primary health care includes the promotion of health, the prevention of illness and injury, early detection of problems, and cure and rehabilitation. It strives to make available relevant, affordable, accessible, acceptable, and appropriate resources to achieve the state of health described above.

Eight essential requirements (WHO-UNICEF, 1978) are given priority within primary health care:

The education of the community concerning prevailing health problems and the methods of preventing and controlling them

The promotion of adequate supplies of food and of proper nutrition

Adequate supply of safe water and basic sanitation

Maternal and child health, including family planning

Immunization against the major infectious diseases

Prevention and control of locally endemic diseases
Appropriate treatment of common diseases and injuries
Provision of essential drugs

This preliminary list addresses the most significant health problems internationally; if implemented, it would save countless lives and improve the quality of life for the majority of the world's population. Appropriate technology and knowledge exist to address these problems today. Yet the health of the world's population is in decline, as emphasis remains with cure and research on curative aspects of health problems, with minimal attention paid to prevention and the range of factors that contribute to the etiology of poor health.

Primary health care is not restricted to the above list but should address the prevalent problems within a nation. In developed nations, diseases of contemporary lifestyles include heart disease and stroke, cancer, injury and accidents, diabetes, disability, mental illness, communicable diseases (sexually transmitted diseases), degenerative diseases of aging, substance abuse, and respiratory disease—the major causes of sickness and death. The disenfranchised within developed nations—for example, indigenous populations and the poor—experience the ills of both developing and developed nations. Primary health care strives to address the discrepancies within society, to reduce significant differences in morbidity and mortality, the rate of illness, and prevalence of health risk factors between socioeconomically advantaged and disadvantaged peoples, including children, youth, women, migrants, aboriginal people, the elderly, the un- and underemployed, the rural poor, and inhabitants of urban slums (WHO, 1986).

Health cannot be achieved by the health sector alone (Ebrahim & Ranken, 1988). The current health care system, dominated by institutionally based, specialized care under the control of regulated professionals, technology, and medicine, is only one component of the health sector within societies. Primary health care involves, in addition to the health care system, all related sectors at national, provincial/state, and local levels, in particular agriculture, animal husbandry, food, industry, education, housing, public works, communications, and other sectors, and all levels of government, with the coordinated efforts of all those sectors required in order to ensure that people will optimize their health and well-being.

Primary health care is an intersectorial and interdisciplinary, collaborative, and coordinated approach to health, addressing the underlying factors that are the barriers to achieving health:

Disregard for the environment
Neglect of prevention in health
Inadequate resources for health promotion
Financial constraints
Segmented and compartmentalized services
Lack of intersectional commitment to health
Poverty and social alienation
Inappropriate health education for health and medical professionals

Professionals from a wide spectrum of disciplines including government officials, health workers, economic planners, agricultural workers, teachers, engineers, environmental specialists, the media, and others require relevant education about the factors affecting health and about the approach to health taken within primary health care, so that they can successfully collaborate with the community, voluntary agencies, and self-help groups and work in a partnership with the community. Primary health care ensures

> that people will use much better approaches than they do now for preventing disease and alleviating unavoidable illness and disability, and that there will be better ways of growing up, growing old, and dying gracefully. And it means that health begins at home and at the workplace, because it is there, where people live and work, that health is made or broken. And it means that essential health care will be accessible to all individuals and families in an acceptable and affordable way, and with their full participation. (Mahler, 1982)

TRADITIONAL HEALTH AND HEALING

The construction of primary health care is grounded in the history of humanity. Humankind has always cared for its members, attempted to live in relative harmony with the environment on which it depends for survival, and cared for the injured, ill, and dying, curing illnesses through remedies and actions developed within social and cultural contexts. Several specific remedies considered valuable in contemporary biomedical treatment, such as opium, quinine, and digitalis, were not discovered by scientific research but by traditional practitioners of medicine (Mutalik, 1983).

Likewise, social justice, a cornerstone of primary health care, has been addressed through the teachings of Abraham, Krishna, Moses,

Zoroaster, Buddha, Christ, Muhammad, and other prophets, and in such writings as the Talmud, Koran, the Vedas, and the Old and New Testaments. Oral and written histories have transmitted knowledge about health, healing, and healers through time. The teaching of the elders has prevailed until this century, and that teaching continues within societies that have not been separated from the past by colonialism, industrialization, and technology. Contemporary scientists and scholars document that the wisdom of the elders within indigenous and Western societies is not diametrically opposed but shared cross-culturally, linking relationships between humans, nature, and the environment (Knudtson & Suzuki, 1992).

Traditional healers and indigenous pharmacopoeias continue to be dominant in health care in many parts of the world. In the last decade of the twentieth century, there is a reappraisal of practices that have existed for centuries: humoral therapy, spiritism, Ayurvedic medicine, medical astrology, traditional Chinese medicine, acupuncture and moxibustion, allopathic medicine, homoeopathy, naturopathy, divination and exorcism, hypnosis, Yoga and meditation, herbal medicines, traditional psychiatry, traditional midwifery and contraception, autogenetic training, biofeedback, reflexology, shiatsu and *do-in,* T'ai Chi, and more. The challenge now is to integrate these influences within the philosophy, policies, and practices of Western medicine, which will require imaginative promotion, development, and use of traditional medicine as a vital component of primary health care (Mutalik, 1983).

For most of the world's population, health is not divided into wellness and illness, or mental and physical aspects. Developing a realistic approach to traditional medicine is required to ensure that it not only acts as a complement to existing modern systems but is functionally integrated into the larger health system. Promoting the integration of proven knowledge, skills, practice, and procedures of traditional medicine into the health care system is required. The primary health care approach is based on integrated community development. It would be only logical that these systems, which were born at an early stage of civilization and which have nurtured and sustained communities through the vast expanse of time, should fit well into a community development endeavor that includes health and health care as essential components (Mutalik, 1983).

Biomedical science has become the traditional medicine of industrialized societies and, as such, is a newcomer to the world of medicine. Because of its reliance on experts and institutions and its focus on the individual and not the collective, it is failing to respond to the needs of the majority of the world's population. Institutionalized care (hospitals) creates dependency as people are treated out of the context of their social world, their family, and other social supports, making health a commodity that can be managed and delivered by experts (NCEPH, 1992). This approach to medicine is being challenged to lessen its control and to work alongside people and the vast array of approaches to health and healing that exist worldwide. Primary health care offers this option as it is dispensed in accordance with the norms that govern the life of the population. It is based not only on scientific knowledge and appropriate health technology but also on practices that are traditionally accepted and have been found to be effective in each particular community, practices that are desired in communities that find Western medicine limited in its response to their needs.

FORGING PARTNERSHIPS FOR THE FUTURE

Health for all refers to community involvement rather than community participation, as the latter implies a passive rather than active role in health-related activities. This collaborative approach requires communication and knowledge to be multidirectional, not unidirectional as is common in the dominant health delivery system, and the forging of a horizontal partnership in place of the top-down, vertical approach pervasive in the mainstream health care delivery system. Active participation of people in the assessment, planning, implementation, and evaluation of health activities requires control over resources and decision making, an empowerment that necessitates flexibility and innovation and that is responsive to the changing health needs of people, giving consideration to the socioeconomic and cultural characteristics of the community (WHO, 1977).

Community involvement in health is described as a process whereby people, both individually and in groups, exercise their right to play an active and direct role in the development of appropriate health services, ensuring the conditions for sustained better health and supporting the empowerment of communities for health development (WHO, 1991). Consumers participate actively in their own health care to the degree with which they are comfortable and are supported in doing so. This includes the identification of problems and needs; the planning, management, and evaluation of health policy, services, and programs; and input into the educational training of health professionals. This active participation enables people to develop knowledge and skills and to gain confidence in their ability to influence their own lives. Participation should help people gain greater control over the factors affecting their health, by making their own decisions, organizing their own activities, and taking greater responsibilities, which will require massive decentralization in decision making and a reallocation of material and financial resources (Hill, 1986).

Primary health care is ultimately about processes including collaborating, participating, consulting, educating, facilitating, learning, detecting, promoting, preventing, rehabilitating, providing, exploring, negotiating, cooperating, caring, understanding, discovering, sharing, enabling, and empowering (Mardiros, 1994). This list is not inclusive. The processes demonstrate that it is not so much what is done but how it is done that is the purview of primary health care. Focusing on processes to respond to needs implies that there is a belief in people and in their individual and shared wisdom as resources and not as obstacles in the fostering of health and well-being. Furthermore, as communities are heterogenous, holding a variety of health ideologies, these ideologies need to be negotiated. That is, there needs to be a give-and-take within the various cultural and social systems, legitimizing interdependence and mutual contribution toward improving health (Hill, 1986).

Political and economic processes contribute to, perpetuate, and maintain the poor health status of the majority of the world's population and restrict the choices of people in developing nations. Responding to primary health care requires relevant education that is holistically oriented and includes the study of health within a global context. It requires a redistribution and reorientation of power and resources toward the sustainability of the factors that contribute to the health of the world's population (Ebrahim & Ranken, 1988). Control of health activities is placed in the hands of those whose health is being acted upon and within contexts that are meaningful to people. Health professionals learn to work with people to help them meet their health needs and to identify strategies for responding to health-related matters. Sustainability in health can only occur if solutions to problems and preventative measures are grounded in the lives of people.

Health professionals, bureaucrats, and politicians must adapt to newly evolving roles and responsibilities, and there must be a willingness to develop new relationships among health disciplines, related sectors, and consumers, resulting in a shared control of resources related to health (Ebrahim & Ranken, 1988; Mull, 1990). Conflicts of interest and counterproductive ideas and attitudes deriving from elitism, vested interests, and class distinction are some of the obstructions that occur in any health establishment. Attention is thus taken away from the need for structural changes in society and for the redistribution of wealth and resources (Muller, 1983).

SUMMARY

As people look more deeply into the reasons for their ill health, they recognize that sickness, disease, and malnutrition are merely symptoms of a deeper malady stemming from social inequality, economic exploitation, and political oppression. Primary health care in the true sense threatens inequitable socioeconomic or political structures. It implies a redistribution of resources, responsibility, and power of a much more radical kind than is generally realized or accepted. Primary health care means shifts in power from top to lower levels of government administration, from the government itself to people's organizations, from military to civilian administrators, from doctors to paramedics, from health professionals to ordinary people, from men to women (Werner, 1977, 1982).

In developed nations, we have opted to put our health into the realm of the health care industry. We seek quick fixes to complex problems and technological solutions to universally experienced common problems of suffering and illness. Specialists continue to receive disproportionate funding in search of remediating the ills of the (Westernized) world, while the nonbiophysiological underlying social and economic determinants of health at the community level continue to receive limited attention.

We have confused health with medicine and have accepted medicine as health care. Medicine as we know it has assumed a powerful place in the lives of all. Yet, medicine, as we have come to realize, is not all-curing and omnipotent. It is failing us because all of us have expected more than it can deliver. It holds limited power to offset the consequences of major health-destroying factors of industrialized society such as alcohol, tobacco, illicit narcotics, pesticides, and infant formula; unnecessary, dangerous, and overpriced pharmaceuticals; arms and military expenditures; and international money lending, as these are multibillion-dollar industries (Werner, 1994).

Biomedical health care is only one small component of the total that relates to health as an inseparable part of life. The failure of the biomedical model to prevent illness, promote health and well-being, and even to intervene when disease occurs (its strongest point) is increasingly noted in developed, industrialized societies. The etiology of poor health is intricately interwoven with all other facets of life. Health is neither measurable nor objective, and the meaning of health varies across the life span of any one person and across gender, culture, age, economy, and education. If this view is held to be true, then empirical science is restricted in its current impact on health. Health is a human condition that others can foster but not deliver (Johnston & Rifkin, 1987; Morley et al., 1983). The challenge is, then, to work toward the health of all through an integrated approach that gives recognition to the complexity of global experience of health and well-being.

REFERENCES

Behrhorst, C. (1975). The Chimaltenango development project in Guatemala. In K. W. Newell (Ed.), *Health by the people* (pp. 30-52). Geneva: World Health Organization.

Ebrahim, G. J., & Ranken, J. P. (Eds.). (1988). *Primary health care: Reorienting organisational support*. London: Macmillan.

Hill, C. E. (1986). Translating primary health care policies to the local level: A comparison of rural communities in the United States and Costa Rica. In C. E. Hill (Ed.), *Current health policy issues and alternatives* (pp. 123-144). Athens: University of Georgia Press.

Johnston, M. P., & Rifkin, S. B. (1987). *Health care together*. London: Macmillan.

Knudtson, P., & Suzuki, D. (1992). *Wisdom of the elders*. Marrickville, NSW: Allen & Unwin.

Last, J. (1987). *Public health and human ecology*. Norwalk, CT: Appleton & Lange.

Mahler, H. (1982, June 8). *Essential drugs for all*. Address given by the Director General of the World Health Organization to the Eleventh Assembly of the International Federation of Pharmaceutical Manufacturers' Associations, Washington, DC.

Mardiros, M. (1994). Qualitative research, primary health care, and the community. In C. Cooney (Ed.), *Primary health care* (pp. 131-147). New York: Prentice Hall.

Morley, D., Rohde, J., & Williams, G. (Eds.). (1983). *Practising health for all*. Oxford: Oxford University Press.

Mull, J. D. (1990). The primary health care dialectic: History, rhetoric, and reality. In J. Coreil & J. D. Mull (Eds.), *Anthropology and primary health care* (pp. 28-47). Boulder, CO: Westview.

Muller, F. (1983). Contrasts in community participation: Case studies from Peru. In D. Morley, J. Rohde, & G. Williams (Eds.), *Practising health for all* (pp. 190-207). Oxford: Oxford University Press.

Mutalik, G. S. (1983). Organizational aspects. In R. H. Bannerman, J. Burton, & C. Wen-Chieh (Eds.), *Traditional medicine and health care coverage* (pp. 281-289). Geneva: World Health Organization.

National Centre for Epidemiology and Population Health. (1992). *Improving Australia's health: The role of primary health care* (Final Report). Canberra: The Australian National University.

Newell, K. (1975). *Health by the people.* Geneva: World Health Organization.
Werner, D. (1977). *Where there is no doctor.* Palo Alto, CA: Hesperian Foundation.
Werner, D. (1982). *Helping health workers learn.* Palo Alto, CA: Hesperian Foundation.
Werner, D. (1988, April). Empowerment and health. *Contact.*
Werner, D. (1994). Health for no one by the year 2000: The high cost of placing national security before global justice. In K. Wotton et al. (Eds.), *Basic concepts of international health module.* Ottawa: Canadian University Consortium for Health in Development.
World Health Organization (WHO). (1977). *The role of the nurse in primary health care* (Scientific Publication No. 348). Washington, DC: Pan American Health Organization.
World Health Organization (WHO). (1986). *Basic documents.* Geneva: Author.
World Health Organization (WHO). (1986). *Resolution of the World Health Assembly,* 34-36. Geneva: Author.
World Health Organization (WHO). (1991). *Community involvement in health development: Challenging health services* (Report of a WHO study group). Geneva: Author.
World Health Organization-United Nations International Children's Emergency Fund (WHO-UNICEF). (1978). *Primary health care.* Geneva: World Health Organization.

17 Intersectoral Health Care Delivery

CONSTANCE M. McCORKLE

Within a given cultural configuration—whether modern or traditional—largely the same fundamental medical theories and techniques, pharmacopoeia, and so forth are applied to human and nonhuman patients.[1] This congruency is hardly surprising because everywhere, down through history and still today, the medical arts for *Homo sapiens* and for their food, work, and later, pet animals, have evolved together.[2] Thus, the science/ethnoscience of medicine is much the same across patient species within every culture. In modern Western medical contexts, however, health care services and their clinical delivery systems are dichotomized in two sectors: human medicine versus veterinary medicine. Likewise, most Western cultures today draw a sharp line between practitioners in these two sectors, broadly dividing them into medical doctors versus veterinarians, according to the species they treat.

Not so for the majority of traditional or non-Western medical systems, however. They instead parse the clinical universe and its practitioners first by professional specialization: herbalists, bone setters, surgeons, midwives, acupuncturists, masseuses, and so forth. Thus, the same traditional health workers typically treat *both* humans and their livestock or other animals—much as the veterinarian of yore often did in rural areas of the Western world.

AUTHOR'S NOTE: This chapter draws on the work of D.V.M./Ph.D. Calvin Schwabe and on recent papers by and discussions with D.V.M. David E. Ward and his colleagues at the Food and Agriculture Organization. Comments by D.V.M./Ph.D. Tjaart Schillhorn van Veen are also gratefully acknowledged.

Such distinctions mirror more general differences in worldviews between Western and non-Western cultures. The former have long subscribed to an anthropocentrism that sets human beings above and apart from all other animals. But this is not the case for the majority of non-Western cultures. They hold more zoocentric or ecocentric worldviews, which class certain animal species as a sort of people, too, and/or which see humans, like animals, as part of nature as a whole (Shanklin, 1985).

For health care delivery, these different worldviews have different outcomes. Anthropocentrism leads to a dualistic system in which, as noted above, practitioners cater exclusively to *Homo sapiens* or exclusively to nonhuman species. Moreover, the two clienteles are served at separate facilities. In contrast, other worldviews lead to more synthetic delivery systems in which practitioners and often locales are one and the same for all species, varying only according to treatment type.

The present chapter argues that, especially for remote or rural peoples of the Third World, an intersectoral approach partly modeled along the lines of traditional, non-Western patterns for the joint delivery of basic health care services to both humans and animals would be more appropriate and feasible than attempting to impose a dualistic Western-style structure. The chapter also argues for intersectoral synergism of another sort. That is, the marriage of informal and formal, traditional and modern medical sectors by including traditional/local practitioners and effective ethnomedical practices as integral parts of such a delivery system (Last, 1990; McCorkle, 1994).

HUMAN AND ANIMAL, TRADITIONAL AND MODERN MEDICINE

Approximately 80 percent to 90 percent of the world's population still rely mainly on informal local practitioners and "folk" medicine for the bulk of their human health care needs (Bannerman, 1983; Duke, 1992, p. 59; WHO, cited in Plotkin, 1988, p. 260). In some nations, as much as 40 percent of all formal-sector personnel serve urban communities that include no more than 5 percent of the citizenry; and 85 percent of all doctors and 100 percent of all pharmacists may be found in the cities (Schwabe, Schwabe, & Basta, 1994). In the area of obstetrics alone, traditional practitioners (midwives) may be responsible for up to 90 percent of all births (Bannerman, 1983). By and large, the same kinds of observations and figures also apply to veterinary services in the Third

World—where, by the way, virtually all rural communities keep livestock of one sort or another. As a rule of thumb, whether for humans or animals, Third World people turn to modern, formal-sector services only after exhausting traditional, informal ones.

For the foreseeable future, this situation is likely to undergo little change. Whether in the human or the animal health sector, along with development exports, Third World governments have increasingly despaired of extending even basic health care packages modeled strictly along modern Western lines to all their human and livestock population. This despair is engendered by the soaring costs of high-tech medicine, plus the expense of conventional Western systems for its delivery to burgeoning numbers of people and animals—all in a global climate of skyrocketing national debt, shrinking public exchequers, and stagnating economies.

Extension of conventional medical/veterinary services is particularly difficult and costly in Third World nations where the necessary infrastructure (roads, clinics, labs, cold chains, etc.) is poorly developed and where much of the populace and their livestock reside in remote, rural areas or may be nomadic or transhumant. Problems of service delivery to such groups are often exacerbated by a multitude of other factors. To name just a few:

A shortage of competent health care workers willing to accept postings in remote areas with few amenities or among groups they consider backward or primitive[3]

Recurrent civil or political strife that disrupts delivery systems

Bureaucratic bloat and corruption that leave ever fewer operating funds

Such difficulties have stimulated both medical and veterinary scientists and development personnel to take a harder look at the utility—indeed, the imperative—of building on and working with existing local or traditional health care resources, particularly in non-Western contexts. These resources can be conceptualized as consisting of two types:

Software, or sociological resources, in the form of traditional practitioners and any associated apprenticeship systems or informal practitioner networks, plus locally constituted (interhousehold, community, ethnic, gender, paraprofessional) organizations for the mobilization of human or livestock health care action.

Hardware, or (ethno)technological resources, in the form of traditional therapies and prophylaxes that are demonstrably effective. These may include:

herbal medicines and home remedies; traditional surgical, vaccination, manipulatory, and other treatment techniques; holistic folk health-management practices; and so forth.

In its Alma Ata Declaration (WHO, 1978a), the World Health Organization concluded that it is necessary to draw on all such resources if universal coverage in basic *human* health care is ever to be achieved (Akerele, 1985; WHO, 1978a, 1978b, 1990, 1991a, 1991b, 1993; Zhang, 1994). Familiar software and hardware examples given in support of this conclusion are China's "barefoot doctors" campaign and the acupuncture techniques of traditional Chinese medicine. Subsequently, WHO established a worldwide network of Collaborating Centers for Traditional [human] Medicine; and in 1993 the U.S. National Institutes of Health created a new Office of Alternative Medicine to evaluate promising ethnomedical therapies. Meanwhile, there has been an explosion of publications, international meetings, and conferences on traditional human health systems, their *materia medica*, and practitioners, with respect to their potential contributions to universal health care.[4]

Concerted attention to local-level involvement in the delivery of *animal* health care also began about the mid-1970s, notably with World Bank and other livestock development projects in Africa (e.g., de Haan & Bekure, 1991; de Haan & Nissen, 1985; Sollod, Wolfgang, & Knight, 1984). Likewise for systematic attention to traditional, ethnoveterinary medicine and, to a lesser extent, its practitioners. (For references to pioneering initiatives in ethnovetinary R & D, cf. Mathias-Mundy & McCorkle, 1989; McCorkle, 1986; also McCorkle, 1995; McCorkle & Mathias- Mundy, 1992; McCorkle, Mathias, & Schillhorn van Veen, 1996). Particularly groundbreaking work in this subject was done by the Food and Agriculture Organization (FAO, 1980, 19841, 1984a, 1984b, 1986, 1991a, 1991b, 1992). Subsequently, private voluntary and nongovernmental organizations (PVOs, NGOs) rapidly expanded implementation of numerous paraveterinary or "barefoot vet" programs all around the world (McCorkle & Mathias, in progress).

However, not until about the mid-1980s was much consideration finally given to the joint delivery of human and livestock health care and related services (e.g., Schwabe, 1984; Schwabe et al., 1994; Ward, Ruppanner, Marchot, & Hansen, 1993). Only more recently still have discussion and action been taken on linking informal, ethnoveterinary practices and practitioners with more formalized systems of veterinary medical practice (e.g., Grandin, Thampy, & Young, 1991; International

Institute for Rural Instruction, 1995), as is already under way in human medicine.

POTENTIALS AND BENEFITS OF INTERSECTORAL HEALTH CARE DELIVERY

The potential advantages of concerted coordination across and among health care sectors—human and animal, traditional/informal, and modern/formal—are multifold. This is particularly true for poor nations, where much of the populace is rural, where people and livestock live dispersed across vast spaces, and/or where there is a long-standing tradition of medical practitioners' treating both humans and animals. At a minimum, intersectoral coordination may include the following:

- Medical-related infrastructure, logistics, matériel, and ancillary personnel
- Recruitment of practitioners
- Training for all levels and types of practitioners, and other kinds of information dissemination to them
- Treatment options
- Strategies for winning client credibility in, and thus use of, the health care services being offered
- Epidemiological intelligence systems

Infrastructure, Logistics, Matériel, and Ancillary Personnel. For example, when it comes to establishing fixed or mobile health clinics, diagnostic labs, cold chains, drug procurement/supply/control systems, and so forth, the cost savings and efficiencies to be garnered from intersectoral integration are patent. Far fewer buildings, vehicles, lab outfits, refrigeration units, computers and record-keeping systems, telephones, and what-have-you will be required if the two sectors share them. Support staff requirements (e.g., cold depot managers, procurement officers, accountants, drivers, mechanics, and so on) can be utilized economically in this way, too.[5]

Intersectoral mobile clinics offer especially tantalizing possibilities. Such clinics are expensive to operate, if only in terms of vehicles and fuel. But they make for greatly expanded coverage of people or animals who live too far distant to be able to afford travel to a fixed clinic or to reach such a facility in time to solve a pressing health problem. However, such groups *may* be able to make it to one of the points on a mobile unit's regular route. Unfortunately, few if any Third World governments or private-sector entities would be able to support a dual network of such clinics. But with intersectoral coordination in the form of mobile units staffed by an interdisciplinary or multipurpose medical/veterinary team, more such services could be offered to rural people and their livestock.

In short, coordination solely along such relatively simple lines as those sketched above could go far toward overcoming the not-uncommon situation in which merely the infrastructural, logistic, and communication costs of getting services out to only animals or only people exceed the cost of the treatments rendered—with the sad consequence that often no treatment at all is tendered.

Recruitment of Practitioners. In the Third World, ratios of medical doctors to the population regularly range between 1 to 10,000 and 1 to 20,000 (e.g., Bodeker, 1994; Zhang, 1994); in the livestock sector, similar magnitudes can be assumed to hold for doctors of veterinary medicine (DVMS). In contrast, ratios for traditional/informal-sector practitioners range between 1 to 100 and 1 to 200. The message in these figures should be obvious. It is essential for Third World nations to recognize and draw upon this broad base of software if they are to have any hope of getting even basic health care services to the majority of their citizenry and livestock (cf. again WHO, 1978a, 1978b).

Many nations have already taken steps in this regard, by acknowledging alternative or traditional healers' associations. In some cases, these associations have been linked with formal-sector medicine in one or another arena, such as training (below) or drug control, oversight, and patient-referral systems (cf. Last, 1990). So far, however, few countries have recognized in any formal or semiformal way the existence of traditional healers for livestock (one example is found in Nuwanyakpa, De Vries, Ndi, & Django, 1990) or the fact that in rural areas, local health care workers often attend both humans and animals. Thus, these multifunctional software resources are not fully exploited.

One can only echo the words of Schwabe (1993) that "this is especially tragic in poorer countries struggling to utilize very limited manpower and other resources most effectively" (p. 126). The tragedy lies in the fact that, without acknowledgment and support, such software resources are fast disappearing—and along with them, their invaluable hardware knowledge of unique techniques, botanicals, and other medicinal agents of vast potential benefit to *all* species. As underscored in publications and conferences too numerous to list here (see the references in McCorkle, 1995), the loss of such local/indigenous knowledge (and often also of its accompanying biological diversity) is nothing less than apocalyptic. Sadly, Western educational and cultural imperialism has led more and more young people to deprecate and abandon the traditional medical/veterinary knowledge and practices of their elders. Ironically, this is occurring in tandem with a groundswell of First World interest in alternative medicine and its practitioners—as the present volume attests.

To the extent that ethnomedical software and hardware in the form of known and respected traditional healers and proven traditional treatments can be recognized and brought into play alongside formal sector medicine, losses in vital medical/veterinary personpower, skill, and knowledge can be stemmed. At the same time, recruiting these resources as part of the national health care team would increase public recognition, remuneration, and status for them. This can in turn encourage existing practitioners to continue—and more youth to enter—what may become partly techno-blended but still localized health care professions. Such strategies can also stimulate more ready recourse to a range of health care services for people and their animals, insofar as providers are then composed of familiar, respected, affordable, same-culture practitioners and practitioner networks (see "Service Credibility and Utilization" below).

Training and Information Dissemination for Practitioners. Because medical and ethnomedical concepts and general treatments or treatment types are substantially similar for humans and livestock, where training in one sector is planned for practitioners (whether they are from the formal or informal sector), it costs little more to extend training in the other as well. Say, for example, that instruction is being given to increase local practitioner skills at bone setting, obstetrics, vaccinations, injections, dosage calculations, or what-have-you—but all for use in human health care. In such cases, training could also efficiently include the appropriate application of the same techniques to livestock. Or vice versa.

Also, whether in training or other kinds of information dissemination, it would cost little more to note the indication and posology of drugs for all pertinent species of patients, given that a great many of both traditional herbal and modern commercial treatments are administered for similar purposes in humans and (at least mammalian) livestock. The point in all the foregoing is to make practitioners and treatment information polyvalent, so they can do double duty as needed.

Treatment Options. Such cross-training of health workers can also be extended to instruction in both informal- and formal-sector medical/

veterinary treatment. For instance, all of the modern-sounding techniques just cited above (bone setting, obstetrics, vaccinations, drug therapy) also have their correlates in most ethnomedical traditions. This offers yet another kind of intersectoral benefit.

To wit, a greater choice of treatment options can be offered to clients, depending on the pragmatics of the situation. Poor rural people may be unable to afford expensive commercial drugs, professional fees, hospital stays, sophisticated surgical procedures, and so forth. Or there may be no time to access such goods and services before a health problem becomes irreversible. Or such resources simply may not exist anywhere in the region. Or people may not trust themselves or their animals to unfamiliar practitioners and techniques (next section).[6] In these situations, nearly as good, just as good, or sometimes even better remedies, health care providers, outpatient and home-care treatment regimes, modest surgical interventions (or even alternatives to surgery) can often be found in the informal sector.

Take the case of drug therapy, for example. It is no accident that at least a fourth of all prescription medicines in use in the Western world today were first known in traditional medicine (Cox & Balick, 1994). Innumerable herbal drugs for both humans and animals have been—and almost daily still are being—demonstrated effective for the conditions they are traditionally used to treat. Moreover, traditional remedies may produce fewer or more benign side effects, or they may provide desirable synergistic effects (Bodeker, 1994). Sometimes traditional/informal medical resources and responses may surpass modern Western ones in other ways, too. The renowned bone setters of pastoral Africa are a case in point; they are often able to treat complex fractures in both humans and livestock that their formally trained counterparts despair of. To take another example, ethnoveterinary medicine for camels can successfully address many diagnostic and therapeutic needs of these astonishing creatures better than can Western veterinary medicine.[7]

This is not to say that informal/traditional medicine is perfect. Sometimes the action of useful herbal drugs may be limited in comparison to their more potent Western commercial equivalents. For instance, a traditional anthelmintic (dewormer) may have a kill rate of only 60 percent to 80 percent instead of 90 percent to 100 percent; or an indigenous vaccination technique may offer protection in only 50 percent of cases. Nevertheless, the larger point remains that taking whatever beneficial medical action one can is unquestionably preferable to doing nothing at all. Certainly, 80 percent or 50 percent is better than 0 percent.

At the very least, just as informal-sector practitioners can be mobilized and trained in basic techniques of modern medicine, formal-sector health care workers should be trained in valid ethnomedical options so they can offer these to their patients when circumstances permit little else.

Fortunately, many medical schools and colleges of veterinary medicine both in the First and Third Worlds are now adding (or restoring) courses in herbal medicines or traditional farm-and-home health care management to their curricula. Meanwhile, a variety of development organizations have begun compiling and extending information on traditional alternatives for both humans (e.g., WHO, 1990) and livestock (e.g., IIRR, 1995).

Service Credibility and Utilization. Various studies and reports suggest that rural peoples may be more likely to access formal-sector medical services for humans when these are extended alongside veterinary services, whether via mobile or even fixed clinics. Aside from the convenience factor, this phenomenon probably also reflects the fact that—as noted in the introduction to this chapter—in most traditional systems the same panoply of practitioners serve all species. Thus, by analogy, rural clients who are already familiar with and value local formal-sector *veterinary* services are more apt to have confidence in, and therefore to use, *human* health care services recommended or extended to them through the same personnel or facilities.

One example of this kind of positive "credibility spillover" from veterinary to human medicine is dual vaccination programs for both children and livestock. Such programs have achieved child vaccination rates that far outstrip national averages when this service is extended alone (Schwabe et al., 1994). Moreover, findings from such experiences suggest that in combined medical/veterinary delivery, a portion of the revenues from veterinary services can be used to defray the expenses of extending low- or no-cost health care to humans. This is important because sometimes impoverished rural people who feel they cannot afford medical attention for family members *will* pay for veterinary care. Many Third World rural families subsisting at the edge of survival are faced with such heart-breaking health care choices, because their only way to pay for an individual's special medical expenses may be to sell off animals that are the whole household's fundamental means of economic support and food security.[8]

By winning over a larger (and paying) clientele, intersectoral service delivery might also attract more formal-sector medical workers to rural areas, where they would then be on tap to treat cases of human illness that home remedies and traditional practitioners cannot always effectively address. In fact, a majority of rural dwellers in the Third World may never have seen a nurse, much less a doctor or a hospital. But not so for their local (including formal-sector) veterinary practitioners. Indeed, for many rural groups the veterinarian may be the only well-educated "outsider" medic they ever encounter where they live (Schwabe et al., 1994).

Epidemiological Intelligence. If, as suggested above, people and their livestock are attended jointly by an intersectorally coordinated health care system, bonus benefits for public health can result. Much more prompt and effective measures for the identification, treatment, and control of zoonoses (diseases transmissible between humans and animals) can be taken. Although formal-sector medical and veterinary services in the Third World have historically collaborated in tackling such dramatic zoonoses as rabies, coordination has often been less than ideal (Schwabe, 1980).

Clearly, there is scope for far more such collaboration—and not just with regard to zoonoses. Epidemiological surveillance for *all* disease threats to humans and livestock can be conducted jointly, with the same cost savings and efficiencies as those noted for other aspects of medical infrastructure, logistics, and so on. Only half the number of trained scouts, vehicles, and so forth would be required to reconnoiter and report on patterns of disease incidence in far-flung rural areas.

Indeed, this function could be folded in with other coordinated efforts, like the multipurpose mobile units mentioned earlier. Alternatively, local software in the form of traditional medical/veterinary practitioners and paraprofessionals can be trained and motivated to collect and record epidemiological data. It has been demonstrated that even illiterate personnel can fill this role, using simple pictographic record sheets (Sollod & Stem, 1991). Furthermore, investigations by the International Laboratory for Research on Livestock Diseases suggest that sensitive ethnomedical questionnaires can be useful for rapidly estimating variable disease risk. Such methodologies could partly substitute for more accurate but expensive laboratory diagnostic surveys in providing early warning of disease threats (Delehanty, 1996).

In sum, a growing body of research indicates that, with such strategies, epidemiological intelligence can be obtained more quickly, accurately, and cheaply than in conventional schemes relying only on a distant and disinterested cadre of civil servants (e.g., Baumann, 1990;

Zessin & Carpenter, 1985). This can only benefit poor nations' public exchequers and populace.

HEALTH CARE FOR *ALL*

As numerous experts have observed, when applied to rural areas of the Third World, the modern Western model of dualistic health care delivery to humans and their animals has rarely worked well, for a host of reasons. Some consensus is now emerging that what is needed instead is a more synthetic and integrative vision of "one medicine" and, with this, of joint human/animal health care delivery. Taking a cue from traditional, non-Western medical/veterinary paradigms, such a vision includes new (or really, sometimes very old) tools and ways to integrate across human and animal health care sectors. This implies a thorough "rethinking of Western models and anthropocentric biases," a rethinking that should incorporate "traditional healers . . . as part of the primary health care delivery team" (Ward et al., 1993, pp. 61, 62) along with useful traditional/informal-sector treatments.

Not to do so seems at best nonsensical and at worst socioeconomically reprehensible. Third World nations in particular need to find every possible way to get the "biggest bang for the buck" out of their health care dollar. Without greater intersectoral coordination—medical/veterinary and formal/informal—billions of humans and their animals (and thus, again, humans) will continue to suffer needlessly.

NOTES

1. This statement and many of those in the following section admittedly represent broad generalizations to which many caveats can be found. But for the purposes of this chapter, they are sufficiently accurate.

2. Indeed, much of humankind's early knowledge of medicine derived from empirical observation of animal anatomy, physiology, pathology, ethology, and so on, during hunting or ritual sacrifice, slaughter, practical necropsy, and butchering (Schwabe, 1978; Schwabe & Kuojok, 1981). Animals continue to serve us as medical models in the laboratory; in the field, study of their feeding behaviors can suggest new drugs for human use; animal illnesses also often provide the first alert of environmental health threats to humans (Schwabe, 1993).

3. See McCorkle, 1995, for a succinct discussion and additional references to these and still more problems in the livestock sector, all of which are duplicated in the human health care sector as well.

4. These have involved such entities as arboreta and botanical gardens, environmental and development NGOs and PVOs, cultural and other research institutes, both established and venture-capital pharmaceutical firms, the U.S. government's National Institutes of Health, Canada's International Development Research Center, representatives of the U.S. Department of Agriculture, the Pan-American and World Health Organizations, the World Bank, advocacy groups such as the World Council of Indigenous Peoples, and numerous universities. A number of such events have featured the active participation of traditional healers and spokespersons. Significantly, the International Congress on Traditional and Folk Medicine is currently in its ninth year.

5. The author cannot help but recall the many townships she has visited around the Third World in which the Ministry of Health and the Ministry of Livestock (or Agriculture, the Veterinary Service, or what-have-you) each maintains a pathetically equipped office and lab facilities, poorly stocked or outdated drug stores, and so on, each with its full complement of support personnel idling about for want of fuel. Alternatively, one service may be flush with such amenities and the other floundering. In either case, the situation cries out for intersectoral coordination and complementarity.

6. This often occurs when formal-sector health care providers are from a different ethnic-linguistic group and especially if they are traditional enemies or oppressors of the clients they seek to serve.

7. See Mathias-Mundy and McCorkle, 1989, and McCorkle and Mathias-Mundy, 1992, for more references and greater detail on these and still other examples.

8. Such vital livestock resources include, for example, the work oxen, camels, water buffalo, and so on, that patiently plow the fields, mill the grain, haul the wood and water, transport farm inputs to fields, and carry the crops (and the family) to market; the milch cows and dairy goats that can be relied upon both for daily nutritional inputs of much-needed high-quality protein and maybe even for some surplus dairy products to sell for a little cash; and, of course, the critical mass of breedstock to ensure the continuity of all these critical animal resources.

REFERENCES

Akerele, O. (1985). The WHO traditional medicine programme: Policy and implementation. *International Traditional Medicine Newsletter, 1,* 1, 3.

Bannerman, R. H. (1983). The role of traditional medicine in primary health care. In R. H. Bannerman, J. Burton, & C. Wen-Chieh (Eds.), *Traditional medicine and health care coverage* (pp. 318-327). Geneva: World Health Organization.

Baumann, M. P. O. (1990). *The nomadic animal health system (NAHA-System) in pastoral areas of central Somalia and its usefulness in epidemiological surveillance.* Master's thesis, University of California-Davis School of Veterinary Medicine.

Bodeker, G. (1994). Traditional health knowledge and public policy. *Nature and Resources, 30*(2), 5-16.

Cox, P. A., & Balick, M. J. (1994). The ethnobotanical approach to drug discovery. *Scientific American, 271,* 82-87.

de Haan, C., & Bekure, S. (1991). *Animal health services in sub-Saharan Africa: Initial experiences with alternative approaches.* Washington, DC: World Bank.

de Haan, C., & Nissen, N. (1985). *Animal health services in sub-Saharan Africa* (Technical Paper No. 44). Washington, DC: World Bank.

Delehanty, J. (1996). Methods and results from a study of local knowledge of cattle diseases in coastal Kenya. In C. M. McCorkle, E. Mathias, & T. W. Schillhorn van Veen (Eds.), *Ethnoveterinary research & development*, pp. 229-245. London: Intermediate Technology Publications.

Duke, J. A. (1992). Tropical botanical extractives. In M. Plotkin & L. Famolare (Eds.), *Sustainable harvest and marketing of rain forest products* (pp. 53-62). Covelo, CA, and Washington, DC: Island Press for Conservation International.

FAO. (1992). *Traditional veterinary medicine in the Philippines*. Bangkok: Author.

FAO (based on the work of J. V. Anjaria). (1984a). *Traditional (indigenous) systems of veterinary medicine for small farmers in India*. Bangkok: Author.

FAO (based on the work of P. Buranamanus). (1984c). *Traditional (indigenous) systems of veterinary medicine for small farmers in Thailand*. Bangkok: Author.

FAO (based on the work of S. B. Dhanapala). (1991b). *Traditional veterinary medicine in Sri Lanka*. Bangkok: Author.

FAO (based on the work of D. D. Joshi). (1984b). *Traditional (indigenous) systems of veterinary medicine for small farmers in Nepal* [Reprinted in 1991]. Bangkok: Author.

FAO (based on the work of M. Maqsood). (1986). *Traditional (indigenous) systems of veterinary medicine for small farmers in Pakistan*. Bangkok: Author.

FAO (based on the work of S. Poedjomartono). (1991a). *Traditional veterinary medicine in Indonesia*. Bangkok: Author.

FAO (based on the work of C. G. Sivadas). (1980). *Preliminary study of traditional systems of veterinary medicine*. Bangkok: Author.

Grandin, B., Thampy, R., & Young, J. (1991). *Case study: Village animal health care—A community-based approach to livestock development in Kenya*. London: Intermediate Technology Publications.

International Institute for Rural Reconstruction (IIRR). (1995). *Ethnoveterinary medicine in Asia; An information kit on traditional health care practices*. Silang, Cavite, The Philippines: Author.

Last, M. (1990). Professionalization of indigenous healers. In T. M. Johnson & C. F. Sargent (Eds.), *Medical anthropology: Contemporary theory and method* (pp. 349-366). New York: Praeger.

Mathias-Mundy, E., & McCorkle, C. M. (1989). *Ethnoveterinary medicine: An annotated bibliography* (Bibliographies in Technology and Social Change, No. 6, Center for Indigenous Knowledge and Agricultural and Rural Development). Ames: Iowa State University Research Foundation.

McCorkle, C. M. (1986). An introduction to ethnoveterinary research and development. *Journal of Ethnobiology, 6*, 129-149.

McCorkle, C. M. (1994, March 2-4). *Intersectoral action and policy directions in traditional health systems for humans and animals*. Paper presented to the International Workshop on Traditional Health Systems and Public Policy, International Development Research Centre, Ottawa.

McCorkle, C. M. (1995). Back to the future: Lessons from ethnoveterinary RD&E for studying and applying local knowledge. *Agriculture and Human Values, 12*(2), 52-80.

McCorkle, C. M., & Mathias, E. (in progress). *Paraveterinary health care*. London: Intermediate Technology Publications.

McCorkle, C. M., Mathias, E., & Schillhorn van Veen, T. W. (Eds.) (1996). *Ethnoveterinary research & development*. London: Intermediate Technology Publications.

McCorkle, C. M., & Mathias-Mundy, E. (1992). Ethnoveterinary medicine in Africa. *Africa: Journal of the International African Institute, 62*, 59-93.

Nuwanyakpa, M., De Vries, J., Ndi, C., & Django, S. (1990). *Traditional veterinary medicine in Cameroon: A renaissance in an ancient indigenous technology*. Unpublished manuscript, Heifer Project International, Cameroon.

Plotkin, M. J. (1988). Conservation, ethnobotany, and the search for new jungle medicines: Pharmacognosy comes of age . . . again. *Pharmacotherapy, 8*, 257-262.

Schwabe, C. W. (1978). *Cattle, priests, and progress in medicine*. Minneapolis: University of Minnesota Press.

Schwabe, C. W. (1980). Animal disease control, Part II: Newer methods, with possibility for their application in the Sudan. *Sudan Journal of Veterinary Science & Animal Husbandry, 21*(2), 55-65.

Schwabe, C. W. (1981). Animal diseases and primary health care: Intersectoral challenges. *WHO Chronicle, 35*, 227-232.

Schwabe, C. W. (1984). *Veterinary medicine and human health* (3rd ed.). Baltimore: Williams & Wilkins.

Schwabe, C. W. (1993). Interactions between human and veterinary medicine: Past, present, and future. In *Advancement of veterinary sciences: The bicentenary symposium 1991* (pp. 119-133). Oxon, UK: Commonwealth Agricultural Bureaux International.

Schwabe, C. W., & Kuojok, I. M. (1981). Practices and beliefs of the traditional Dinka health healer in relation to provision of modern medical and veterinary services for the southern Sudan. *Human Organization, 40*, 231-238.

Schwabe, C. L., Schwabe, C. W., & Basta, S. S. (1994). *Vaccination of children and cattle in pastoralist Africa: Practical intersectoral cooperation*. Unpublished manuscript.

Shanklin, E. (1985). Sustenance and symbol: Anthropological studies of domesticated animals. *Annual Review of Anthropology, 14*, 375-403.

Sollod, A. E., & Stem, C. (1991). Appropriate animal health information systems for nomadic and transhuman livestock populations in Africa. *Revue Scientifique et Technique de l'Office International des Épizooties, 10*(1), 89-101.

Sollod, A. E., Wolfgang, K., & Knight, J. A. (1984). Veterinary anthropology: Interdisciplinary methods in pastoral systems research. In J. R. Simpson & P. Evangelou (Eds.), *Livestock development in sub-Saharan Africa: Constraints, prospects, policy* (pp. 285-302). Boulder, CO: Westview.

Ward, D. E., Ruppanner, R., Marchot, P. J., & Hansen, J. W. (1993). One medicine—Practical application for non-sedentary pastoral populations. *Nomadic Peoples, 32*, 55-63.

WHO. (1978a). The Alma Ata conference on primary health care. *WHO Chronicle, 32*(11), 431-438.

WHO. (1978b). *The promotion and development of traditional medicine: Report of a WHO meeting* (WHO Technical Report Series, No. 622). Geneva: Author.

WHO. (1990). *The use of traditional medicine in primary health care: A manual for health workers in South-East Asia*. New Delhi: Author.

WHO. (1991a). *Guidelines for the assessment of herbal medicines*. Geneva: Author.

WHO. (1991b). *Report of the consultation to review the draft guidelines for the assessment of herbal medicines*. Munich: Author.

Zessin, K-H., & Carpenter, T. E. (1985). Benefit-cost analysis of an epidemiologic approach to provision of veterinary service in the Sudan. *Preventive Veterinary Medicine, 3*, 323-337.

Zhang, X. (1994, March). WHO's policy and activities on traditional medicine. In A. Islam & R. Wiltshire (Eds.), *Traditional health systems and public policy: Proceedings of an International Workshop, Ottawa, Canada* (pp. 139-142). Ottawa: IDRC.

18 Ethnobotany

Linking Health and Environmental Conservation

MICHAEL J. BALICK

The philosophies of environmental conservation and health care have much in common, with many lessons for contemporary society. As the human body must be in balance, so must the individual be in balance with the environment. Tragically, many contemporary peoples are not. In many parts of the world, the ecocide is apparent, differing only in degrees of injury. Environmental devastation resulting from human-induced actions such as overdevelopment, excessive industrial pollution, and the uncontrolled migration of people to urban areas is symptomatic of a widespread insult to the earth. People are ultimately a part of their environment, an environment that reflects the health of its inhabitants.

Ethnobotany, the study of the relationship between plants and people, is one example of an interdisciplinary science that can yield positive benefits to human health while supporting conservation. The linkage between ethnobotany, health, and conservation gives rise to a number of important policy questions involving community, business, and government interests at local, regional, and international levels. In traditional medicine and the herbal industry, the yields are immediate, and the economic impact on the individual, community, and region can be quite significant. Who pays for and who benefits from the collection and use of known medicinal plants can to a large degree determine the availability of these plants into the future—and the sustainability of their cultivation.

THE SCIENCE OF ETHNOBOTANY

In the past few decades, the discipline of ethnobotany has undergone great evolution in its methodology and focus, as well as its application. Traditionally, ethnobotanical studies were carried out by systematic botanists whose goal was to produce lists of useful plants of a particular tribe or region. Most of these studies were presented in encyclopedic form. Ethnobotanical inventory is still very important, as such a small fraction of the total information that exists on the utility of plants has been catalogued. Recently, however, the interdisciplinary approach has become more important in ethnobotanical research, involving the close collaboration of botanists, pharmacologists, anthropologists, chemists, nutritionists, economists, conservationists, policymakers, ecologists, and those in many fields.

One result of this new approach has been the application of ethnobotany to public policy questions; for example, in the areas of health and ecosystem conservation. Ethnopharmacological studies initiated by Dr. Paul Alan Cox (1990) and colleagues in Samoa have resulted in the conservation of significant areas of endangered Samoan rain forest, as well as the identification of a potent anti-HIV compound. Ethnobotanical studies in Madagascar, coordinated by Dr. Nat Quansah (personal communication), take place in forest reserves and seek to establish a sustainable dynamic between the people's use of the area and the biological integrity of the protected ecosystems.

THE LINK BETWEEN MEDICINAL PLANTS, DRUG DEVELOPMENT, AND CONSERVATION

It is usually assumed that the discovery of a new plant drug will ultimately be of value to conservation efforts, especially in rain forest regions. This notion is based on the profit potential and economic impact, as well as the feeling that governments and people will somehow place greater value on the resource if it or its derivatives can produce a product with a multinational market. The distribution and potential of medicinal plants to support conservation can be viewed from three perspectives: regional traditional medicine, the national and

TABLE 18.1 Economic Value of Plant Medicines and Their Potential Value for Conservation

Sector	*Distribution of Economic Benefit*	*Amount of Taxes Collected*	*Pitfalls*
International pharmaceutical industry	Upper end of economic spectrum	Substantial	Overharvest Synthesis (if no provision for benefits included) Plantations outside area of discovery
National and international herbal industry	Full spectrum of economic system	Medium	Overharvest Plantations outside area of discovery
Regional traditional medicine	Lower end of economic system	Small	Overharvest (sustainability)

international herbal industry, and the international pharmaceutical industry (Table 18.1).

Within each level, the distribution of economic benefits varies greatly. In traditional medical systems, the economic benefits accrue to professional collectors, who sell the plants to traditional healers, or to the healers themselves. The local and international herbal industries produce value for a broad range of people and institutions, including collectors, wholesalers, brokers, and companies that produce and sell herbal formulations. Proportionally, the bulk of the economic value in the international pharmaceutical industry goes to the upper end of the economic spectrum, at the corporate level, as well as to those involved in wholesale and retail sales.

A comparison of the market value of these products reveals an interesting point. The value of traditional medical products, which are used by billions of people around the world, is billions of dollars each year. Whether or not it is comparable to the $80 billion to $90 billion of global retail sales of pharmaceutical products has not been calculated, to the best of my knowledge. However, it can be argued that commerce in traditional plant medicines, consisting primarily of local activity such as previously described, constitutes a significant economic force. If it is assumed that 3 billion people use traditional plants for their primary health care, and each person uses $2.50 to $5 worth annually (whether harvested, bartered, or purchased), then the annual value of these plants could range between $7.5 billion and $15 billion, a sum that is significant and comparable to the two other sectors of the global pharmacopoeia. It is roughly estimated that the international herbal industry is about 10 times the size of the U.S. herbal industry, the value of which is about $1.3 billion annually (M. Blumenthal, personal communication).

An interesting perspective emerges when the tax yields to government are compared. Obviously, in traditional medical systems, taxes are neither assessed nor paid. The international herbal industry is subject to taxes, including those levied at the point of sale and on corporate profits. Governments benefit most from taxes through commerce for therapies produced and sold by the international pharmaceutical industry.

Those who promote the linkage between conservation and the search for new pharmaceutical products often fail to point out that the time frame from collection of a plant in the forest to its sale on the pharmacist's shelves is eight to twelve years, and that programs initiated today must be viewed as having long-term benefits, at best. An exception to this are agreements such as that between Merck, Sharp, and Dohme and INBio, the National Biodiversity Institute of Costa Rica (Gamez, Piva, Sittenfeld, Leon, & Mirabelli, 1993). This agreement provides a substantial "up front" payment from Merck for infrastructure development at INBio and for the national parks system in Costa Rica, and it may provide a model for such North/South collaborations in the future.

The potential for strengthening conservation efforts ranges from low to high, depending on whether or not the extraction of the resource can be sustainably managed over the long term or is simply exploited for short-term benefits by collectors and an industry that have little interest in ensuring a reliable supply into the future. Conservation potential is minimal if the end products are derived from synthetic processes or from plantations developed outside of the original area of collection. To address this issue, the National Cancer Institute's Developmental Therapeutics Program seeks to ensure that the plant's primary country of origin will have the first opportunity to produce the plant should commercially valuable products arise as a result of their program.

Table 18.1 also summarizes the pitfalls inherent to each level, including overharvesting, synthesis with no provision for benefits, land tenure issues and, as previously mentioned, plantations established outside of the range of the species. In any attempt to plan for the maximum conservation potential of a discovery, these pitfalls must be kept in mind.

Harvest itself is not without pitfalls. One of the primary concerns about extraction is sustainability. A case in point is the extraction of a drug used in the treatment of glaucoma, pilocarpine (Pinheiro, 1995). The source of pilocarpine is several species of trees in the genus *Pilocarpus* that occur naturally in the northeast of Brazil: *P. pinnatifolius, P. microphylla,* and *P. jaborandi.* Leaves have been harvested from the trees for many decades, usually under subcontract from chemical companies. Limited attempts at sustainable management were undertaken in the 1980s but, for the most part, harvest continued in a destructive fashion. Extinction in many areas—at the population level—has been the fate of these plants. Finally, over the past few years, cultivated plantations of *Pilocarpus* species have been developed, which will reduce the value of the remaining wild stands and eliminate any incentive for conserving them.

THE BELIZE ETHNOBOTANY PROJECT

The Belize Ethnobotany Project (BEP) was initiated in 1988, as a collaborative endeavor between the Ix Chel Tropical Research Foundation, a Belizean nongovernmental organization headed by Dr. Rosita Arvigo, and the Institute of Economic Botany of the New York Botanical Garden (Balick, 1991). The main goal of the project has been to conduct an inventory of the ethnobotanical diversity of Belize, a country with significant tracts of intact forest. The project has carried out dozens of expeditions to various locales and has collected some 3,600 plant specimens as of early 1995, about 50 percent of which contain ethnobotanical data. The specimens have been deposited at the Belize College of Agriculture and Forestry Department, as well as The New York Botanical Garden and U.S. National Herbarium. A database has been established at The New York Botanical Garden, with planned distribution to several computer facilities within Belize. The BEP involves gathering traditional knowledge provided by more than two dozen colleagues who are traditional healers of Mopan, Yucatec, Kekchi Maya, Ladino, Garifuna, Creole, East Indian, and Mennonite descent.

Through a contract with the U.S. National Cancer Institute (NCI), the project has provided some 2,000 bulk plant samples to the NCI for screening in their human cancer and HIV Developmental Therapeutics Program (DTP). Samples, each weighing about 500 grams, have been collected and dried at low heat, then shipped to the NCI's testing facilities in Frederick, Maryland. Although NCI scientists have expressed interest in some of the species collected to date, more comprehensive studies have not identified a particular plant with a novel compound for advanced development in the DTP. However, in the future, as more and more species are put through the two HIV screens and 40 human cancer screens, we expect that greater interest in some of the species will be shown.

DEVELOPING A FOREST-BASED TRADITIONAL MEDICINE INDUSTRY

As discussed above, one of the primary dilemmas in the development of a program for extraction of nontimber forest products has been the long history of overcollecting the resources, with a resultant decline in these resources, as well as the export of raw materials for processing to centers and countries far from their origins. Rattan is a classic example of this overexploitation, with people in producing countries who are closest to the resource receiving the smallest percentage of the profits involved in its manufacture into high-quality furniture.

In Central America and elsewhere, locally developed brands of commercialized traditional medicines are now being marketed. A key difference in these types of endeavors is that the value-added component of the product is added *in the country of origin* of the raw material. As these product brands develop, and as new brands and products appear based on the success of the original endeavors, greater demand for ingredients from rain forest species will result. This could contribute to preservation of tropical forest ecosystems, but only if people carefully manage the production or extraction of plant species that are primary ingredients in these products. In addition, it is expected that small farmers will cultivate some of the native species, for sale to both local herbalists and commercial companies.

To address the latter possibility, our work in Belize has included a project with the Belize College of Agriculture (BCA), Central Farms, learning how to propagate and grow more than twenty-four different plants currently used in traditional medicine in that country. Hugh O'Brien, Professor of Horticulture at BCA, has coordinated this effort, which has included the genera *Achras, Aristolochia, Brosimum, Bursera, Cedrela, Croton, Jatropha, Myroxylon, Neurolaena, Piscidia, Psidium, Senna, Simarouba, Smilax, Stachytarpheta,* and *Swietenia.*

ESTABLISHING AN ETHNOBIOMEDICAL FOREST RESERVE

The concept of the extractive reserve as a tool for conservation has received a great deal of attention over the past few years. Many of these reserves are tracts of forest where nontimber forest products can be harvested by local individuals or groups who, theoretically, have a stake in the preservation of their biological integrity (Allegretti, 1990). Products such as rubber, Brazil nuts, copal resin, plant oils, fruits, fiber, construction materials, foliage and house plants for the florist trade, and other items have been selected for harvest and marketing from extractive reserves in the Amazon, Central America, Asia, and Africa. Numerous perspectives on these resources, both positive and negative, have been highlighted recently (Browder, 1992; Ryan, 1991).

In June 1993, a 6,000-acre lowland tropical forest government-owned reserve was established for the extraction of medicinal plants, teaching, and apprenticeship, with financial support from The Healing Forest Conservancy and the Rex Foundation (Balick, Arvigo, & Romero, 1994). This particular forest, in the Yalbak region of Belize, contains a broad diversity of medicinal plant species. Also within its borders are many species of animals, including jaguar, tapir, peccary, howler monkeys, and numerous other mammals, birds, and reptiles. A unique feature of this reserve is that it has been designated for the extraction of medicinal plants used locally as part of the primary health care network. Accordingly, this type of extractive reserve was classified as an *ethnobiomedical forest reserve* (Balick et al., 1994), a term intended to convey a sense of the interaction between people, plants, animals, and the health care system in the region.

One objective of the reserve is ethnobotanical and ecological research, designed to identify the plant resources it contains and develop appropriate technologies for their sustainable extraction. David Campbell and his students from Grinnell College (Iowa) have constructed ecological transects in selected parts of the reserve to serve as long-term study sites. Some of these transects will monitor extraction, whereas others monitor changes in the native vegetation. Ethnobotanical inventories have begun to catalog economically important plants in the reserve, as well as in the surrounding Cayo District. Other scientists will be invited to participate in these studies.

It will be years before this first ethnobiomedical forest reserve can be judged a success or failure. A great deal of work must go into developing the management plan and finding the financial and human resources to implement it. Land-use pressures surrounding the reserve, specifically logging and agriculture, as well as sociological and political factors, could endanger the long-term existence of the reserve. However, in Belize there is a great deal of optimism and support for this innovative reserve, much of it at the grassroots level.

Reserves for protecting medicinal plants have recently been established in other areas of the world, such as India, in an effort to ensure the supply of these important species.

CONCLUSION

Revitalization of interest in traditional medicine can be a powerful force in promoting conservation, contributing to local economic development, and improving the primary health care delivery system. There is great advantage to all in linking once-disparate constituencies such as conservationists and health care workers. Future efforts in these fields, in order to ensure success, will involve an approach using teams of investigators and implementers from varied backgrounds. As limitations of resources and time increase their pressures on global programs, such efforts will become even more necessary.

REFERENCES

Allegretti, M. H. (1990). Extraction reserves: An alternative for reconciling development and environmental conservation in Amazonia. In *Alternatives to deforestation: Steps toward sustainable use of the Amazon rain forest* (pp. 252-264). New York: Columbia University Press.

Balick, M. J. (1991). The Belize ethnobotany project. *Fairchild Tropical Garden Bulletin, 46*(2), 16-24.

Balick, M. J., Arvigo, R., & Romero, L. (1994). The development of an ethnobiomedical forest reserve in Belize: Its role in the preservation of biological and cultural diversity. *Conservation Biology, 8*(1), 316-317.

Browder, J. O. (1992). Social and economic constraints on the development of market-oriented extractive reserves in Amazon rain forests. *Advances in Economic Botany, 9*, 33-41.

Cox, P. A. (1990). Ethnopharmacology and the search for new drugs. In D. Chadwick & J. Marsh (Eds.), *Bioactive compounds from plants* (Ciba Foundation Symposium 154, pp. 40-47). Chichester, UK: Wiley.

Gamez, R. A., Piva, A., Sittenfeld, E., Leon, J., & Mirabelli, G. (1993). Costa Rica's conservation program and National Biodiversity Institute (INBio). In W. V. Reid, S. A. Laird, C. A. Meyer, R. Gamez, A. Sittenfeld, D. H. Janzen, M. A. Gollin, & C. Juma (Eds.), *Biodiversity prospecting: Using genetic resources for sustainable development* (pp. 53-67). Washington, DC: World Resources Institute.

Pinheiro, C. U. (1995). Saving the leaf that saves the eye. *Ophthalmology World News, 3*(1), 24.

Ryan, J. C. (1991). Goods from the woods. *Forest Trees and People, 14*, 23-40.

19 The Herbal Alternative

JAMES DUKE

How many times has your doctor prescribed fiber, vitamins, and/or minerals for you? Chances are good you were given a synthetic pill containing a strong chemical compound. Because we can synthesize, economically at least, fewer than 10 percent of the phytochemicals used in modern prescription drugs, there's at least one chance in four your doctor prescribed a pill that contained a natural chemical compound from a higher plant, a second chance in four that it came from a fungus or animal (Duke, 1991). But that pill will have the isolated chemical—the "silver bullet"—usually omitting the multitude of compounds that accompanied the chemical in nature.

Nature's compounds and their allies are so complex as to befuddle the pharmaceutical profession. The synergisms, agonisms, and antagonisms of the hundreds of compounds found in a single herb are enough to confound research on their biological activities. For just two compounds, there is an infinite number of combinations, and each living cell is estimated to contain somewhere between a thousand and ten thousand enzymes, to count just one group of specialized compounds. Compounds in herbs of the same species may vary in quantity by one or two or more magnitudes. The methods of preparing extracts or decoctions of the herbs may introduce one or two or more magnitudes of quantitative variation. The next herbal tea made of a different individual of the same herbal species may have differing proportions in all these compounds. Hence, even with inferred checks and balances, reproducible scientific results are not as likely as when single compounds are studied.

This, coupled with the difficulty in patenting natural products, much less plant species, makes the simple synthetic compound more attractive for scientific evaluation. So we take one compound or so from the plant, usually one or more active ingredients, leaving behind hundreds of compounds that accompanied the one we extract. All the fiber, minerals, vitamins—and usually the alkaloids, glycosides, and more obscure secondary metabolites—are thrown away so that we will get the purified silver bullet. We may be discarding our best medicines in our search for those purified compounds.

If your physician has diagnosed your ailment properly (and you suffer from only one ailment and are not deficient in any of the minor or major nutrients, vitamins, and/or minerals), chances are good that the silver bullet will help. Most of the people who go to the doctor are going to get well, even without the silver bullet. These people might just as well have taken the herbal shotgun shell, assuming it is innocuous and judiciously taken.

If you were to take a calculated risk and consult with an herbalist you trusted, you might get an herb, with all its vitamins, minerals, fiber, and a whole host of bioactive compounds, usually herbs that humans have been using for millennia. On the other hand, your medical doctor might even say that most Americans get too many vitamins. But if you smoke (more than 25 percent of Americans do) or drink too much (more than 10 percent of Americans do), you may be short on a few vitamins and minerals. And if your diet parallels that of half of Americans, you don't get enough fiber. If you are old, and nearly a quarter of us are, you may be short of vitamins or minerals, for example, the calcium and iron so frequently found in herbs, especially in the leaves. The more than half of us who are female may suffer anemia during many moons of our lives, anemia that may call for iron and vitamins B_6 and B_{12}. If you are under stress, and perhaps another quarter of us suffer stress today, that, too, may be depleting you of certain vitamins.

In spite of these unfavorable odds, or perhaps because of them, middle-class Americans are becoming more and more judicious about such matters as diet, exercise, and alternative medicines. They don't want the wrong herb or the wrong synthetic. They are leaning toward more natural dyes, antioxidants, foods, and so on, but they are being discouraged as they seek out natural herbal medicines. There are many examples of counterproductive interventionism in alternative herbal and/or food "farmacy" therapies by an agency (the FDA) that blithely allows cigarettes and alcohol to kill hundreds of thousands of Americans. Old-fashioned root beer is still outlawed, although the safrole in it rendered a can of root beer less than one tenth as carcinogenic as ethanol renders a can of ethanolic beer (Duke, 1991). Perhaps the worst example was documented on *60 Minutes* (December 1, 1991). There it was shown that, thanks largely to behind-the-scenes lobbying of the Drug Enforcement Administration, the country was about to eliminate the use of herbal *cannabis* for the side effects of chemotherapy. It was to be replaced by a synthetic dear to the pharmaceutical industry's heart. The only catch was that the nonherbal alternative (Zofran) would cost $600 a day. Worse, it requires hospitalization for intravenous feeding. How many Americans can afford $600 a day, plus hospital costs?

According to Sen. David Pryor (D-AR), drug prices in the United States are 50 to 60 percent higher than they are in other industrialized countries. The average American takes seven prescriptions per year (about $275 a year, more than the per capita gross national product in Haiti) (*Austin American-Statesman*, May 25, 1992). Increasingly, more and more Americans will be unable to afford modern pharmaceuticals, many of which were developed with taxpayer money, while the profits accrue to the pharmaceutical industry. The American consumer is swept into the pockets of the pharmaceutical industry, one of the most profitable in the United States.

We want the best medicine, be it synthetic or natural. How will we know which is best, the synthetic or the natural? We won't. Unless you, the reader, convince your congressional representatives to stand up to the pharmaceutical lobby, which might not encourage preventive medicine. Economics leads the pharmaceutical firms to prefer a semisynthetic derivative or synthetic to the natural product. Today, according to pharmaceutical industry estimates, it costs $500 million to prove a new drug safe and efficacious ("Vital Statistic," 1993). Drug companies are therefore more interested in developing unnatural drugs that can be better protected by patents. To use an old and frayed example: What drug company wants to invest $500 million to prove an herb like feverfew, which you and I could grow at home, can prevent migraines? How would they get their $500 million back if we raised homegrown feverfew and self-medicated? And how much would they lose in sales of remedial migraine medications if this herb prevented 70 percent of migraine headaches?

We don't know the answers to these questions, and we won't know. Unless we bend the ears of an intelligent member of Congress. It behooves Congress and its constituents to insist that we learn whether the herbal alternatives are safe and efficacious. In some cases, I predict the herbal options will prove both safer and more efficacious, not to mention cheaper, than the overexpensive synthetic options. Ask your representative: Who benefits most from preventive medicine, the consumer, the government, the medical establishment, or the pharmaceutical industry? Clearly, the doctors and pharmaceutical industry stand to lose if preventive medicine prevails. But the government and the tax-paying consumer gain. Then why is most government funding earmarked for curative medicines, the efficacy of which is too often measured in days added to a miserable, uncured life?

As it stands today, the Food and Drug Administration (FDA) prohibits the sale of herbal alternatives if there are any preventive or curative messages implied. These herbs could save thousands of lives. The FDA tolerates tobacco while prohibiting the sale of licorice or lobelia to help people stop using tobacco, or antioxidant teas or even carrots to prevent lung cancer, or willowbark to prevent heart attack. As it is today, the FDA tolerates the sale of killer alcohol, while prohibiting the sale of evening primrose to curb the alcohol habit or milk thistle seed or dandelion flowers to prevent cirrhosis, or antioxidant teas to prevent oral, kidney, or liver cancer (Duke, 1996). They tell us that, without scientific proof of their efficacy, these herbs cannot be sold with health messages. Are they helping the American consumer or the pharmaceutical industry? Are we missing some of the safer, more effective herbal drugs because of this paranoid myopia, coupled with the high cost of proving a new drug safe and efficacious? Yes, we are.

Don't despair. Write a personal letter, not a form letter, to your congressional representatives. Let them know that the costs of modern pharmaceuticals are slipping out of economic reach of more and more of their constituents. Tell them you think the American consumer and the world need and deserve answers to the above questions. Request legislation that would require a pharmaceutical firm, in any new synthetic drug trial, to compare its new drug, not only with a placebo, but also with one or two of the better herbal alternatives. Urge your congressional representative to give the herbal alternative a chance to help poor and wealthy alike avoid economic strangulation by a greedy pharmaceutical industry. Put the burden of proof of empirical herbal effectiveness on the agency that confiscates an inexpensive, long-standing, and empirically proven botanical, while favoring the exorbitant synthetics, as well as expensive, unproven, or unnecessary interventions like angioplasties, bypasses, chemonucleolysis, caesareans, hysterectomies, and the like. These cause thousands of deaths a year. How many herbal fatalities were there in the last decade?

According to the late Rep. Ted Weiss (D-NY), more than half (102 of 198) of the prescription drugs approved by the FDA between 1976 and 1985 caused serious reactions that later caused the drugs to be relabeled or removed from the market. Fatal drug reactions have been estimated to occur in 0.1 percent of hospital patients and 0.01 percent of patients who have surgery. This means one in a thousand people admitted to hospitals for medical rather than surgical reasons will be killed by the medicine. Among the general population, elderly people (65 or older) are affected by adverse drug reactions at nearly twice the rate of others (160 per million as opposed to 85 per million people) ("Prescription Drugs," 1990).

Roughly 3 percent to 8 percent of patients hospitalized in the United States will suffer a bacterial infection during their stay. Of an estimated 4 to 8 million patients infected, Centers for Disease Control estimates that infections contracted in a hospital are related to one hundred thousand deaths each year. The *Chemical Marketing Reporter* states that such infections are the primary cause of deaths in intensive care units ("Intravenous Antibiotic," 1985).

Julian Whitaker, M.D., surveys many treatments that are more lethal than the diseases they treat. For example, a million angiograms are given a year, 90 percent of which are unnecessary, and 0.1 percent to 0.5 percent of which result in death. Nearly three hundred thousand people have $15,000 in angioplastic procedures a year, and 2 to 4 percent die during the procedure or during the first year after it. As many as 44 percent of bypass patients don't need the surgery and might be better off with a combination of drugs, diet, and exercise. Five percent of bypass patients die as a result of the surgery (Whittaker & Roth, 1989). The Bjork-Shiley heart valve, never reviewed by the FDA, has killed 240 people. There's no way to find and warn the eleven thousand or so Americans who don't know their heart valve is a Bjork-Shiley (Finch, 1992).

Another example is seen in the treatment of arthritis. Estimates are that the nonsteroidal antiinflammatory drugs used to treat arthritis cause perhaps two hundred thousand cases of gastrointestinal bleeding each year, leading to ten thousand to twenty thousand deaths ("Searle Ulcer," 1989). Yet, the herbal industry is forbidden to make curative claims for the treatment of arthritis or any other ailment. Is the pharmaceutical industry, sanctioned by the FDA, killing as many as twenty thousand people a year, while it perhaps alleviates the symptoms of, but fails to cure, arthritis?

A California study cited in the *Chemical Marketing Reporter* ("Drug Ads," 1992) indicated that 92 percent of drug advertisements in leading medical journals fail to comply with FDA regulations. After examining 109 advertisements in 10 medical journals in 1990, the study found an average of 4.3 cases of inadequate or misleading information *per adver-*

tisement. Half of the ads had little or no educational value, 60 percent contained poor or unacceptable scientific references, 38 percent lacked information on safety, and 28 percent failed to disclose side effects or contraindications. Meanwhile, FDA commissioner Dr. David A. Kessler expresses the hope that the industry will examine its marketing practices more closely and recommit itself to giving consumers accurate, nonmisleading information about products.

If Dr. Kessler is going to let the multibillion-dollar pharmaceutical fox guard the chicken coops (advertising is a multimillion-dollar business in itself), should he not extend the same privilege to the depauperate botanical (herbal and food farmacy) industry. No. We fear not. Favoring the Goliath Pharmaceutical Industry, the FDA attacks the Davidian botanical industry with rules, confiscations, and midnight marauding raids. The empirically proven botanicals should be considered innocent until proven guilty. Let the FDA or some responsible government agency prove the botanicals safe or unsafe, efficacious or inefficacious. For now, the botanical industry has to spend all its money on lawyers trying to protect it from the Goliath, the FDA, and vested interests. Ask your congressional representative for proof that the expensive synthetic medicine the FDA approves is safer and/or more efficacious than the much cheaper and empirically proven botanical. We really deserve to know, not just assume, which is better and safer—the herbal or the synthetic.

REFERENCES

Drug ads are faulted in study: Noncompliance with rules found. (1992, June 8). *Chemical Marketing Reporter, 241*(23), p. 4.

Duke, J. (1991). Promising phytochemicals. *The Journal of Naturopathic Medicine,* 2(1), 48-52.

Duke, J. (1996). *Green farmacy*. Emmaus, PA: Rodale.

Finch, S. (1992, July/August). *Beyond breast implant—what else haven't they checked out?* Boulder, CO: Time Publishing Ventures.

Intravenous antibiotic is approved to treat hospital-acquired infections. (1985, May 13). *Chemical Marketing Reporter, 227*(19), p. 7.

HHS official charges *GAO* misleads on drug side effects. (1990, June 4). *Chemical Marketing Reporter, 237*(23).

Searle ulcer drug okayed; major market is predicted. (1989, January 2). *Chemical Marketing Reporter, 235*(1), p. 3.

Vital statistic: Disputed cost of creating a drug. (1993, November 9). *Wall Street Journal.*

Whitaker, J., & Roth, J. (1989). *Reversing health risks: How to get out of the high risk category for cancer, heart disease, diabetes, and other health problems.* New York: Berkley Books.

20 You Are What You Eat

ROBERT RODALE

What is now seen as the alternative in agriculture will soon become conventional.

Why do I make that prediction? The answer is simple. A powerful group of forces is rapidly pushing trends in the direction of a regenerative food system. After roughly fifty years of almost total opposition from the government, academia, and business, the push for change has suddenly burst free from the crushing burden of uninformed disapproval that kept most people from taking alternatives seriously for so long. It's like the Berlin Wall coming down. Suddenly farmers are free to tread anywhere in the realm of agricultural ideas.

At the same time, throughout the United States, Europe, and much of the rest of the world, consumers are ready for revolt. For a long time, consumers have been outsiders in the food system. Now, they are rapidly gaining power by voting with their food dollars and becoming active—in fact, dominant—players in directing agricultural practices and policies. The "wall" separating consumers from influence on farm methods is coming down.

CONSUMER POWER

The technological force that is changing our outside environment is also altering and reducing the value of our food. Speaking plainly, we

---

AUTHOR'S NOTE: Adapted with permission from Rodale Press. 611 Siegfriedale Road, Kutztown, PA, 19530-9749.

are falling victim to a form of internal pollution, just as we have to external pollution. The production of food itself has been changed through mechanization and chemical manipulation. And we have become separated from the crop in the field by a massive complex of food processing involving not only machines and chemicals but packaging, storage, and selection procedures that often work to lower the nutritional value of food.

Organic gardeners and health-oriented people have long objected to machine-handled food. But in the United States, our arguments have been countered by industry claims that Americans are the best fed people on Earth. Now we have solid evidence of internal pollution that cannot be refuted by broad claims that supermarket food is the best available.

Anyone who shops in supermarkets can see the change that has come about in the way food is presented to the customer. But it has taken studies by the government and by first-rate scientists like Roger Williams to prove that all the glamor and superficial prettiness of packaged supermarket food is producing a poorer diet. Years ago when you went into a food store, you saw few foods in pretty boxes and packages but plenty of items close to the state in which they came off the farm. Even the smell was different. Instead of sniffing the disinfected, deodorized scent of the supermarket, you could feast your nostrils on the aroma of cured meats, raw soap, and ripening fruit in season.

The only trouble with food then was that it required plenty of work to get it ready to eat. There were no instant foods. Coffee not only had to be percolated at home, it sometimes had to be roasted and ground, too. The food companies were on the right track when they took over the coffee roasting and grinding chores, but they have gone too far beyond that in search of ways to do the consumer's work and turn a profit in the bargain. Food, like our environment, has become something to be exploited. The result is internal pollution. In addition to the chemicals put into food during processing, the internal pollution consists of an excess of food energy (calories) in relation to real food value (protein, vitamins, and minerals).

Unfortunately, once people get in a rut, they have trouble getting out. Nobody likes eating chemical-laden food, but few have sufficient motivation to make the little extra effort to get better food. They don't realize how deep in the rut they are. They read the list of chemicals on a package of processed food, and those long names zip over their heads. They don't begin to understand what those chemicals are doing there in the food.

What bothers me most is the feeling in the food trade that the old traditions are gone, that anything goes as long as people like the taste and can't tell the difference between what you are selling and real food.

You are what you eat. And the average American is eating food that is increasingly doctored with chemicals and decreasingly of any substantial nutritional value.

The best way to counter this assault on well-being is to grow as much food yourself as you possibly can. Most people find it difficult or impossible to grow all their own food, but almost anyone with access to a plot of land can grow some. That way, you know what you are putting into your soil and what is getting on your plants. You control all the processing steps and can use the food fresh.

FARMING SYSTEMS

Farms are whole systems. Farmers are the last working generalists in our society, operating and usually understanding their own personal production systems. They can't wait for the "experts" or government to save the day. Farmers are quickly generating practical solutions to problems, such as pesticide residues and groundwater pollution, that government and industry seem unwilling or unable to deal with. The innovative power of individual farmers is tremendous and is doing more to solve basic production and other problems than any of the experts give them credit for. Largely on their own, farmers are cutting production costs, improving product quality, and lessening their impact on the environment.

The conventional U.S. agricultural research establishment, after making big productivity gains in the 1950s through the 1970s, is now a disaster zone. The agricultural universities are so fragmented and superspecialized that there is almost no way they can bring their narrow ways of thinking to bear on whole farm systems. Either that will change drastically in the near future or agricultural universities and ag science establishments in general will continue to shrink, both in size and in reputation.

The prestige of agricultural scientists is quite low today, compared with the respect and rewards society accords to other scientists. I would even say that agricultural scientists are near the bottom of the heap. At the top are physicians, molecular biologists, and certain medical specialists. They are the ones who get most of the big offices and large paychecks. Occasionally they are even treated as celebrities.

It was not always that way. Think of Washington and Jefferson, the U.S. founding fathers. They were thoughtful, analytical farmers. Most leaders of society either knew farming well or were naturalists or generalists in the best sense. Those who could lead others toward better production on the land were held in high esteem.

We have a relationship of close accountability with nature. Our incomes go up when the way we work fits the requirements that nature gives us. And our bank accounts get smaller when our farming methods fall out of step with the resources nature provides us. Nature—which is defined in the dictionary as the creative and controlling force in the universe—has sent the world a message:

> I have been around a long time and will be here for many millions more years. And I will continue to make resources available for the use of all living creatures and plants. But you human beings are getting very numerous and are taking more all the time without giving back things that I can recycle and purify. So it's time you start using my resources in a different way. Be more gentle. Don't try to dominate me. Especially, learn to farm more sustainably. Get together with people from all over and start to work on new ideas.

PART III

New Paths: Toward an Ecology of Health

21 Health and Self-Mastery

The Ecology of Personal Power

PHIL NUERNBERGER

The current debate about health care has little if anything to do with health. It is first and foremost a struggle for control and money, as entrenched powers—medical, economic, political, legal—shamelessly fight to protect their own selfish interests. Second, it is a debate about how to spend money on disease. But no matter how sophisticated the delivery systems, how coordinated managed care services become, or how we structure insurance, disease will always be costly. Redistributing the costs doesn't change this fact. It is like debating what color to paint an elephant at feeding time. It really doesn't matter which colors we use; the fact still remains that we must *feed* the elephant. Sophisticated delivery systems do not keep the executive or the plumber from having a heart attack, nor does managed care give our children the inner strength necessary to resist the pressure to take drugs.

The real problem we face is how to create a healthy world, free of physical, mental, social, and environmental disease. In the United States, we have no choice but to provide the best possible medical services equally for every citizen. But when you cut right to the issue, being healthy has little to do with doctors and health insurance. On a personal level, it is a matter of our living habits—what, when, and how we eat, whether or not we exercise, our emotional habits, even our beliefs. On a social level, it is a matter of whether or not we respect and care for each other, and whether or not we create families and neighborhoods that are free from poverty and violence. On an environmental level, it is determined by whether or not we respect the integrity of our ecosystem and create organizations that support individual, societal, and environmental health and well-being. At all levels, it is a matter of knowledge and skill.

Health involves all aspects of our life. Just as we cannot separate health from diet, exercise, and emotions, we also cannot separate it from violent or toxic environments. Nor can we separate our individual health from the health of our families or the environment. Few of us, however, have the authority, position, or power to create changes throughout the society or the environment. We do have the authority and power to become healthy ourselves, and in that way, we begin to transform society. The health of each dimension of society rests on the physical, mental, and spiritual health of the individuals who constitute it and thus live within a personal, socioeconomic, and environmental context. It is who we are as individuals that determines whether or not we are healthy as individuals, whether or not our families and our society are healthy, and whether or not we create a healthy environment.

As individuals, and together as a collective force, we are ill-prepared to meet the challenges we face. Our health reflects our lack of self-knowledge, self-discipline, and skill. Instead of responding effectively and confidently to the pressures and challenges of modern life, we find ourselves playing the role of victim. We feel powerless and ineffectual because we *are* powerless and ineffectual. We have made a lifestyle of giving away responsibility: for our health, to the health professionals; for our communities, to the politicians; and for the environment, to those whose only goal seems to be money. In every case, we have become so preoccupied with our technology that we increasingly ignore the nearly infinite power of our own minds and resources.

A PROBLEM OF IGNORANCE

There are few things more personal than our health. Yet how much do we really know about how body and mind work together to create health or disease? Unless you are a health professional or biological scientist, your education probably stopped after the mandated high school health class taught by the assistant basketball coach. Most of us know more about how our automobile works than we do about our own bodies and minds.

The foundation of power is knowledge. We have enormous technical and scientific knowledge about the external world. Doctors are very sophisticated in their material knowledge, but they aren't any healthier than the rest of us. In all probability, the psychiatrist would commit suicide before you would, and your doctor will die at a younger age than you. Knowing what medications to use to treat high blood pressure doesn't prevent one from getting it. Knowing that tension and stress can lead to high blood pressure doesn't keep one from being tense and stressed out. If we haven't the skill to stay relaxed under pressure, to manage our emotional reactions, or to keep ourselves from worrying, then even the best information about disease does very little good.

We are abysmally ignorant of our own inner realities as to how body, mind, and spirit work together. Yet our inner realities determine whether or not we are healthy, whether or not we love and respect each other, whether or not we respect and care for our environment. Knowledge, without the ability to use it, is useless. Along with self-knowledge, we must have skill. We know that to become a skilled tennis player we must practice tennis. To become a skilled surgeon, we must practice surgery. But what do we practice if we want to become a skilled human being? We don't even think in these terms, yet this is the very task we face.

YOGA—THE SCIENCE OF SELF-MASTERY

We cannot create health at any level until we can master *ourselves.* Health—whether personal, social, or environmental—demands knowledge and skill. Many systems of self-mastery—and perhaps the most sophisticated—Yoga, Taoism, Zen, martial arts—come from the East. In spite of tremendous scientific, medical, religious, and social prejudice, these introspective sciences are being used in Western society with great effect. The clinical programs of Ornish (1990) and Kabot-Zinn (1990), as well as others less well-known, have proven the practical benefits of training in self-mastery. As one of the most sophisticated disciplines in self-mastery, yoga science provides a comprehensive understanding of human behavior. More important, it provides the practical tools and techniques so necessary for developing knowledge, skill, and self-discipline at all levels of our reality—social, physical, emotional, intellectual, and spiritual.

Contrary to popular misconceptions, Yoga is not a religion nor a philosophy. It is an introspective science sharing the same critical elements of any science: empirical evidence, rigorous observation and experimentation, and verification through experience. Western scientists use their minds to study external phenomena. The yogi, an introspective scientist, studies the source of knowledge itself, the human mind that constructs the knowledge. The entire realm of human behavior and capacity is the field of study. The body and mind are the laboratory, self-knowledge and self-discipline are the foundation, and the outcome is complete knowledge of human activity, from the most mundane physiological function through subtle mental/emotional activities, to the highest expression of our spiritual Self.

The goal of yoga science is self-mastery, the maximum development of human potential through self-knowledge and self-discipline (skill). Both are necessary. Self-knowledge without the skill to manage our resources turns us into paper tigers. We know who we are but don't have the capacity to *do.* On the other hand, self-discipline without self-knowledge leads to egoism and fanaticism, where our skills are driven by our desires and fears.

Above all, Yoga is practical, providing both the knowledge and techniques we need to take control of our life, our health, and our destiny. We can use this practical knowledge to create health for ourselves, our communities, and our environment.

A MAP OF THE TERRITORY

As an introspective science, Yoga provides a practical analysis of the different dimensions of our personality. These dimensions, referred to as *koshas,* or sheaths, are seen as coverings of different density that surround our spiritual core, or Self. The spiritual Self is regarded and individualized pure Consciousness and corresponds roughly to the individual soul of Western religion. Within each dimension are power functions that provide us with different forms of knowledge and skill. The more aware we are of these dimensions and power functions, the more effectively we use them to create a healthy mind and body. Although we discuss these dimensions and functions as separate factors, bear in mind that our mind always functions as a whole. We cannot separate mind and body, mind and spirit, or intellect and emotion. They all exist as integral parts of the whole person.

The first and most primitive sheath or dimension is the physical body. The body plays the role of facilitator, and effort is made to gain conscious control of the natural resources of the body in order to maintain a healthy system. For our purposes here, we can identify two primary power functions: an innate capacity for health and a capacity to gather and provide information. The body's capacity for health is based on inner balance and harmony between the various physiological systems. When we mismanage our internal systems, we become imbalanced and experience stress. If we ignore the symptoms of imbalance, we eventually end up with disease.

Our body is also a valuable resource for information and knowledge. Like a sophisticated receiver, it picks up and responds to a variety of signals from the environment. The more sensitive we are to these responses, the more effectively we deal with the world. We understand others more completely, make better decisions, and communicate more effectively. We also use our body's sensitivity to access the knowledge in our unconscious mind. How often have you heard someone say "that doesn't feel right to me" or "something smells funny about this." Our body is directly connected to our entire mind. Subtle states of knowledge, such as instinct and intuition, all have their physical expression. But these messages are often subtle and can be easily distorted by stress and confused with fears, wants, and desires. The healthier we are, the more sensitive we are to our body, the more effectively we use our body to make the right decisions for ourselves.

The second dimension is the energy sheath. This is the life force energy, called *prana,* which supports the physical structure. Prana plays a critical role as the mediating link between the body and mind. The spectacular control of physiological functioning demonstrated by Swami Rama at the Menninger Clinic is a result of knowledge and mastery of this dimension (Encyclopedia Britannica, 1973; Green & Green, 1974, 1977). Just as blood, nerves, and glandular discharges are distributed throughout the body, this life force energy is distributed through specific channels. Eastern systems of health and medicine provide sophisticated descriptions of these energy channels. Japanese and Chinese medicine refer to the energy as *Ki* and *Chi* respectively. They refer to the energy channels as *meridians* and use them as the template for acupuncture. Yoga science calls these same energy channels *nadis* and has sophisticated techniques to develop awareness and control of them.

The primary function within the energy dimension is the breath. Yogis use the breath to gain direct, conscious control of the autonomic nervous system. This allows them to control the internal organ systems enervated by the autonomic system. The yogis have never forgotten that the natural mechanism of breathing is the diaphragm. And proper diaphragmatic breathing is necessary for a healthy body and calm mind (Rama, Ballentine, & Hymes, 1979). Unfortunately, most of us breathe with the chest, which is why chest breathing is called normal. Chest breathing is the body's emergency breathing mechanism. What we refer to as normal breathing creates a chronic fight-or-flight alarm reaction and maintains chronic stress in the body. It also creates unnecessary strain on the cardiovascular system, leading to heart and vascular disease. The high incidence of heart and vascular disease that we suffer in our society is intimately connected to this unhealthy habit of chest breathing (Nuernberger, 1992).

The next three dimensions are concerned with the structure and function of the mind. Yoga science does not confuse the mind with the brain, which is an organ of the body. This is radically different from Western science and medicine, which not only basically ignores the mind but often denies its existence. Eastern introspective sciences have a sophisticated understanding of the mind. More important, they provide the systematic methods by which to bring this powerful reality under conscious control and use its full capacity.

The third dimension is the sensory mind, the most familiar part of our mind. The function of our sensory mind is to collect, organize, and interpret sensory data. This dimension serves as our personal reality generator. In the yogic view, we have total responsibility for creating our personal world of meaning. Four very powerful functions operate within this dimension: perception, habits, language, and emotions. Our emotions, past experiences (memory), beliefs, expectations, worries and fears, and desires and wants, as well as constitutional and genetic factors, the state of our health, stress, and environmental and social factors, all affect our sensory mind. As you might expect, this is a very busy, noisy dimension.

Although all functions are important, two functions—habits and emotions—play crucial roles in our health as well as in the development of self-discipline. It is obvious that our habits—lifestyle, physical, and emotional habits—play key roles in determining whether or not we have stress and develop psychosomatic disease. Habits are also the foundation of our self-discipline and skill. If we use these intelligently, we can develop and sustain the skills necessary for personal mastery and a high level of health. No less important are emotions, which energize our behavior. Powerful emotions, such as fear and self-hatred, are destructive not only on a personal level, but also in our communities and our society as a whole. When the emotions are severely distorted, as they are in abused children (the physical and emotional abuse created by poverty, by a lack of loving and supportive parents and family, or by an indifferent, self-centered society), they always lead to dysfunction and disease.

We know we should be emotionally mature and self-disciplined, but no one shows us how to accomplish that. Our education does not train the whole person. It does not provide the knowledge or skills we need for self-management. We do not teach our children how to use their inner resources. We fill their minds with facts and theories but hold out as models those whose egocentric greed brings them the most money, the most fame, the most power over others. Controls exerted by family, religion, and community, when directed by emotionally mature, disciplined, and loving individuals, are powerful influences. But in our materialistic society—where both parents work, where income and possessions are more important than quality of life, where 25 percent of children under six live in poverty—these influences have nearly disappeared. Even where positive influences still exist, the overwhelming pressure of materialism, its corrupting influence on political and economic leadership, the rise of religious fanaticism, the glorification of violence and greed in our mass media, and other influences provide powerful countermodels. The heroes of our modern culture, characterized by greed, self-centeredness, and egotism, hardly provide the models of emotional maturity needed for a healthy mind and society.

When we enter the fourth dimension, a powerful but subtle sheath called discriminating mind, we leave the noisy and disturbance-prone regions of our sensory mind, energy, and body and enter realms where stress and disease do not exist. The fourth dimension is where the energy of the mind is first modified into knowledge states that we eventually experience as thoughts, images, and sensations. The power function of this dimension is discrimination. To discriminate means to distinguish between things, to discern cause/effect relationships. Discrimination is the basis for clarity of thought and our ability to think things through. In its pure form, discriminating knowledge is unlimited by the sensory or the perceptual functions of the sensory mind. It is thus free of the limitations of time/space and pain/pleasure created by the sensory mind in order to structure our perceptions. With the sensory mind, we see the world as we have learned to see it. With the power of discrimination, we see the world as it is.

This pure knowledge is called *intuition* by yoga science. We have all experienced the power of this knowledge. Recall a time when you were about to do something that you had planned for several days. You were sure of your choices; even your friends had agreed that this was the right thing to do. But right before you began, a very quiet, subtle thought passed through your mind and said better not do this. You paused for a moment but went ahead with your plans anyway. Three days later, after everything had fallen apart, you said to yourself, "I knew I shouldn't have done this." And you *did* know, you simply didn't listen to your intuition. This very powerful tool is subtle, easily hidden by the noisy sensory mind. But with training, we can learn to access this powerful resource and use it as a conscious skill to guide our decisions.

The fifth and final dimension of the mind is called the balanced mind. It is the most subtle level of the personality. Yoga science considers this sheath the purest condition of the mind, before knowledge has even formed. Only the ego function exists to maintain boundary. As there is no modification of the mind's energy field (which the yogi calls knowledge), there is no stress within the field, and consequently, there are no distortions or conflicts. When we become conscious of this level of our mind, we experience it as bliss. This does not mean happiness or pleasure; it refers specifically to the experience of freedom from all inner conflicts, desires, wants, needs, fears, or anxieties. At that moment, we are entirely at peace with the world and with ourselves. This tranquility is the critical power function of this dimension.

This experience is not uncommon. It happens to us all occasionally when we are out for a walk and respond to the calm and beauty of our surroundings. It is that feeling of great harmony or contentment, that sense that all is right with the world. This inner harmony isn't created by a change of external conditions but rather by the quieting of a distracted mind. What we experience is our own inner balance and harmony, our own inner bliss. The practical outcome is unlimited and genuine self-confidence, an ever present source of strength for the personality. The conscious ability to access this very subtle resource provides us with psychological balance and a profound equanimity, the ability to face whatever life has in store with a clear and confident mind.

CULTIVATING THE SPIRITUAL SELF

There are two general functions of the mind, the ego and our memory. The ego creates boundaries, providing a unique center on which all other mind operations depend. Without the limiting frequency of the ego, the energy field called mind would dissipate and could not retain a cohesive form. We experience this function as a sense of *I-ness*, a central identity for the personality. The ego also serves a management role, supervising and integrating all dimensions and functions in order to sustain and enhance the total organization of the personality.

The memory function is actually more than just short-term or long-term memory. It also includes the template function that structures the shape of the energy field we call *mind*. The experiences we have modify the energy field of our mind, literally shaping the overall structure of the field itself. This not only determines how we interpret our reality but even what experiences are possible for us to have.

But the most powerful resource of all has nothing to do with our mind and body. It is the spiritual core, the Self that uses mind and body as a tool. There are many ways that we talk about this reality. Some speak of the power of the human heart. Others use religious terms such as the soul. It doesn't matter what we call it, or even what we believe. What is critical is that we experience this unlimited strength within ourselves—that we learn to use the selfless, unlimited love, joy, and tranquility that this experience provides in our daily lives.

This spiritual Self is beyond the personality structure and cannot be known or understood by the mind. That doesn't mean that we cannot experience or understand it. There is a great body of mystical knowledge and wisdom that is most often ignored, particularly by academics and scientists. This knowledge is not intellectual or rational but stems from the deepest insights and intuition into the very nature of life itself. It is Truth experienced within a variety of cultures and times, but each expression is fully coherent and consistent with all others.

Spiritual knowledge is singularly experiential. Yoga science, as well as other introspective disciplines, provides a systematic developmental process to expand personal awareness in order to experience this spiritual core Self. This experience is called *samadhi* and grounds our identity in the spiritual Self. This experience alone frees us from the fears, desires, and limits of the ego-self, giving us the freedom to love without dependency, to experience compassion for others, and to share in the joy of life. How one chooses to express this experience is irrelevant. The critical factor is the experience of this unlimited knowledge, love, and joy.

SKILL: THE SYSTEMIC DEVELOPMENT OF SELF-DISCIPLINE

Self-knowledge is only the beginning of self-mastery. The map described above is only useful to the degree that we also develop our ability to use the resources of mind, body, and spirit. The power of Yoga lies not in its analysis but in its practical and systematic approach to the development of personal skill. To that end, there are a number of different subsystems within yoga science. For example, *karma yoga* has a focus on the development of personality through selfless service; *hatha yoga* places its emphasis on training the body to train the mind and spirit; *nada yoga* uses sound; *kundalini yoga* is an advanced practice involving breathing and concentration exercises to awaken the powerful spiritual energy force; *jnana yoga* develops the mind through refined logic; *bhakti yoga* is the yoga of devotion. As the individual becomes more skilled, there are more sophisticated approaches, such as the Samaya school of *tantra yoga.* There are different branches of yoga science because there are different personalities and different needs. But each leads to a systematic development of individual personal strengths.

Probably the most practical approach, particularly for Westerners, is *astanga yoga,* the classical system of Yoga as defined by Patanjali, the codifier of yoga systems. Astanga means eight limbs, representing eight areas of focus. These provide a holistic, systematic, and practical approach to self-mastery. Astanga yoga is a blueprint for creating healthy people and a healthy society.

CONCLUSION

The essentials remain the same in all the different introspective disciplines and traditions. Whether we say "know thyself" or "be still and know that I am" or "Yoga is the cessation of the modifications of the mind," these statements all refer to the same freedom—the freedom from the tyranny of ignorance and fear, from stress and disease. We cannot mandate health through rule or law or congressional action, nor by scientific experiment, philosophical reasoning, or sermons. We certainly cannot solve our health problems by fighting over money and power. But we can create magic when we become masters of ourselves.

I do not share the pessimism expressed by others, but I know that we cannot achieve our potential without effort. There are no easy answers, no magic crystals, no fast-food solutions. But with the tools of yoga science and other introspective disciplines, and with patience, practice, and effort, we can create a health for ourselves, for our society, for our environment. We have the power, we have the resources—now, we must make the effort and become masters of ourselves.

REFERENCES

Encyclopedia Britannica. (1973). *Britannica yearbook of science and the future.* Chicago: William Benton.

Green, E., & Green, A. (1974). The ins and outs of mind-body energy. In *Science year: The world book of science annual* (pp. 137-199). Chicago: Fields Enterprises Educational Corp.

Green, E., & Green, A. (1977). *Beyond biofeedback.* San Francisco: Robert Briggs.

Kabat-Zinn, J. (1990). *Full catastrophe living.* New York: Delta Books, Dell.

Nuernberger, P. (1992). *Increasing executive productivity.* Englewood Cliffs, NJ: Prentice Hall.

Ornish, D. (1990). *Dr. Dean Ornish's program for reversing heart disease.* New York: Ballantine.

Rama, S., Ballentine, R., & Hymes, A. (1979). *The science of breath.* Honesdale, PA: Himalayan Publishers.

22 Addiction and Recovery for Individuals and Society

JIM JOHNSON

Compulsive drug use is not only one of the most physically destructive human behaviors, it has also become very destructive of society, and, despite statistical ebbs and flows, is generally on the increase.[1] Like clinical depression, addiction appears to have a number of possible causes, including genetic, social/environmental, psychological, and physiological factors. Of particular relevance is that significant increases in drug use and drug dependency have become virtually synonymous with rapid development and the concomitant disintegration of traditional human societies (Milam & Ketcham, 1983).

Arguably the most effective treatment for drug addiction is participation in Twelve-Step recovery fellowships such as Alcoholics Anonymous and Narcotics Anonymous. This examination considers how the successful treatment of addiction through these recovery fellowships may suggest broader solutions for many social problems that are either partially or wholly caused by social disintegration.

THE NATURE OF ADDICTION

Although much has been learned in recent years, addiction remains a fairly mysterious behavioral dysfunction. The physical side of addiction is fairly well documented, and some important advances have been made in the development of medical treatments. However, even those who specialize in the medical treatment of addiction admit that successful, long-term recovery is largely dependent on psychological and environmental factors (Milam & Ketcham, 1983, pp. 34-46).

Well-adjusted people use emotional discomfort as a guide for appropriate behavior: for example, learning to respond to feelings of guilt by curtailing unethical practices, or to feelings of fear by avoiding dangerous situations. In short, people need fully functioning emotions in order to meet the demands of everyday life. As our society's relationship to alcohol suggests, drug use is effective as a short-term alleviator of emotional distress; as a way of easing the pain of life's difficulties, it seems to work. Although most addicts initially use drugs recreationally, their drug use, as with most compulsive behaviors, tends to develop into an unconscious and maladjusted response to emotional discomforts (Gore, 1993).

Over time, instead of treating unpleasant emotions as important "feedback" from the environment, an addict erroneously makes it a habit to stifle them or seek distraction as the most effective way to respond. In the absence of firm guidance and healthy role models, this "pseudo-coping skill" sinks deeply into the behavioral patterns of the individual over time, to the point that it becomes a virtually natural and unconscious response—a psychological addiction—greatly exacerbating whatever physical dependence on drugs the individual has already developed (Gore, 1993).

Although addicts may ostensibly use drugs for escape from life's darker emotions and situations, compulsive drug use does much more than "kill the pain." When addicts chronically numb their negative feelings with drugs instead of truly owning emotional discomfort, they deprive themselves not only of much of life's richness but also of the mechanisms they need to move through everyday living.

OBSTACLES TO TREATMENT

Reacting to stress and emotional pain with drug use can result in significant long-term damage to one's mental health, physiological health, family, friendships, career, romantic relationships, and financial status. Nonetheless, several factors complicate the detection and treatment of drug addiction:[2]

1. *Fear of Change*: In spite of the magnitude of personal wreckage already experienced, an addict's instinctive fear of change may still obstruct both the recognition and the treatment of the problem. Only when their personal lives have degraded significantly may typical addicts begin to suspect that something is wrong. Even when the damage has been tremendous, addicts may be reluctant to suspect that their most basic, unconscious, and apparently successful method of coping with the pain of life may itself be the culprit.

2. *Familiarity*: The daily "familiar pain" of addiction, reinforced by the overwhelming and immediate euphoria of drug use, is much more attractive to addicts than the prospect of the unpredictable pain of a normal emotional life, without drugs. This is the "vicious circle" of addiction, in which the most natural response of addicts is to pursue short-term relief, even though they may be fully aware that they are deepening the long-term problem.

3. *Alienation*: Also, the disorientation and embarrassment of fundamentally reorienting their relationship to life's discomforts is often overwhelming; dependency on drugs with severe physical withdrawal symptoms makes recovery even more difficult. Most addicts report feeling a sense of alienation from others, even from a very early age. Although the causal relationship to actual addiction may be in question, there is little doubt that this perception discourages the development of confidants and persuades many addicts that no one else has ever experienced or will understand their condition.

4. *A Long Road Ahead*: Even when addicts accept their condition and become more committed to pursuing treatment, their difficulties have only begun. Although many nonaddicts assume that the agonizing process of initial withdrawal is the worst part, this stage is, in fact, often the least difficult. Once "clean," addicts begin to confront years—perhaps decades—of emotional and psychological underdevelopment. This intensely difficult process of "growing up late" and "facing life on life's terms" can take many years. Because most nonaddicts are unable to comprehend this ordeal, a recovering addict's friends, relatives, and even professional counselors are often quite limited in their ability to support the addict seeking to stay clean.

ADDICTED SOCIETY: AN OVERVIEW

Up until recent history, almost all people lived in small villages or tribes and maintained relative intimacy with nature. Generations tended to live together, survival was a shared responsibility, and behaviors were guided by innumerable cues from sunlight, weather, and other natural forces. In a very real sense, each human was inseparable from both the tribe or village and the natural environment. The development of agricultural techniques brought great changes to social organizations and humanity's relationship to the Earth, but intimacy with the land and climate remained essential, and the fundamental economic unit was still tribal.[3]

With the advent of industrialization, however, human societies reoriented around factories and urban centers; the environment became artificial and polluted, and most remnants of tribalism vanished from people's lives. Survival became dependent on the ability of a human being to act as a semi-intelligent machine on an assembly line or behind a desk. The nuclear family became the largest typical social unit, with many people living alone in apartment buildings. Suburbia was born, with its pseudo-natural, sterile, carefully managed "ecosystems." Predator/prey relationships, the weeding out of the weak by disease, and other aspects of Earth's natural rhythms were lost from the daily human experience (Lenski & Lenski, 1987).

Early nomadic peoples traveled as tribes and maintained the consistency of familial ties. With the alienation of humans from the earth-bound, tribally oriented framework of society came a completely new class of problems. The endless transition of modern times, the constant uprooting and dispersal, inevitably lead to emotional strife and disorientation. This is a wholly unnatural sort of challenge, something for which tribal creatures have never had the opportunity to develop coping mechanisms. Stripped of their natural social context, people tend to lose their sense of identity with other people and, consequently, become more likely to engage in gratification at the expense of others (Lenski & Lenski, 1987).

The search for relief from this psychic pain of the lost tribe leads to excessive forms of distraction and gratification. Most notably, drug abuse and addiction itself have become much more common. Part of this may be due to the increased availability of drugs, as well as increased availability of cash from industrial labor. A more significant contributing factor, however, is the emotional strain and stress incurred by an uprooted people engaged in dehumanizing work (Lenski & Lenski, 1987, pp. 347-349).

The pursuit not only of drugs but also of money, power, sex, beauty, status, food, entertainment, consumer goods, unrealistic degrees of security, and a host of other "fixes" has become an undisputed by-product of industrialization, which sometimes manifests itself in a ruthless and indiscriminate fashion. Compared with their tribal ancestors, many people living in industrial society exhibit behaviors strikingly similar to those of drug addicts. Corporations and marketing industries feed on these compulsions, not only by providing the goods but also by simultaneously reassuring consumers that what they are buying will actually make life better (Gore, 1993).

Thus, society mimics the vicious circle of addiction. Whole populations suffering (consciously or unconsciously) from the loss of their landed traditions seek short-term escape and distraction; the long-term unfulfilling nature of this lifestyle inspires a still more desperate pursuit of anything that can provide distraction and relief, further distancing individuals from the environmental feedback that could actually help them the most (Gore, 1993).

RECOVERY FELLOWSHIPS: THE REINVENTION OF TRIBALISM

Perhaps the fastest growing social change movement in recent history is that of the Twelve-Step recovery fellowships (Alcoholics Anonymous General Services Office, personal communication, May 5, 1995).[4] The first fellowship, Alcoholics Anonymous (AA), was started in 1935; as of January 1, 1995, there were more than 89,000 AA meetings worldwide. Because membership is anonymous, it is difficult to estimate the exact numbers, but best estimates indicate that more than 2 million addicts from all walks of life are currently seeking recovery in AA. A major fellowship known as Narcotics Anonymous (NA) was founded in 1953, its purpose being to broaden the perspective of AA to all drugs, advancing the concept of a "disease of addiction" not specific to any one substance. In early 1995, NA reported more than 20,000 active meetings, with an estimated 450,000 active members.[5] Attempts to treat other self-destructive behaviors, such as compulsive gambling, anorexia nervosa and compulsive spending, have resulted in the creation of dozens of other spin-off fellowships (Wuthnow, 1994).

The fundamental purpose of the fellowships is addiction recovery through self-help, and many sources indicate that they have proven to be a more effective long-term treatment than any method developed by the medical or mental health professions.[6] However, the implications of their rapid, widespread acceptance and remarkable degree of success range far beyond recovery from drug addiction. The success of the recovery fellowships is a direct result of their partial re-creation of humanity's original tribal social structure; such a structure is effective in neutralizing the primary causes of drug addiction, namely, the social disintegration and environmental disengagement inherent in industrialized society (Wuthnow, 1994).

THE TRIBAL SOLUTION

Analyses of methods of addiction recovery often overlook or minimize the sense of community and belonging that the fellowship provides, even though it may be the most obvious difference between the fellowships and other forms of treatment. In fact, this aspect of recovery fellowships is of enormous significance in their effectiveness. Far more than being a simple morale booster, this community environment represents "the lost tribe" in the racial memory of many recovering addicts—a tribe that is painfully and unconsciously missing from their everyday lives.

A look at the history of AA itself provides compelling evidence of this "power of the tribe." In what is generally considered to be the first AA meeting, the two cofounders of AA met when one of them desperately sought out the company of another struggling alcoholic as a means of overcoming the compulsion to drink. By honestly discussing their plight with one another, *both* men were able to overcome the compulsion to drink. This was long before the Twelve Steps of AA were written. These two men brought their amazingly simple tactic for staying sober to other alcoholics seeking sobriety, and many more found that simply keeping company with one another could blunt the intensity of their addiction (*Pass It On*, 1984).

Additional evidence that the tribe is the primary tool of recovery for drug addicts lies in the fact that many fellowship members never follow the suggested program of "getting a sponsor" or "working the Steps," and virtually none do until they have been clean for several weeks or longer. Yet they are able to stay clean, at least initially, simply by attending meetings. In the early years of AA, before the recovery experiences of successful members were translated into the Twelve Steps, literally all members who found recovery did so by simply attending meetings. Many members of the fellowships don't seem to understand this power; they talk about "the feeling of love in the room" and attribute it to "the miracle of the program," never realizing that they are rediscovering the form of social organization that comes most naturally to human beings (fellowship members, personal communications, February 1992 to May 1995).

In the company of other addicts seeking recovery, members have the opportunity to lose their sense of isolation by listening to others who have experienced the same depths of pain, confusion, insanity, shame, and guilt. As members take turns speaking and listening to each other in meetings, they learn from each other's mistakes and can exchange affirmations that they are only sick people, not evil people. Because the only requirement for membership is a desire to stop using drugs, the fellowships represent an atmosphere of relatively unconditional acceptance; race and class boundaries typically evaporate, and it is not unusual for professionals and homeless people to sit side by side (Wuthnow, 1994, pp. 163-188).

The recovery meetings represent a near ideal-environment for addicts to effectively assume personal control of their lives and actions. This affirmative and supportive environment can provide gentle and loving feedback on behaviors and habits, in a way that is particularly easy for addicts to accept. Coping with emotional pain and overcoming fear of change become shared experiences. There are many role models of successful recovery from which to choose in learning how to break the vicious circle of habitually numbing life's discomforts. Appreciation for the instructive pain of aware living is cultivated, and the relatively normal tribulations and tragedies of life contribute to the development of personal character and philosophy, just as they do with "normal" people. Addicts learn to appreciate the essential role of emotional pain as one of life's many teachers.

This type of environmental feedback and assistance in rehabilitation is not only essential for addicts to recover successfully, it also represents the antithesis of dehumanized, impersonal, indulgent consumer society. Given enough exposure to this contemporary equivalent of a tribe,[7] the "unbearable" quality of the addict's life fades away, undermining the fundamental impulse to use drugs. Without even realizing it, the recovery fellowships have partially reinvented the native social ecology of human society. The remarkable degree of success that they have experienced, in an area in which virtually all other social innovations have fallen short, is but one example of the enormous contemporary potential of this original social order.

PROBLEMS WITH THE FELLOWSHIP MODEL

Of course, there are problems and shortcomings with the recovery fellowships. In some ways, they are downright controversial; this section can provide only a brief overview, but there is an abundance of material on the subject by both fellowship advocates and opponents.[8]

Perhaps the most widely held misconception is that the Twelve-Step recovery programs are religious in nature. Indeed, AA was initially influenced by the Oxford Group, a first-century Christian organization (*Pass it On,* 1984). However, AA's founders wanted AA to appeal to addicts of any metaphysical or religious affiliation, and they specifically articulated their intent to reach atheists and agnostics within the context of their existing beliefs (*Pass It On,* 1984).

One very early member of AA, an atheist, indicates that the fellowship was initially quite nonreligious. He recounted how the AA fellowship took on religious overtones only when it grew significantly in membership, indicating that new members "brought religion with them when they came in" (Harold L., personal communication, September 5, 1993). The NA literature echoes this sentiment by referring to the program as "spiritual, not religious" (Narcotics Anonymous, 1988). Although many members, perhaps even a majority of the fellowship, may be religious, the program itself is clearly not intended to be. Also, the literature of both NA and AA repeatedly refer to use of the fellowship itself as a "higher power," illustrating that many members differ from the mainstream in their definition of *God,* in that they are not referring to a Supreme Being (Narcotics Anonymous, 1988; see also *Twelve Steps,* 1981).

Another frequently voiced criticism of recovery fellowships is that they exhibit cultish behavior.[9] These tendencies, however, involve a small minority of cases in a generally unstructured, decentralized social organization of millions of people. Early members of AA were actually quite foresighted in their handling of these problems, addressing these cultish tendencies wisely by implementing the Twelve Traditions early on in the development of the fellowships. These principles outline a decentralist, nonauthoritarian model for the fellowship and establish a democratic service structure and complete autonomy for each group (*Twelve Steps*, 1981; see also *It Works*, 1993). Given this structure, cultish behavior on the part of any group tends to remain confined within that group, and it is unlikely to spread throughout the entire program. For this reason, one writer and ex-AA member expressed great admiration for the spirit and practice of the Twelve Traditions in a work that was otherwise harshly critical of AA (Bufe, 1991).

The autonomy of each group gives rise to many and varied subcultures within the fellowships; in a large urban area, one may find at least a few groups that can appeal to practically anyone, professional, blue-collar, gay/lesbian, teenager, punk rocker, hippie, atheist, agnostic, or what-have-you. In fact, the recovery fellowships are compelling examples of how large-scale, functioning anarchy is actually possible and can even prove to be a more effective method of social organization than hierarchical organizations (Bufe, 1991; Wuthnow, 1994). At the very least, their structure provides a means by which nonreligious addicts may comfortably find recovery, ensures the availability of options to any cultish tendencies groups may develop, and constitutes an enduring tool for addressing the many other challenges of addiction.

AN EMERGING "TREATMENT" FOR DISINTEGRATED SOCIETY

Natural selection suggests that, eventually, humans will adapt (or not) to being uprooted and dispersed, but by what means? And in the meantime, what social mechanisms facilitate this adaptation and help people to overcome the disorientation and emotional strife of endless transition?

As previously described, there are many analogies to be found by comparing the addict's relationship to life with humanity's relationship to modern society. Likewise, the widespread, successful use of a tribal social model as a successful treatment for addiction (even if it is unintentional re-creation) also suggests an effective method by which entire populations may more effectively and less painfully adapt to rapidly changing social, environmental, and economic conditions. In fact, there is already an apparent trend toward neotribalism that may be observed in a wide variety of social and economic contexts.

There is a burgeoning "small groups" phenomenon in the United States.[10] An astounding four out of ten Americans regularly attend at least one small group's meetings. There are approximately a half million groups described as "self-help," with an estimated 8 to 10 million members. Many other types of groups exist. Groups are formed around a wide variety of needs and topics, including political and current events discussion groups, book discussion groups, sports/hobby groups, Bible study and Sunday school groups, anonymous recovery/Twelve-Step groups, therapy groups, and groups focusing on issues specific to women, men, young people, singles, and couples. Small-group membership is relatively evenly distributed across classifications of age, gender, education, income, geographic region, and population density.

The small-group movement helps people adapt to a rapidly changing world by providing a supportive community. When members are asked what types of needs they are seeking to meet through small groups, primary responses are to share deep feelings, to find others with like values, to discuss beliefs and values, to secure help in time of need, to grow spiritually, and to gain relief from loneliness and/or depression (Wuthnow, 1994, p. 53). About 80 percent felt that groups helped them to apply ideas to their lives; 78 percent found significant value in hearing others tell stories about "what worked and what didn't" (p. 259).

Also significant to the argument that small groups help people make broader social changes is that 62 percent of members surveyed worked with their group to help others outside the group. Furthermore, 56 percent reported becoming more interested in social justice, and 45 percent became more interested in social and political issues (Wuthnow, 1994, p. 320). Clearly, these groups support people in becoming more interested and active citizens and encourage them to face society's problems.

In contrast to cultish tendencies, dogmatic morality and institutional loyalty are uncommon in small groups; a majority of members indicated that spiritual beliefs were private and personal, that their own beliefs were not dependent on involvement in any organization, and that "it doesn't matter what you believe, so long as you are a good person." About 51 percent of members surveyed described their group's degree of respect for different points of view as "good," and 38 percent described it as "excellent" (Wuthnow, 1994).

Although some groups are oriented toward casual interests or leisure activities, these appear to be in the minority. Indeed, the historical vanguard of this movement is the Twelve-Step recovery fellowship, which has had great success tackling the problem of addiction where other approaches have failed. Addiction has not only cost untold thousands of lives but has also wreaked inestimable havoc on families, employers, and society at large. Given the successes of recovery fellowships, there are clearly some essential social functions that small groups can perform much more effectively than large institutions and specialized professionals.

The importance of participatory democracy-in-practice in the small-group setting cannot be underestimated. Debating eloquently, learning to listen, creatively exploring issues and ethical dilemmas, tolerating and valuing dissenting views, all with a mix of diverse personalities—this is Democracy 101; the analytical and communication skills learned here significantly enhance the ability to comprehend, and the willingness to confront, society's larger challenges.

CONCLUSION

The condition of an individual addict is comparable to that of modern industrial society; likewise, the addict's recovery in the neotribal environment of a recovery fellowship can be correlated to how our troubled society may gain useful insight from these remarkable programs. Our civilization's most compelling issue, the burgeoning environmental crisis, is inextricably linked to both the cause and the cure of humanity's difficulties; the nature of our relationship with our planet is at the very heart of our destructive behaviors, not only as individuals, but as entire cultures as well.

By reinventing humanity's original tribal social model in myriad forms and applications, we are helping each other to adapt to our society's rapid changes, and, perhaps, to slow them down. We are rebuilding the fundamental infrastructure of community that is the core of every culture's true strength. By encouraging the formation of autonomous groups networking in a decentralized fashion, we help to secure a safer, more stable social environment for ourselves and for future generations.

NOTES

1. Although accurate surveys are notoriously difficult, the general consensus is that the increasing sophistication of trafficking organizations, supply lines, and the

culture of drug use itself is making more drugs and more kinds of drugs available. For a historical overview of the social cycles of drug use, see Musto, 1987.

2. The testimonials of recovering addicts are a highly valued part of the literature of the recovery fellowships and provide compelling evidence of the personal challenges facing even addicts with substantial "clean time." In particular, see Narcotics Anonymous, 1988. A medical overview of these problems and how they can impair treatment is found in Milam and Ketcham, 1983.

3. An excellent presentation of industrialization's effects on humanity and society is provided in Merchant, 1990. A sociological perspective that firmly links the deterioration of organic human society with the onset of industrialism is found in Lenski and Lenski, 1987.

4. The recovery membership figures included are really "guesstimates." Both Service Offices cite many unregistered groups. A random sampling by the author of two Narcotics Anonymous Service Committees revealed that over 80 percent of active groups were unregistered, and fewer than 10 percent of registered groups were defunct.

5. Author's estimate, based on the ratio of groups to members in AA.

6. AA included in their original text the testimonials of prominent doctors and psychiatrists lauding the efficacy of the program; see *Alcoholics Anonymous*, 1992.

7. It is not the intent of this examination to trivialize the role of the Twelve Steps and the Twelve Traditions in the lives of recovering addicts; in fact, it is these twenty-four principles that articulate the actual organizational structure and underlying principles of recovery. But it is also apparent that the most vital element in addiction recovery is the social framework of decentralized, autonomous, nonauthoritarian tribes. This is the primary reason for the phenomenal success and growth of the recovery fellowships.

8. See, for example Bufe, 1991. For an AA view on how they successfully cope with these problems, see *Twelve Steps*, 1981. For a work that emphasizes AA's strengths while straightforwardly detailing its drawbacks, see Milam and Ketcham, 1983.

9. In fact, a small, cultlike subset of AA has arisen known as "structured AA" or "Orthodox AA," practicing dress codes, gender separation, and other hierarchical forms of social organization (Marcus E., personal interview, February 4, 1994).

10. See Wuthnow, 1994. Because of the decentralized and relatively informal nature of small groups, demographic evaluations are notoriously difficult to conduct; however, Wuthnow's work was carefully executed and is probably the most extensive research conducted on this topic to date.

REFERENCES

Alcoholics Anonymous. (1992). New York: AA World Services.

Bufe, C. (1991). *Alcoholics Anonymous: Cult or cure?* San Francisco: Sharp Press.

Chomsky, N., & Peck, J. (Eds.). (1987). *The Chomsky reader.* New York: Pantheon.

Gore, A. (1993). *Earth in the balance: Ecology and the human spirit.* New York: Plume.

It works: How and why (1993). Van Nuys, CA: World Service Office.

Lenski, G., & Lenski, J. (1987). *Human societies: An introduction to macrosociology.* New York: McGraw-Hill.

Merchant, C. (1990). *The death of nature: Women, ecology, and the scientific revolution* (2nd ed.). San Francisco: Harper & Row.

Milam, J., & Ketcham, K. (1983). *Under the influence: A guide to the myths and realities of alcoholism.* Seattle: Bantam.
Musto, D. (1987). *The American disease.* New York: Oxford University Press.
Narcotics Anonymous. (1988). Van Nuys, CA: World Services Office.
Pass it on (1984). New York: AA World Services.
The triangle of self-obsession (1993). Van Nuys, CA: World Service Office.
Twelve Steps and Twelve Traditions (1981). New York: AA World Services.
Wuthnow, R. (1994). *Sharing the journey.* Ontario: Free Press.

23 Learning to See New Landscapes

The Canadian Outward Bound Wilderness School

PHILIP BLACKFORD
STEPHEN COUCHMAN

The real voyage of discovery lies not in seeing new landscapes but in having new eyes.

—Marcel Proust

Originally, the expression *outward bound* referred to a time when sailors headed for open sea, leaving behind the safety of a familiar harbor. Today, at more than thirty Outward Bound schools around the world, it means leaving the comfort and security of family and friends to undertake a challenging voyage of experience, adventure, and self-discovery.

Outward Bound is a nonprofit educational organization, formulated around an interpretation of the educational philosophy of German educator Dr. Kurt Hahn (1886-1974). Hahn's educational philosophy was founded on the utopian vision described in Plato's *Republic.* He was impressed by Plato's notion of nurturing the development of traditional

Athenian civic virtues in a "healthy pasture" removed from the corrupting influences of modern society (James, 1980).

Hahn's first school was established in 1920. Germany had been ruined by the First World War. The social climate was one of dissolution and despair. Salem School was intended as a force for social and political regeneration. Its purpose was "to train citizens who could, if called upon, make independent decisions, put right action before expediency and the common cause before personal ambition" (Hahn, quoted in James, 1980, p. 19). Hahn's goal was to ensure "the survival of an enterprising curiosity, an undefeatable spirit, tenacity in pursuit, readiness for sensible self-denial and, above all, compassion."

Hahn later went on to establish a number of other innovative and influential organizations, including Gordonstoun School in 1934 and the Federation of World Colleges in 1962. But Outward Bound is his best-known and most enduring legacy.

The first Outward Bound school was founded in 1941 in the tiny Welsh seacoast town of Aberdovy. In the early days of the Second World War, many young recruits to the British merchant marines were succumbing to the hardships they faced when forced into lifeboats in the North Atlantic. Often, their senior colleagues were surviving the ordeal. It was felt that although the younger men might be more physically fit, their older compatriots had at least two advantages. First, they had been through difficult times before and were more psychologically prepared; they knew how to access personal reserves of tenacity and perseverance. Second, they knew the advantages of teamwork and were aware, from experience, that their chances of survival increased dramatically when they worked together.

The initial Outward Bound program was very specific in its purpose. It was a response to an immediate and critical set of circumstances. Even so, Hahn was clear that the Outward Bound training should focus not so much on technical skills as on developing those personal skills of self-reliance, tenacity, and teamwork. Laurence Holt, Hahn's partner in the venture, articulated their shared vision: "The training at Aberdovy must be less a training *for* the sea than *through* the sea, and so benefit all walks of life" (Holt, quoted in Miner & Boldt, 1981, p. 33).

Outward Bound has changed tremendously since those first British sailors arrived in Aberdovy more than a half century ago. The more than thirty Outward Bound schools now scattered around the world have all developed their own unique character. Several years ago, a Canadian journalist exploring the origins of Outward Bound remarked,

> There is no blueprint, no set of instructions on how to run an Outward Bound school. I tried to puzzle this out in the schools I visited and came up with a comparison to Common Law. Guided by precedent, successive waves of practitioners have absorbed the basic thinking and adapted it to the special circumstances of each new school. (Wilson, 1985, p. 5)

The Canadian Outward Bound Wilderness School (COBWS, or COBWEBS, as it is affectionately known) is by no means the largest or most affluent Outward Bound school in the world. It is, however, unique. The school's main summer site is the most remote Outward Bound base in the world. An hour and a half north of the Trans Canada highway near Thunder Bay, Ontario, Homeplace is separated from Hudson's Bay by a single railway line, a few logging roads, five or six small Aboriginal communities, and several thousand square kilometers of forest, lakes, and rivers. During the day, you can watch rain squalls sweep across the lake. At night, with no significant sources of artificial light for more than a hundred kilometers in any direction, you can paddle out from shore and watch the stars, meteors, and northern lights reflected in the silent black water.

COBWS has also acquired a reputation within Outward Bound as having a particularly strong orientation to community. Although promoting the skills of working and living together is an important component of all Outward Bound programs, COBWS seems to have singled out this aspect of Hahn's philosophy for special attention. It may have something to do with the school's remoteness. Staff living and working at the school must rely on each other for social as well as professional interaction. And, most certainly, the first staff of the school set a tone early on of community and consensus. This emphasis on community underlies a significant characteristic of the school, which is that COBWS is quite possibly the most diverse Outward Bound school in the world.

In essence, this diversity stems from the belief that no matter who you are—how young or old, rich or poor; whatever the color of your skin or the level of your physical abilities—you have something to gain from participation in an Outward Bound program. As is the case at all Outward Bound schools, COBWS strives to involve a wide cross section of participants. Subsequently, the school recognizes the special needs of individuals. To provide for these needs, the school has developed three program areas.

The largest and most well-known of these are the open enrollment programs. As the name suggests, these programs are available for any individual who wishes to experience Outward Bound. Through the Center for Change, COBWS also provides a wide variety of programs for corporations and organizations. These groups, who are most often experiencing a transition or dealing with difficult issues, or who may simply wish to explore the further potential of their business, find that the communications, group dynamics, and team-building approach of the school can have a significant positive impact on the culture of their organization.

Finally, the school is extremely proud of its Community and Health Services Programs. These programs, which now account for more than a quarter of the school's work, are intended to make the Outward Bound experience available and accessible to a wide range of people who might not normally consider a learning experience of this sort. As part of this program area, COBWS runs courses for troubled youth, women who have experienced violence, older adults, aboriginal participants, and people with differing physical abilities.

It is important to point out that it is not the school's intention to segregate these individuals from the regular stream of courses. Many individuals who might fall into one of these groups choose each year to participate in standard courses. However, the school found that by offering special programs, it could sometimes entice participants to join who would not normally "take the leap." At the same time, it was felt that richer experiences might be provided for some by creating an environment of heightened emotional safety or by framing a course within a particular context, be it developmental, cultural, or simply shared experience.

> Often during the day I find myself thinking about the great feelings of camaraderie with the other women, and I glow all over again as I remember the wonderful feats I accomplished up there. Each day I remember something positive about my Outward Bound experience, whether it be words of praise or a simple smile of a good friend. (*"Women of Courage" participant)*

Although the school provides a variety of programs, instructors never stray far from a methodology that has developed along with the school. The focus of this learning process, which consists of experience and adventure within a holistic context, creates a landscape for change. Regardless of the motivation of individual participants, the process through which they explore themselves and their relationship to the world is remarkably similar.

CREATING A LANDSCAPE FOR CHANGE

"The greatest challenge you'll face at Outward Bound was the one you overcame in arriving here today." These are often the first words a student hears on arriving at COBWS. Tired after a long journey to an unfamiliar place, bitten by mosquitoes and blackflies, and asked to pack all their worldly possessions into a small sack, many participants would likely climb right back into the van for a trip home if it were not for a deep-seated spirit of adventure and a desire to explore unknown places within themselves and the world around them.

Often, people choose to take an Outward Bound course at an important transition point in their lives, such as finishing school, ending a relationship, or changing jobs. Regardless of the circumstances, more than anything else, the greatest tool for growth is an individual's eagerness to create such an opportunity. Once an individual identifies the will to change within herself or himself, the greatest challenge has been overcome.

The Outward Bound process assumes that learning takes place when people engage in and reflect on experiences in challenging environments. Participants are presented with a series of increasingly difficult physical and mental problems, none designed to be beyond their capacity. By confronting difficult tasks, they must call on forgotten or hitherto unrecognized reserves of ingenuity, strength, perseverance, and compassion. By rising to meet these unavoidable challenges, students learn the necessity and the rewards of working well with others. Through direct experience, Outward Bound students are presented with irrefutable evidence that they can succeed far beyond preconceived expectations.

EXPERIENCE

The foundation for learning at Outward Bound is experience. There are no textbooks at the school, nor are there any chalkboards (which is probably for the best because there are no walls). Lessons in geography are learned while participants find their way through the woods, and classes in physics are taught over the din of foaming white water. Rather than being passive receptacles of information, participants are encouraged to learn for themselves the skills they will need to accomplish the many challenges placed before them during the course of the program.

Some of these skills, such as how to paddle a canoe in a straight line, pack a wannigan, use a map and compass, and cook lump-free oatmeal, represent technical knowledge. Mastery of these skills is necessary for the group to be able to travel safely and comfortably through the wilderness. At the same time, less tangible but ultimately more important goals such as trust, teamwork, communication, and consensus building, are addressed.

The foundation for this model of education is expressed in the work of the educational theorist David Kolb:

> Experiential learning occurs through a four-stage cycle; immediate concrete experience is the basis for observation and reflection. These observations are assimilated into a "theory" from which new implications for action can be deduced. These implications or hypotheses then serve as guides, interacting to create new experience. (Chickering, 1977)

Through the course of an Outward Bound program, participants are presented with a series of problem-solving experiences. After each experience, time is given for reflection and group discussion. During these sessions, participants have an opportunity to discuss personal perspectives on the activity and to critique the working relationship of the group in preparation for increasingly difficult tasks to come. In this way, the focus is not on the successful completion of individual tasks, but on the ability of the group to learn to work together effectively. Each of us has strengths in one or more of the stages of the learning cycle Kolb describes. Some of us are better thinkers; others are better doers. Some of us feel most comfortable in learning environments that allow us to watch and reflect; others prefer to tinker with a problem. In a sense, the four stages of the experiential learning cycle also represent four somewhat distinct learning styles. One of the beauties of Kolb's model in a community setting is that it allows for all participants to play a role in the learning process. Most formal educational environments favor a cognitive approach to learning. In experiential learning, the ability to think abstractly is valued equally with an orientation to experiencing things firsthand, the ability to observe and reflect, and a willingness to test out new assumptions through experimentation.

It is important to realize that learning by experience is a much more fundamental, and for most, accessible learning strategy than the more conceptual approach favored throughout much of the world. In fact, an experiential approach to learning was, until relatively recently, the more common mode of learning.

Think of the time in life when learning is most intense: infancy and early childhood. How do young children accomplish the Herculean tasks of learning to walk, learning a language, learning the principles of cause and effect? They do it through experience. As adults, there is no reason why this mode of learning cannot and should not remain useful.

Historically, until well into the eighteenth century and certainly prior to Gutenberg's printing press, most of the world's people were information poor but experience rich. People learned what they needed to know through trial and error and by listening to elders, whose life experience was of great value. As society changed, the need to educate people for different tasks through book learning increased. The process has continued to this day. We now live in a society that is information rich but experience poor.

Through presenting challenges in a variety of ways, Outward Bound encourages participants to develop a balanced approach to learning and to recapture the value of experience in understanding the world. At the same time, participants are able to rely on the strengths of other group members.

These various experiences can provide for powerful learning. However, the *metaphors* of experience elicit even deeper, more lasting lessons. The assumption is that, under stress, individuals behave in roughly the same way, whether they are at Outward Bound or at home. A corporate group that fails to complete an initiative because everyone is talking at once provides insight into an unsuccessful business deal. The young student who found being stuck on a ledge fifty feet off the ground to be the best time to express how peer pressure had so often led him into "impossible" situations is also experiencing the power of metaphor.

Although there are no guarantees that such events will ensure change, highly charged experiences like rock climbing or carrying a canoe across a long swampy portage are not easily forgotten. The memories and the meaning individuals invest in them remain crystal clear for years to come. It has been suggested that metaphors like these can carry "a depth and complexity of meaning as therapeutically potent as any insight gained from the more conventional psychotherapeutic approaches practiced by mental health professionals" (Couchman, 1995).

ADVENTURE

I found the whole experience to be terrific. I began to realize that I had been setting the unnecessary limits on my own capabilities. My attitude changed. I'll never put off accepting a challenge again, because I did things on my course that I never dreamed I could do.

When was the last time you had an adventure? When was the last time you did something out of the ordinary, risked uncertain outcomes, or accepted unforeseen or unknown challenges? For many people, the spirit of adventure is something left to the very young, the foolhardy, and *National Geographic* photographers. It is an approach to life abandoned sometime between the ages when you stopped climbing trees and started using credit cards.

For many, the idea of adventure has a macho stigma. Too many Hollywood movies have portrayed the rough and tough adventurer, out to win against the wilderness. In this light, an adventure is a test of physical endurance, extreme discomfort, and sheer pigheadedness. However, when speaking to those who have climbed the highest mountains, paddled the longest rivers, sailed oceans, and crossed Arctic waters, what becomes clear is that to be an adventurer is to find peace of mind. Rather than displaying great machismo, adventure requires and promotes more philosophical strengths such as self-actualization (Hirsch, 1992). Boldness and self-confidence are crucial components to achieving great feats, but they are always tempered by a sense of humility that comes from experiencing the power of nature. In the context of Outward Bound, it is adventure that most helps participants overcome old notions of what is and is not possible. In turn, this leads to extraordinary feelings of empowerment and an increased sense of one's own capacities.

The metaphor of a camera serves us well in illustrating the role of adventure at Outward Bound. As children, we begin seeing the world through an almost limitless, wide angle lens. Over time, however, most of us begin adjusting the focus. Partly out of necessity (there is just too much going on today for most of us to be able to handle life at full throttle) and partly due to the pain and frustration that often accompany maturation, we begin to narrow our attention, interest, and expectations. Although this may not be all bad, it can mislead us into believing that many of our limitations are, in fact, externally imposed. Through adventure, we allow ourselves to be open to possibilities that are outside the scope of our day-to-day lives.

Tom Price (n.d.) affirms this belief that the most valuable element in the spirit of adventure is the childlike quality of wonder:

> The traveler who, gazing upon the new vista, is not struck by a feeling of wonder and wild surmise will soon settle down and cease his adventuring. Darwin's voyage in the Beagle stimulated him to such a sense of wonder that its impetus carried him through thirty years of dedicated toil, a

> life-long adventure of the mind. It is a childlike quality, but it can be possessed alike by Einstein or by Wordsworth's "Idiot Boy" for it is not a question of intelligence. It is a kind of extreme mental health. The total absence of it, I suppose, is acute depression. One of the great tasks of education is to sustain this childlike sense of wonder into adulthood, and if possible throughout life. (p. 90)

Adventure can sometimes carry with it a flavor of recklessness and egoism. At Outward Bound, however, the role adventure plays in the learning process is, instead, tied closely to Kurt Hahn's understanding of the central argument of Plato's *Republic;* namely, that human perfection cannot be realized outside of a perfect society. Hahn believed that the purpose of adventure in personal development was to unlock individual capacities, which could then be used to help create a just and harmonious society.

> The individual student comes to grips with what must be done to create a just society, within which a human being might aspire to perfection. Here is the true, unadvertised peak climb of an Outward Bound course. An inner transformation precedes outward conquest. This is why Hahn placed compassion above all other values of Outward Bound, for it among all emotions is capable of reconciling individual strength with collective need. (James, 1980, p. 19)

LANDSCAPE

The physical space that COBWS occupies is a vital component to the programs provided. Aesthetic beauty and a sense of space and place, along with the powerful lessons taught by wind, rain, lightning, and beaver swamp, are an important part of the school's approach to learning. Matched with this appreciation for the physical world, COBWS attempts to create programs that provide a safe environment for participants to explore their lives.

Most people are familiar with the term *landscape* as it refers to physical settings or their representations. Social commentators, such as Zukin (1991), have expanded the term to include both physical surroundings and an ensemble of material and social practices. In this sense, a theme park such as Disney World is both a physical landscape and a social construction loaded with meaning.

The landscape of our daily lives is a testament to ever increasing alienation. On a physical level, the horizon, consistently obstructed by overpowering buildings, limits our sense of space and place. On a cognitive level, surviving in today's world is largely an exercise in filtering a constant flow of information: television, work, meetings, military coups, the national debt, ozone depletion. In contrast, the "real reality" of a wilderness experience allows individuals to reconnect with vital, sensual information that, according to Bill McKibben (1992, pp. 233-249), is vital to the knowledge of ourselves as human beings. Simply the act of being in a natural environment—of seeing from horizon to horizon without obstruction—places one in a different relation to the world. At the same time, knowing that all you need to survive and live comfortably for three weeks is located in the canoe you are sitting in is extremely reassuring. It is freeing to be rid, even for a brief time, of all the baggage we have accumulated in our lives. Among other things, it allows us the freedom to explore those things that are truly important to us.

> Imagine you are 60 km back in the wilderness. A summer storm strikes. You've had the good sense to set up a secure camp beforehand. At that moment, a hot meal in a bowl and a cup of tea overwhelm thoughts of designer clothes, the latest CD equipment, the reupholstering of the sofa in a more contemporary color pattern. It amazes me how simple it is to live life comfortably. (Couchman, 1995)

The physical landscape of wilderness has a powerful impact on participants on an Outward Bound program. At the same time, the program attempts to engage individuals on all levels—physical, intellectual, emotional, and spiritual. The program is designed to provide for the entire landscape of individual learning. In understanding this landscape, it is important to recognize that the components of personal development are not separated but are simultaneously integrated into every aspect of the program.

The transference of experience back into everyday life is the final crucial step in the learning process. Outward Bound provides its participants with a significant learning experience based on a landscape of adventure and experience in a powerful natural setting. However, ultimately it is up to individuals to use that learning back in the world with which they are most familiar.

For the more than fifteen thousand COBWS participants who have left the security of family and friends to undertake a challenging voyage of experience, adventure, and self-discovery, the effectiveness of experiential learning is quite real. The memories of breakfast in the early morning mist, aching muscles after a long day's paddle, and the peacefulness of solo time are forever etched in their memories. They are reservoirs to be drawn on for strength through life's many experiences. At Outward Bound, the experience of significant personal achievement leads to feelings of empowerment and mastery. To accomplish what a day earlier was thought to be impossible is to see the world anew. It is to begin with the courage to risk and the confidence to try again.

> Be tough yet gentle
> Humble yet bold
> Swayed always by beauty and truth.
>
> Bob Pieh (1916-1993), founder
> of the Voyageur and Canadian
> Outward Bound Wilderness Schools[1]

NOTE

1. This quotation has long been attributed to Pieh, who died on September 18, 1993. His daughter, Wendy, herself a moving force in Outward Bound, said she believed he had written the short poem.

REFERENCES

Chickering, A. W. (1977). Kolb's experiential learning theory. In *Experience and learning*. Change Magazine Press.

Couchman, R. (1995). *Some reflections on the role of Outward Bound in promoting change.* Unpublished manuscript.

Hirsch, J. (1992, December). The ecology of an adventure. *Recreation Canada*, pp. 14-15, 32.

James, T. (1980, Spring). Sketch of a moving spirit: Kurt Hahn. *Journal of Experiential Education*, 17-22.

McKibben, W. (1992). *The age of missing information.* New York: Random House.

Miner, J., & Boldt, J. (1981). *Outward Bound U.S.A.* New York: William Morrow.

Price, T. (n.d.). Adventure by numbers. *Colorado Outward Bound School Staff Manual.*

Wilson, R. (1985, Fall). Kurt Hahn and the legend of Outward Bound. *Mountain News*, *3*(4), 5.

Zukin, S. (1991). *Landscapes for power: From Detroit to Disney World.* Berkeley: University of California Press.

24 Humor and Healing

Or, Why We're Building a Silly Hospital

HUNTER "PATCH" ADAMS

The arrival of a good clown exercises more beneficial influence upon the health of a town than of twenty asses laden with drugs.

—Dr. Thomas Sydenham,
seventeenth-century physician

Humor is an antidote to all ills. I believe that fun is as important as love. The bottom line, when you ask people what they like about life, is the fun they have, whether it's racing cars, dancing, gardening, golfing, or writing books. Philosophically speaking, I'm surprised that anyone is ever serious. Life is such a miracle, and it's so good to be alive that I wonder why anyone ever wastes a minute.

Anyone who has picked up a copy of *Reader's Digest* in the last forty years knows that "laughter is the best medicine." In spite of the empirical nature of this truth, the mainstream medical literature hasn't refuted it, as far as I know. The late Norman Cousins (1979) wrote eloquently about having laughed himself back to health after suffering from a serious chronic disease. The experience had such an impact on him that he changed careers late in life to help bring this information to the health care profession. Jokes seemed so important to Sigmund Freud (1960) that he wrote a book on the subject. But we don't need professionals to tell us about the magnetism of laughter. With great insight, we call a funny person "the life of the party."

Humor has been strongly promoted as health-giving throughout medical history, from Hippocrates to Sir William Osler. As science became dominant in medicine, subjective therapies like love, faith, and humor took a backseat because of the difficult task of objectively investigating their value. I am astounded that anyone feels the need to prove something so obvious. When individuals and groups are asked what is most important for good health, humor invariably heads the list, even over love and faith, which many people feel have failed them. Few people deny that a good sense of humor is essential in a successful marriage. All public speakers recognize that humor is essential in drawing attention to what they are saying.

People crave laughter as if it were an essential amino acid. When the woes of existence beset us, we urgently seek comic relief. The more emotions we invest in a subject, the greater its potential for guffaws. Sex, marriage, prejudice, and politics provide a bottomless well of ideas; yet humor is often denied in the adult world. Almost universally in the business, religious, medical, and academic worlds, humor is denigrated and even condemned, except in speeches and anecdotes. The stress is on seriousness, with the implication that humor is inappropriate. Health education does little to develop the skills of levity. On the contrary, hospitals are notorious for their somber atmosphere. Although hospital staff members may enjoy camaraderie among themselves, with patients their goal seems to be to fight suffering with suffering. What little humor there is occurs only during visiting hours.

Although humor itself is difficult to evaluate, the response to humor—laughter—can be studied quite readily. Research has shown that laughter increases the secretion of the natural chemicals catecholamines and endorphins, that make people feel so peppy and good. It also decreases cortisol secretion and lowers the sedimentation rate, which implies a stimulated immune response. Oxygenation of the blood increases, and residual air in the lungs decreases. Heart rate initially speeds up and blood pressure rises; then the arteries relax, causing heart rate and blood pressure to go down. Skin temperature rises as a result of increased peripheral circulation. Thus, laughter appears to have a positive effect on many cardiovascular and respiratory problems. In addition, laughter has superb muscle relaxant qualities. Muscle physiologists have shown that anxiety and muscle relaxation cannot occur at the same time and that the relaxation response after a hearty laugh can last up to forty-five minutes.

Physiologically, humor forms the foundation of good mental health. Certainly the lack of a good sense of humor indicates underlying problems, such as depression or alienation. Humor is an excellent antidote to stress and an effective social lubricant. Because loving human relationships are so mentally healthy, it behooves one to develop a humorous side.

I have reached the conclusion that humor is vital in healing the problems of individuals, communities, and societies. I have been a street clown for thirty years and a practicing physician for more than twenty, and I have tried to make my own life silly, not as that word is currently used, but in terms of its original meaning. *Silly* originally meant good, happy, blessed, fortunate, kind, and cheerful in many different languages. No other attribute has been more important. Wearing a rubber nose wherever I go has changed my life. Dullness and boredom melt away. Humor has made my life joyous and fun. It can do the same for you. Wearing underwear on the outside of your clothes can turn a tedious trip to the store for a forgotten carton of milk into an amusement park romp. People so unabashedly thank you for entertaining them.

Being funny is a powerful magnet for friendship, life's most important treasure. Nothing attracts or maintains friendship like being a jolly soul. This is as true for my marriage—still fun after twenty years—as for my medical practice or even the chance encounter on an airplane. I know that humor has been at the core of preventing burnout in my life. Finally, as a nonviolent person, I feel that humor has often protected me by deflecting potentially violent situations.

We live in a troubled world. Many aspects of society are unhealthy or even deadly, and large segments of the population live on the edge. If we are to doctor society, we must rely heavily on humor.

A PRESCRIPTION FOR HAPPINESS

The most distressing health problem for many people is the combination of boredom, fear, and loneliness. Our health is damaged most by loneliness and lovelessness; in more than twenty years as a physician,

I have never seen any suffering that begins to touch the horror of loneliness. It has become a private hell that the afflicted do not reveal unless probed deeply. Brief visits to the doctor or superficial conversations will not relieve their suffering. If relationships with our families, friends, and ourselves are not going well, no amount of physical health can compensate.

In our society the gods of money and power have made boredom, loneliness, and fear the context in which many of us live. Our news media—newspapers, TV, and radio—scream the headlines of pain each day. The news is slanted to cover the ugly, the tormented, the tragic. The camera dissects each traffic accident with surgical precision but reports happy news only in anecdotal asides. If I were to publish a newspaper, I would print mostly happy stories, relegating unhappy ones to the back pages, so that anyone who wanted to "make news" would have to do something funny. Imagine a newspaper that would ecstatically tell of a walk in the woods.

The focus on suffering permeates popular culture. Splashy, commercial television productions promote negative emotions, such as suspicion, envy, and unhappiness. We have become so habituated to pain that many of us believe a happy existence would be undesirable or even boring. This is an interesting paradox. During years of in-depth conversations, I have learned that many people want, even *pine for,* a happier life; yet many do not believe they can *be* happy.

I am interested in happiness because I am a physician. Over the years, I have interviewed thousands of people extensively. Most say happiness is a rare commodity in their lives and can list the few specific times they were happy. People often decline to do things that would make them happy—a physician must completely ignore huge areas of a patient's life because the patient doesn't want to make lifestyle changes. With great sadness, we prescribe treatments that we know will only partly help.

It takes great effort to reject joy and beauty; it is not a passive act. With all the potential for happiness in this world, it is astounding that people are so bored and lonely. I do not intend to trivialize sadness or anxiety but simply to say that we choose these ways of life. People who feel sad tend to blame external events over which they have no control. This is irresponsible. Such individuals become accomplices to the paradigm of pain when they sing out the "script" of victim. Yes, the terrible things that happen *are* painful. Choosing to give up, however, is what makes these experiences continue to wound us.

Viktor Frankl (1962), a survivor of the Nazi concentration camps who knows the importance of freedom of choice, wrote,

> We who lived in concentration camps can remember the men who walked through the huts comforting others, giving away their last piece of bread. They may have been few in number, but they offer sufficient proof that everything can be taken away from a man but one thing: the last of the human freedoms—to choose one's attitude in any given set of circumstances, to choose one's own way.

THE BOTTOM LINE: DOLLARS OR HEALTH?

Our health care system does a terrible job of preventing illness. A large portion of the population is out of shape, overweight, and without assistance in breaking addictions to drugs, alcohol, and cigarettes. A huge segment of the population is bored, lonely, afraid, and in need of help for emotional problems. Sexually transmitted diseases have yet to be brought under control. On the contrary, they are becoming more prevalent—and, in the case of AIDS, more deadly—especially among young people.

One reason we have such a costly health care system is that it offers little if any emphasis on preventive medicine. Relatively little money is spent on preventive medical services, and health insurers give minimal reimbursement for wellness counseling. Hospitals survive and prosper when people are sick; they are not designed to thrive with empty beds when people are healthy.

Overall, there is too little care for the poor and uninsured, and too much care for everyone else. This leads to misuse and waste. Many patients pay such high health insurance premiums that they feel entitled to a $900 high-tech test for their heart, when they have no evidence of heart disease, or a CAT scan for their headaches. A ridiculous proportion of every U.S. dollar spent on health care goes toward administrative and billing costs. These practices use funds that otherwise could provide services for the uninsured.

This malaise is bound to affect health care professionals, both physically and spiritually. America's medical professionals must constantly defend themselves to a public that is unhappy—if not disgusted—with impersonal treatment and an obsession with laboratory values and dollars. Perhaps this is why applications to medical schools have dropped 25 percent during the past five years, and why a recent survey shows that most of the nation's primary care doctors are increasingly sick of their jobs.

The question is no longer whether but *how* change should be brought about. Many of the proposed solutions rely heavily on the federal government to bail the system out. Even if this were desirable, it is not possible. The U.S. government is too debt-ridden to afford it and is likely to remain so. The proposals for financing by corporations, small businesses, risk pools, insurance mechanisms, rationing, payroll taxes, and catastrophic coverage plans, to name only a few, are also unworkable as long as medical services are so grossly overpriced.

The bottom line is to control health care costs and the greed that drives them up. Who is to blame? Doctors are an easy target, but what about health insurance companies? Hospitals? Drug manufacturers? Pharmacists? Politicians who do nothing to help? Lawyers who sue for malpractice? Patients who hire them? The rest of us who tolerate and thereby condone this wretched system?

Health care in the United States is sick and in danger of dying. All of us know it. Prominent medical journals devote numerous articles and editorials to fixing the system or finding alternatives; politicians base their campaign platforms on health care issues. But the discussions of solutions don't get to the roots of the problem; the existing system focuses on sickness, not wellness, and health care costs too much and is available to too few. The poor suffer most of all.

What is needed is a drastic rethinking of the problem. Rather than trying to quick-fix the crumbling health care system, we need to create solutions that will excite both patients and caregivers. We must, in a mutual, multidisciplinary effort, tear down what hurts us and go on to heal a profession of healers. We must take medicine out of the business sector and recognize that greed and selfishness have placed society—and its health care system—in great peril. Our citizens need to feel a sense of belonging and of community. By attending to all members of society, improved health care could help unite society.

CREATING THE ULTIMATE FANTASY HOSPITAL

One of the most puzzling aspects of the discussion about "the health care crisis" is a paucity of description by health care professionals of their ultimate fantasy hospital. Has anyone or any study asked doctors and nurses to fully describe their ideal clinic or hospital? Is it discussed in hospital cafeterias? At medical student Saturday seminars? Or at meetings of the American Medical Association? Is it powerlessness that quiets the dreamer's edge? With the vast majority of staff and patients *not* liking hospitals, why don't they change? Why is the current context held onto so tenaciously?

Can people dare to think up a healing context in which the staff craves to work hard and to which patients and family delight in returning, when sick or well?

Context has been the horror of so much of today's medicine. One can still find the one-on-one intimacy so treasured in medicine, or work with an endearing team, but these are special cases. Even as doctors and nurses have these great moments, they still feel choked by the context of their practice. The administrative context (billing, paperwork, regulations, etc.) and the hospital context (serious, solemn, and unfriendly) are not conducive to a thrilling, thriving practice of medicine. The modern medical context, so criticized in both the lay and medical press, must change. Many new experiments in context are needed to explore this very complicated issue.

GESUNDHEIT INSTITUTE: SEND IN THE CLOWNS

Gesundheit Institute is one such experiment. For twenty-four years, Gesundheit has been in the pursuit of its ideal medical/hospital context. The initial stimulus was to create a model that addressed health care delivery as a political act. Gesundheit Institute has never charged money, accepted third-party reimbursement, or carried malpractice insurance. We are committed to creating a medical setting that embodies to the extreme the philosophy that fun and connectedness are as important to health as CAT scans and IVs.

We define *health* as happy, vibrant, maximum well-being. Health care is focused on the patient's relationships to himself or herself and to nutrition, exercise, faith, family, friends, hobbies, nature, wonder, curiosity, service, community, and peace. The primary goals of Gesundheit Institute are to support friendship on the individual level and to build community on a broader social level (for more, see Adams & Mylander, 1993).

Money, debt, and malpractice insurance mock these goals. We believe that our stance on debt and malpractice insurance is therapeutic and necessary if we are to build a healthier society. And for us personally, this position is essential if our practice of medicine is to be joyous. We use love as our most powerful medicine, especially when a patient is dying or dealing with intractable problems and pain. Friendship enhances the delicate use of humor in medical practice. This kind of service cannot be bought or sold. By not charging patients and by having them stay in our home, we are freer to be silly and to build friendships. We also believe that not charging money is very good malpractice insurance. One reason Gesundheit Institute has never appeared in court, I feel sure, is that we don't charge for our services. We certainly have experimented with patients in ways that would make many health care professionals cringe, simply because we draw on all other, alternative healing arts. Yet, no legal action has ever been taken against us since we began to practice back in the early 1970s, when the climate was even more hostile than it is today.

The focus on humor in medicine at Gesundheit Institute has often been declared a major deterrent to our getting funds. Still, I insist that humor and fun (which is humor in action) are equal partners with love as key ingredients for a healthy life. In the twelve years we saw patients during the pilot phase of Gesundheit Institute, we had many opportunities to explore the relationship between humor and medicine. Although we greatly appreciated casual humor, it seemed imperative that we deliberately incorporate it into our day-to-day lives; we found that for an atmosphere of humor to thrive, we had to *live* funny. We learned to first develop an air of trust and love, because spontaneous humor can be offensive, and we wanted it to be taken in the spirit of trying. Cautious people are rarely funny. It soon became clear that silliness was a potent force in keeping the staff together as friends. And as physicians, we began to see the potent medicinal effect of humor on diseases of all kinds.

Humor is all-important for the health of a community, whether a neighborhood, church, club, or circle of friends. It has helped me live communally for more than twenty years. For the first twelve years, we used our home as a free hospital, surrounded by patients who had great mental and physical suffering. The staff stayed without pay or privacy because it was so much fun. We discovered that humor was more than medicine. Humor, maybe even more than love, made our pioneering project work. It empowered us to take the most expensive service in America and give it away for free.

Gesundheit Institute has come a long way since the original thought, back in the early 1970s, that we wanted to love our patients. Throughout our evolution, we have never separated the individual, community, and global levels. We believe that the changes people make toward greater health are also steps toward world harmony. Our collective progress so far with quitting smoking and wearing seat belts is just a warm-up for disarmament. What if there were sustained peace on Earth? What are the side effects of an abundance of fun? Our ambitions are limitless as we explore new ways to embrace health. Our goal is to be a stimulus, a squeaky wheel that attracts attention and expands the health care dialogue.

Many creative people—scientists, engineers, artists—are willing, if asked, to donate goods and services to health care facilities. They would do this, not for high salaries, but for the challenge of working creatively with others in service to society. The Gesundheit Institute demonstrated this on a small scale and will continue to do so. More pilot projects, I am certain, would elicit the service of many great minds and hands, proving that large numbers of people are willing to pursue not fame and fortune, but integrity in the creation of a healthy society.

REFERENCES

Adams, H., & Mylander, M. (1993). *Gesundheit!* Boston: Healing Arts Press.
Cousins, N. (1979). *Anatomy of an illness.* New York: Bantam.
Frankl, V. (1962). *Man's search for meaning.* Boston: Beacon.
Freud, S. (1960). *Jokes and the relation to the unconscious.* London: Routledge & Kegan Paul.

25 Hospice

A Return to Compassionate Care

EDNA McHUTCHION

Health care institutions charged with providing terminal care for the majority of people in Western society recently have come under criticism by the public and by a number of health care professionals (Fraser, 1985; Kubler-Ross, 1969; LeShan, 1977; McHutchion, 1987; Saunders, 1967; van Bommel, personal communication, 1994; Wald, Foster, & Wald, 1980). Adler (1976) described the situation that now exists for dying patients in institutional settings:

> In the twentieth century, home and family have been replaced by nursing home and hospital as the site where most people die. The fear that death will be unnatural and alien is surely accentuated when sickness is accompanied by removal to an unnatural and unfamiliar place where accomplishments, acquisitions, and identity must be left behind. (p. 321)

The philosophy undergirding most health care institutions is said to be based on a belief in the well-being of the whole person, including upholding "quality of life" for the dying. However, the literature and personal experience as a family member and professional caregiver demonstrate a discrepancy between the stated philosophies and day-to-day activities of institutions, particularly in the sphere of terminal care.

The depersonalized clinical routine of the hospital, the institution in which most North Americans die, has been structured to meet professional requirements, rather than the needs expressed by the clients served. This indictment is harsh. However, the clear mission of the acute care hospital is to cure patients by investigating, diagnosing, and treating disease. Too frequently, terminally ill patients for whom there is no cure are perceived as embarrassing and frustrating failures. As a result, no group is more vulnerable or suffers more in this highly technological environment than do dying patients and their families.

As an alternative to institutional care, there is a current move toward having patients die at home. Being actively involved in the care of the dying patient may indeed ease the pain of loss experienced by the family. Care for the dying, however, can be difficult even for experienced professional caregivers who have the support of a multidisciplinary team within a fully equipped hospital. Without an umbrella of care, inexperienced family members, already feeling the stress and pain associated with the loss of someone they love, bear the extra burden of caring for a relative dying at home. The drive toward promoting home as the ideal place to die may in fact be influenced more by economics and the medical profession's reluctance to work with this vulnerable population than by compassionate concern.

Caregivers burn out. Assisted suicide, as practiced in Holland, is gaining momentum as the antidote to experiencing a lengthy, painful dying process. Even the most devoted caregiver may consider this frightening possibility if we as a society have nothing to offer as an alternative.

Roy (1990) reminds us,

> The place of the human species within this planet's biosphere is the first, and often neglected context and reference point. . . . Ethics means taking nothing and no one for granted. (p. 450)

> The time of dying is a time for questions that shake the foundation of one's existence and threaten to expose the emptiness of one's most encompassing dreams. (p. 456)

No wonder we look for the quick fix to suffering. Isolation in a busy tertiary-care setting, or even euthanasia with intent to kill, may be perceived as the only possible alternatives.

The prospect of dying and death is indeed difficult to face. Le Rouchefoucald, a seventeenth-century philosopher, said: "Neither the sun nor death can be looked at with a steady eye." In our society, attitudes toward death swing from denial through ambivalence to a desire to understand and respond to the mystery of death.

The literature on caring for the dying reflects the value-laden, complex nature of death and dying. Aries (1981) noted that in the late twentieth century, death is often perceived to be "an accident, a sign of helplessness or clumsiness that must be put out of mind," or it is circumvented with "rhetoric and beautification" (p. 586). When confronted with the dying patient, however, the caregiver is presented with a dilemma of crisis proportions. The potential is there for lay and professional caregivers to experience the most difficult and/or the best of human experience and emotions. Krishnamurti (1992) writes,

> Death has been one of the problems, probably the greatest problem, in human life. Not love, not fear, not relationships, but this question, this mystery, this sense of ending, has been the concern from ancient times. . . . Dying is something in the future, something of which one is frightened, something that one doesn't want; to be totally avoided. But it is always there.

There is much to be gained by acknowledging the fact that people (we) do indeed die. Denying death does not make the event less likely or, ultimately, less frightening. In fact, by facing the reality of dying and death and seeking to understand the experience, alternative ways of caring may be developed. Hospice care is a viable alternative.

HOSPICE CARE DEFINED

In response to the inadequate and distressing state of terminal care, the alternative concept of care called *hospice* is resurfacing from its ancient origins with renewed vigor.

> Hospice is a program of palliative and supportive services which provides physical, psychological, social, and spiritual care for dying persons and their families. Services are provided by a medically supervised interdisciplinary team of professionals and volunteers. Hospice settings are available in both home and inpatient settings. Home care is provided on a part-time intermittent, regularly scheduled, or around the clock on-call basis. Bereavement services are available to the family. Admission to a hospice is on the basis of patient and family need. (National Hospice Organization, 1981)

Although the National Hospice Organization (NHO) definition addresses some of the key components and strategies of hospice care, it is more congruent with the nature of hospice to describe its origins and development along historical lines. In the next section of this chapter, a description of this old/new way of providing compassionate care evolves. Hospice is presented as a humane, ethical alternative to dehumanized, dispassionate, or frustrated acts of violence toward the weak and vulnerable in our society.

HOSPICE: A HISTORICAL PERSPECTIVE

Stoddard (1978), in her classic book called *The Hospice Movement: A Better Way of Caring for the Dying*, presents a most interesting description of the development of hospital and hospice as two institutions in which terminal care occur. Stoddard describes these two institutions as two divergent branches coming from the same root, the essence of which is captured in the Latin word *hospes*. Hospes means both the host and guest, a process of interaction between human beings.

Stoddard provides an original description of hospice. It is designed "for the ayde and comforte of the poore, skykke, blynde, aged and impotent persones . . . whereyn they may be lodged, cherysshed and refreshed" (from a petition by the citizens of London to Henry VIII, 1538).

The words *hospitality, hospitable, hospice,* and *hospital* are derivations from the root *hospes*. The origin of our health care system was a humane, ethical response to the needs of the vulnerable. However, since the Reformation, the ancient notion of *hospitable care* for the vulnerable has undergone considerable change. In the hospital, the branch that flourished since the Reformation, institutionalized care formerly provided by religious communities came increasingly under government and corporate control. Stoddard (1978) claims that hospital care is so "entangled in bureaucratic procedure demanding so much paperwork of most physicians [and other health care personnel] that time and energy they can give to patients is sorely limited" (p. 53).

As we come to the end of the century, hospitals are under intense scrutiny. Consumers of health care are becoming more demanding of the system. Disenchantment with the established system provides the climate and environment for seeking alternative ways of providing compassionate, holistic care to the sick, poor, aged, and vulnerable among us.

One significant example that was an exception to inadequate hospital care was a hospice founded in Dublin in the late nineteenth century by

Sister Mary Aikenhead. In 1906, another hospice, St. Joseph's Hospice, was established by the English branch of the Dublin Order. St. Joseph's Hospice became a major influence on Cicely Saunders, a pioneer in the field of compassionate care for the dying. Saunders founded St. Christopher's, a hospice opened in 1967 in Sydenham, England. St. Christopher's remains a source of knowledge and skill for hospice practitioners throughout the world.

The work at St. Christopher's Hospice has been the acknowledged basis for much of the recent development of institutional as well as community-based programs designed to care for dying patients and their families. Educated in social work and medicine, Saunders reflects the multifaceted, multidisciplinary foci of hospice care for the terminally ill. A dedicated Christian, she also embodied the total commitment to service and excellence that inspired her mentors and forebears.

Because of the profound and far-reaching influence of St. Christopher's Hospice and its founder, Cicely Saunders, the organizational components of St. Christopher's Hospice are used to provide further information about the hospice concept.

THE ESSENTIALS OF HOSPICE CARE

Like many revolutionary ideas, hospice attracts people of passion and varying backgrounds and beliefs. Although hospice is becoming relatively well-known and practiced throughout the world, there are widely diverging notions of the way that the hospice concept is to be translated into service. As Saunders (1981) notes,

> To many people, a hospice is an institution concerned with the terminally ill, usually cancer patients and their families. That is a simple, neat definition but a limited one. Implicit in the hospice concept is that care should be available to a mixed group of patients with terminal illness or progressive disease when the acute hospital no longer has anything to offer and when the caring responsibility can no longer be met by the family or community. (p. 93)

Because of the differing opinions among professionals and lay people about the structures and processes of hospice care, it is useful to reiterate the elements that have been spelled out by Saunders (1978).

THE ST. CHRISTOPHER'S HOSPICE CONCEPT OF CARE

The Population: Breadth and Depth of Service. An experienced clinical team integrated into the work of the larger medical community is seen as necessary for effective continuity of care. By integrating itself into larger systems, hospice has proven to be influential, for example, in changing some professionals' and lay people's attitudes toward pain management.

Skilled and experienced team nursing is core, and communication within and across disciplines is essential to meet the multivariate needs of patients and families. The interdisciplinary staff meet frequently for discussion. The physician does not relinquish his or her clinical responsibilities, but a member of another discipline may assume leadership for a particular patient and family. In fact the patient/family is considered central, and their decisions, based on "digestible" information, give the team its mandate.

Staff must be prepared for the cost of commitment and the search for meaning that is associated with care of the dying. The rather old-fashioned ideas of altruism and devotion have been outstanding characteristics of past and present hospice caregivers.

The Focus of Care. Understanding control of the symptoms common to terminal illness, especially pain in all its aspects, helps staff to help patients live to their maximum potential. Unexpected remissions and/or the possibility of future active treatments are welcomed by patient and staff alike. Hospice need not connote "death house," although people do indeed die within this system of care. With excellent symptom control and pain management, patients are alert and able to complete "unfinished business" and even to develop new or latent interests. It is notable that physician-assisted suicide does not become an issue for dying patients and families experiencing appropriate hospice care.

Research. Methodical recording and analysis of records are used to monitor clinical practice and, coordinated with relevant research where possible, lead to soundly based practice and teaching. It is the author's belief that research related to hospice follows the service mandate and not the reverse.

Teaching. Teaching in all aspects of terminal care is a hospice mandate—albeit, again, secondary to patient care. Hospice units are a resource, stimulating initial interest, giving experience and tested knowledge to others. Patients' privacy and wishes, however, are central.

Outreach. A home care program, active or consulting and involving all relevant disciplines, is developed according to local circumstance, so that it can be integrated with local services. Partnerships between programs in existence are essential to diminish political struggles in which the patient/family are the inevitable victims.

Evaluation. Hospice care offers help to its patients and families as they seek to understand and exercise appropriate responsibility. Hospice involves them in decisions and supports them in making realistic choices for themselves. The criteria of success are found in what the patient can accomplish in the face of physical deterioration and in how the family lives on. The success of the criteria are evaluated from the patients' and families' perspectives.

Although the foregoing description of hospice care obviously comes through an institutional lens, it is notable that in the early days of hospice development, Saunders saw the relevance of the hospice concept for application far beyond the four walls of the hospital. In speaking of the primary goal of hospice, Saunders (1981) sums up the hospice purpose. She writes,

> [The purpose of hospice is] to provide the efficient, loving care that permits the patient to fulfill his or her remaining time. We try to give, or give back, the sense of community, of belonging, of personal worth that gave meaning to the patient's life—and to our own. The hospice offers hospitality to such a person and to his or her family and friends: if we have done our work well, the lonely journey can be turned into a safe peaceful one. This is equally true of the patient in the bed of a hospital or at home. (p. 93)

To picture the aesthetics and pragmatics of a hospice institutional setting, the following word picture of hospice is presented.

THE IDEAL HOSPICE

The inpatient facility is an aesthetically designed building, linked to other institutions of the health care system by open lines of communication and cooperation. The key concept underlying the design of the building is that the facility is made to meet the comprehensive needs of the terminally ill, not the reverse. The hospice is made pleasing to the senses in every possible way that the architect and gardeners can devise. There are common rooms and open areas where people may come together, and comfortable nooks inside and out where individuals may find privacy if they desire. The windows open out on views that lift the spirit at all seasons of the year. Comfort, beauty, and personal space are words that best describe this hospitable place. The patient's own place is furnished with his or her favorite small personal possessions, as space allows. Comfort and homeyness take precedence over sterile uniformity, and the visitor may be surprised to see colorful afghans covering the beds and perhaps a favorite old recliner chair now outfitted with wheels, conveying its owner to the common room for a midafternoon cup of fresh, hot tea and a bit of gossip with other patients and visitors.

Seasonal flowers from the hospice gardens or greenhouse are on the circular dining room table and in the common rooms. Like so many other special touches, the flowers are arranged by a dedicated and appreciated core of volunteers. Greenery abounds in winter and in summer, pleasing to the eye and a living reminder of the cyclical and yet continuous aspects of all nature. Carefully selected photographs and paintings donated by local artists grace the walls, and there is an ambience of quality and good taste about the place that lifts the spirit. The food is exceptionally good and carefully arranged for individuals who thought that their appetites had disappeared. Favorite dishes are brought in by the family and shared. If indeed the individual is past the need for food, feedings are not forced, but scrupulous attention is paid to providing sips of water or ice chips to alleviate discomfort.

The windows open to catch the breezes and to freshen the air. Cleanliness is a hospice virtue, and constant attention is given to maintaining an atmosphere more redolent of lemon polish and fresh-baked bread than of ether and iodine. Hearing is the last sense to go and may even become particularly acute in the terminally ill; therefore, the building is in a semiresidential area away from the scream of sirens and the buzz of traffic. The hum of a community going about its daily business provides a reassuring sense of inclusion to the terminally ill patients.

Children are allowed, even encouraged, to visit. In fact, day care is provided for staff members' children, and those children may join their parents for lunch in the dining room, bringing a welcome freshness and vitality with them.

At one end of the building, there is a clinic well equipped to handle symptom-relieving procedures such as thoracenteses and paracenteses.

There is also a chapel, a quiet place that invites the patient, family, or caregiver to stop and be refreshed. There is a small room equipped with much-used tapes and musical instruments chosen by a music therapist. Other artistic endeavors are encouraged by an occupational therapist and volunteers from the community who share their talents freely with the patients. There is a conference room equipped with audiovisual aids used for recreational purposes, as well as for seminars and other educational pursuits. Visitors are welcomed from the community and from other centers so that most recent improvements in terminal care can be shared.

People die here. That is expected. But people also live here, some more fully than ever before, and this hospice, rather than being considered a death house by the community, is seen as a place where life is appreciated and even celebrated, a refreshing, reassuring reminder that life may be measured in depth as well as length.

Why then is hospice not more widely accepted as the system of choice for addressing the needs of terminally ill patients? It is helpful to understand elements of resistance before giving in either to accepting the status quo or to being a misunderstood element in the counterculture.

THE INFLUENCE OF MEDICAL SCIENCE

Detrimental to progress is the complacency that comes from the "success" of medical science. At the same time hospice was taking root and spreading quietly but tenaciously, modern medical science did much to influence society's changing attitude toward death. Even with the advent of AIDS, we still believe that we are increasingly in control of life and death. The mortality rate has decreased. More diseases are curable, and for those diseases that have no cure, life can be extended. Medical engineers have devised highly specialized machinery, and pharmacologists and others have developed complex drugs that can be used to prolong lives (or dying) to extraordinary lengths.

Williamson (quoted in Hendin, 1973), a general practitioner, writes about the physician's dilemma and frustration of dealing with death in this technological age:

> I remember when cessation of heartbeat was an observation on which we simply pronounced the patient dead; now this is a medical syndrome known as cardiac arrest, . . . cessation of respiration is a symptom also implying death, which can now be corrected by an ingenious and devilishly efficient machine known as the mechanical respirator. (p. 21)

Kastenbaum (quoted in Hendin) echoes Williamson: "There is simply no place for a human death where the dying person is regarded as a machine coming to a full stop" (p. 88). It is increasingly difficult to know where the machine leaves off and the person begins, to know where life has ended and death occurs.

Because of the escalation of the use of technological means to fight death and to keep people clinically alive, the question arises, what is a timely death? Is there ever an appropriate time to die? Perpetual self-transcendence and prolonged maintenance of youthful strength are attractive notions; however, if these are considered to be life's only goals, mainstream society and medicine appear to be at odds with reality. Before the antidote of physician-assisted suicide becomes the only alternative to this overly mechanized treatment of the dying, hospice must be given the environment to flourish.

CONCLUSION

Hospice is a way of caring for the terminally ill that meets the needs of the patients and families it is commissioned to serve. Hospice philosophy does not deny death but, rather, faces the inevitability of death with an appropriate balance of the best that is known about the art and science of medical care. It allows its patients' families and caregivers a chance to let go, to face the mystery of death with at least a minimum amount of fear and pain, at best in a state of peace and acceptance.

REFERENCES

Adler, C. S. (1976). *We are but a moment's sunlight: Understanding death.* New York: Washington Square Press.

Aries, P. (1981). *The hour of our death.* New York: Knopf.

Fraser, I. (1985). Medicare reimbursement for hospice care: Ethical and policy implications of cost-containment strategies. *Journal of Health Politics, Policy and Law, 10* (Fall), 565-578.

Hendin, D. (1973). *Death as a fact of life.* New York: Warner.

Krishnamurti, J. (1992). *On living and dying.* San Francisco: Harper.

Kubler-Ross, E. (1969). *On death and dying.* New York: Macmillan.

Le Shan, L. (1977). *You can fight for your life.* New York: Jove.

McHutchion, E. (1987). *The family perspective on dying at home.* Unpublished doctoral dissertation.

National Hospice Organization. (1981, November). *Standards of a hospice program of care.* Available from the author.

Roy, D. (1990). Humanity: The measure of an ethics for AIDS. *Journal of Acquired Immune Deficiency Syndrome, 3*, 449-459.
Saunders, C. (1967). *The management of terminal illness.* London: Hospital.
Saunders, C. (1978). *Annual report.* Sydenham, UK: St. Christopher's Hospice.
Saunders, C. (1981, June). The hospice: Its meaning to patients and their physicians. *Hospital Practice*, pp. 93-108.
Stoddard, S. (1978). *The hospice movement: A better way of caring for the dying.* New York: Vintage.
Wald, F., Foster, Z., & Wald, H. J. (1980, March). The hospice movement of health care reform. *Nursing Outlook*, pp. 173-178.

26 Environmental Medicine and Individual Health

WILLIAM J. REA

The study of the effects of the environment on the individual has grown in leaps and bounds over the past thirty years. Environmental medicine's goal is to allow the individual to live in harmony with the environment. This goal has become difficult to achieve due to the ever expanding population, the continuing gross contamination of the environment, the destruction of virgin lands, and the virtual elimination of native populations (who give us glimpses of behaviors tried and developed over centuries that interrelate to their environments).

Through the millennia, human beings have had either to learn how to live in harmony with the environment or perish. Now, with the advent of modern technology, we are able to ignore the environment to a point, but we pay a large price—that of chronic ill health and disease. Over the past thirty years, in our studies at the Environmental Health Center in Dallas (EHC-D), we have found it extremely difficult to find a truly well comparison group of people who have never been sick and medicated or have never taken drugs (for details, see Rea, 1992, 1994, 1996). Most control groups now used in medicine are characterized by "medicated wellness." With such groups as the optimum, most study groups of patients to which they are compared may look similar, thus giving false information. We estimate that the truly well group of people, which, in our opinion, should be used as a benchmark for comparison, includes less than .1 percent of the U.S. population. The goal of environmental medicine specialists is to help their patients attain this level.

This goal would allow individuals to obtain maximum vigor, creativity, and beauty, as well as physical and mental functioning. It is now possible to teach people how to critically evaluate the effects of the environment on themselves, due to creation of less polluted environments and EHC-D studies of more than thirty thousand patients living in them, and in studies by other clinical ecologists of more than a hundred thousand individuals worldwide.

UNDERSTANDING ENVIRONMENTAL FACTORS

The following principles have been learned from the study of individuals in less polluted environments: (a) total environmental pollutant load, (b) total body pollutant load, (c) adaptation, (d) bipolarity of response, (e) biochemical individuality of response, (f) switch phenomenon, and (g) spreading phenomena. Each of these will be discussed separately. If one truly understands these concepts, one can continuously evaluate the surrounding environment as one moves through life, proving cause and effect and thus obtaining optimum function with a disease-free life and nonmedicated wellness.

The *total environmental pollutant load* has more than doubled over the past forty years as our population has increased and mechanization of nature has become nearly complete. The total environmental pollutant load consists of natural pollutants such as marsh (methane) gas (70 percent); odors and emissions from plants, or terpenes (29 percent); volcano ash; sulfur springs; radiation; and other earth products. Man-made pollutants contribute to more than half of the total environmental load. The man-made pollutants are now doubling an individual's environmental load. Our ancestors therefore had much less pollutant load to contend with in maintaining health. Because they ate foods gathered from virgin soil, earlier human beings may have been larger and disease free. These foods were eaten fresh and therefore didn't have the mycotoxins and other contamination or loss of nutrients that occur with preservation.

Man-made pollutants consist of auto exhausts, wastes from refineries and power plants, factory emissions, pesticides, preservatives and additives in foods, and a host of contaminants such as solvents, formaldehydes, fertilizers, oils, gases, phthalates, and other chemicals in water. Studies at EHC-D using a less polluted controlled environment revealed that the individual must be concerned about the total *environmental* pollutant load because if this load is not manipulated carefully in the individual's favor, it could increase the total *body* pollutant load, resulting in organ or system malfunction.

Total body pollutant load is the total of all environmental pollutants that enter the individual through air, food, and water. Total body pollutant load can be divided into three general categories: physical, chemical, and biological substances or conditions. The physical load consists of exposure to heat, cold, light, weather changes, man-made electrical radiation (such as noise, power lines, computers, televisions, etc.), radon radiating from the earth, the moon's magnetic radiation, sun spots, and many other phenomena. Chemicals that may enter the body are now legion, being over sixty thousand that have thus far been discovered or invented. A few of the most recognized include the inorganics such as lead, cadmium, aluminum, arsenic, nickel, titanium, ozone, nitrous oxides, sulfur dioxides, carbon monoxides, beryllium, and so on, as well as the organics such as organochlorine, organophosphate, carbamate and pyrethroid insecticides, car exhausts, formaldehydes, phenols, phthalates (found in plastics), petroleum products, and so on. The biological include bacteria, viruses, parasites, food, molds, and sometimes dust. Any and/or all of these substances can increase the total body pollutant load to the point that the detoxification systems (both the immune and nonimmune systems) cannot keep up with the exposures. Symptoms will occur indicating the onset of ill health. If the load is too toxic or occurs for too long, a fixed-named disease may occur. The timing for this event may be from a few minutes to many years.

The third principle that an individual needs to understand in order to maintain good health is that of *adaptation*. Adaptation is an acute survival mechanism in which the body's immune and enzyme detoxification systems raise to a higher set point in order to counteract the total body pollutant load. When this event happens, people cannot relate their symptoms to specific exposure as was possible in the alarm stage of the event. This inability to further relate cause and effect of specific pollutants to symptoms can allow for more intake of pollutants, thus causing a further strain on the body's detoxification system.

For example, a foul odor comes into the room. It is mildly repulsive to the patient. In the alarm stage, one perceives that the discomfort is caused by the odor and therefore tries to eliminate it. However, if it isn't possible to eliminate the odor, the body accommodates by increasing the output of the detoxification systems, and the odor is masked. If the chemical substance of the odor enters the body, the individual has three choices: eliminate it, use it, or "park" it. The body will accommodate by parking the pollutant in fat tissue, or in the fat of the cell membranes, if all of the pollutant cannot be eliminated or used. This process will increase the total body pollutant load and may eventually increase it until disease occurs.

Once this principle is understood, it can be applied to the advantage of one's own good health. Avoiding a substance in air, food, or water for four to seven days causes de-adaptation to occur. Then the body will revert back to the alarm stage, where cause and effect can again be perceived and proved. Total body pollutant load will decrease, and the individual will begin to feel well. Therefore, if chronic discomfort arises and one suspects, say, water contamination, or food sensitivity, or air contamination, one will avoid suspected causes (e.g., a specific food or a suspected water source) for four to seven days and then expose oneself to the suspected cause. Because the body is in the alarm stage (and not the adapted phase), cause and effect are proved. For example, if a food sensitivity is suspected—say, to beef—avoid it in all forms and then, after four to seven days, eat only organically grown processed beef to eliminate the chemical exposure. If one reacts, eliminate beef from the diet. If there is no reaction, eat commercial beef to see if the additives and preservatives cause the problem. If one suspects the contaminated air at work or at home or in the city is causing the problem, one avoids these areas for four to seven days and, once the symptoms are clear or at a minimum, goes into the area to see if the problem recurs. This is the way one can pinpoint the substances that trigger problems. Often when in an adapted state, the individual becomes addicted to the offending substances and seeks them out because they make them feel good or "normal" temporarily. At EHC-D, we have used this principle and have taught it to our patients thousands of times, and we find that understanding the total body pollutant load and adaptation principles on a personal basis restores and maintains health in the pollutant-overloaded individual.

The next principle that one must understand in order to test and manipulate the near environment for positive maintenance of health is the principle of *bipolarity.* Once the pollutant enters the body, the immune and nonimmune detoxification systems go into action, attempting to combat the pollutant. This often creates stimulatory reactions in the brain, which may be misconstrued as beneficial. If this is the case, the total body pollutant load of the patient will increase. Then if the load is acutely removed or decreased, the individual will have symptoms that last for one or two days, or in some cases longer, due to the slow turning off of the detoxification system. This phenomenon is well-known to people who drink alcohol, smoke cigarettes, or eat chocolate and sugar, and to other food addicts.

Next, understanding *biochemical individuality* is extremely important in evaluating and preventing pollutant overload. This principle says that each individual's uniqueness is manifested in his or her own set of "symptoms" or responses to the environmental load. Therefore, responses will be varied and individualized. For example, Substance A comes into the room and Patient A has no response; B gets a headache; C gets a stomach ache; D gets heart irregularities; E gets asthma; F gets a bladder infection; G gets diarrhea; and H gets menstrual upset. The mechanism of response depends on genetics, the state of nutrition and total body pollutant load in utero, and the state of nutrition and total body pollutant load at the time of exposure. There are more than two thousand metabolic genetic defects that can affect detoxification systems, causing an increase in total body pollutant load. It has been shown that if the mother or father takes in toxic loads, they will be transmitted to the fetus and will increase and cause nutritional depletion. If the pollutant load at the time of exposure is high, the nutrients vital for detoxification become depleted and symptoms occur. This ratio of pollutant overload to adequate nutrients can become abnormal in any organ, thus allowing for different symptoms in different individuals. If a pollutant bothers you and you don't respond as other people do, it may still be a harmful pollutant to you.

The sixth principle used to diagnose pollutant overload and to maintain health is that of the *switch phenomenon*. We have observed this process to occur thousands of times at the EHC-D and warn the individual not to be tricked into believing that the problem is solved if in fact symptoms switch to another organ. In the 1700s, a physician in England by the name of Sauvage noted that patients with psychosis had little asthma or rhinosinusitis. However, when their psychosis improved, their asthma and sinus problems got worse. Often we have seen patients who are medicated for their symptoms (e.g., sinusitis) and improve—only to develop arthritis, premenstrual syndrome, diarrhea, or some other problem. We have also seen altering of a pollutant exposure cause a similar pattern; for example, the odor in the room is masked by a second odor or deodorized. The patient loses the headache only to experience fatigue, muscle aches, asthma, or some other ailment.

The final principle is the *spreading phenomena.* If the offending substances are not eliminated, the localized problem will spread from one organ on to multiple others as the patient gets sicker. When this occurs, the patient may become sensitive to a series of substances, first to those related to the initial offending compound, then to unrelated substances, and finally to foods and common biological inhalants like mold, dust, and so on. Thus, you have two types of spreading, that of sensitivity from one chemical to many and from one organ to many.

DIET AND HEALTH

The other side of the coin in dealing with environmental overload is the individual's state of nutrition. As is shown in the principle of biochemical individuality of response, nutrients are necessary for the body to cope with pollutants. Because our air, food, and water are massively contaminated with pollutants, specific supplementation of nutrients is now necessary for obtaining and maintaining health. One has to realize that food grown with pesticides and artificial fertilizers is depleted of nutrients, and, thus, it is impossible to get enough nutrients for a balanced diet in today's commercial foods.

Many other facts support supplementation. Malabsorption occurs in the gut of the pollutant-overloaded individual; thus nutrients cannot be properly absorbed. Often there are reactions to the acid producer cells in the stomach, and hydrochloric acid is decreased or absent. Therefore, food is not broken down entirely and not absorbed or digested well. In addition, some chemicals outstrip vitamins and minerals for absorption, and therefore the overloaded individual will become deficient. The all-too-common dietary supplements of excess sugar, white bread, coffee, cigarettes, and alcohol will rapidly deplete systems of nutrients. The increased metabolism needed for adaptation and detoxification of chemicals also depletes the individual of nutrients. Finally, it has been shown that many chemicals act as diuretics, causing the release of vitamins, minerals, amino acids, and fats into the urine and/or gut.

These facts support the need for supplementation. The individual will have to search for an environmental medicine specialist because nutrient supplementation is individualized and complicated. Sixty percent of the patients entering EHC-D are deficient of vitamin B_6; 30 percent of B_1, B_2, B_3, folic acid, and vitamin C; 20 percent of vitamin A; 15 percent of vitamin D; and 10 percent of B_{12}. No data are available on vitamin E. However, these statistics reveal that environmentally overloaded individuals need supplementation. Because pollutants tend to damage cell membranes and cause kidney and gut leaks, mineral metabolism is often disturbed. Studies at the EHC-D show magnesium deficiency and chromium deficiency to be the number one and two mineral deficiencies, respectively. However, deficiencies of zinc, manganese, selenium, potassium, copper, and calcium follow. Also due to membrane damage, excesses are often seen in manganese, aluminum, lead, and barium. The latter will cause additional damage to cells. Amino acid deficiencies can also occur, resulting in the need for many of the essential amino acids in addition to glutathione, cysteine, taurine, and methionine. These substances often need to be supplemented for good health. One has to be cautious about supplementation because the pollutant-overloaded individual may be sensitive to the food source from which the nutrients are made and can be made ill by the supplementations themselves.

In summary, in order to obtain and maintain health, one needs to decrease the total environmental pollutant load to decrease the total body pollutant load. This is best achieved by using the principles and facts outlined above, along with good nutrient supplementation, with a varied diet of less chemically polluted foods. The fact that one can prove cause of symptoms and effect of individual and multiple environmental factors is sound. At present, these techniques are only taught in major medical facilities, but it will be necessary to teach every individual in the world. In my opinion and those of my coworkers in this area, this concept should be taught in society to the point that it is better known than the germ theory. Knowledge of how to evaluate the effects of the environment on the individual allows for great independence. It allows individuals to move freely through this complex environment upon the earth, not having to accept anyone's word or propaganda about the safety or efficacy of substances to which one is exposed. One can use one's own God-given sense to record and interpret environmental exposures.

REFERENCES

Rea, W. (1992). *Chemical sensitivity* (Vol. 1). Boca Raton, FL: Lewis.
Rea, W. (1994). *Chemical sensitivity* (Vol. 2). Boca Raton, FL: Lewis.
Rea, W. (1996). *Chemical sensitivity* (Vol. 3). Boca Raton, FL: Lewis.

27 Homeopathy

Cause or Consequence?

WAYNE B. JONAS

Homeopathy is a system for treating individuals with medications that induce a person's body and mind to heal itself. Homeopathy uses a variety of substances derived from plants, animals, minerals, synthetic chemicals, and conventional drugs, all in very small amounts using a special preparation process of serial dilution with succussion or agitation between dilution steps. The homeopathic system outlines specific guidelines for how these medicines are selected and used in treatment so that they stimulate the self-healing properties of an ill person. These guidelines are directed at the total pattern of symptoms a person has rather than a subset of symptoms or assumed cause of symptoms that form the diagnosis. It is directed at stimulating self-healing and so proceeds at the pace the body changes. For functional and psychological symptoms, this may be very rapid. For physiological and anatomical signs and symptoms, this may be slow or not at all. Homeopathy developed from a curious blend of both modern and medieval ideas combined in a type of drug therapy that affects the dynamic process of illness. It is a system that was almost completely abandoned in the West by the turn of the century, and its practice, theory, and science have not advanced much since then. Its emphasis on holism and individualization make it a difficult system to investigate with modern tools that use quantitative and inferential, rather than qualitative and descriptive, analysis.

THE DEVELOPMENT OF HOMEOPATHY

The system of homeopathy was the brainchild of essentially one man named Samuel Christian Hahnemann (1755-1843) (Haehl, 1922). Hahnemann developed this approach over a period of fifty years, and it is a curious blend of medieval ideas of alchemy and vitalism and modern ideas of chemistry and experimentation. Hahnemann was translating an herbal book by a famous British author who declared that a certain herb called China cured malaria because it was bitter. Dissatisfied with this explanation, Hahnemann got the idea to experiment on himself with the herb. He took some China himself and carefully noted all the symptoms that it produced. Many of the symptoms were like malaria, and so he concluded that a drug might cure an illness because it can induce a reaction in the body similar to the reaction induced by the disease. Essentially, Hahnemann implied, the drug acts therapeutically when it produces symptoms in a person without the disease that are similar to those when a person has the disease.

Hahnemann then began to test other drugs with a small group of followers. The drugs were given to healthy people (mostly to themselves and to their relatives or friends) and the symptoms produced were carefully observed and documented. Most of the main homeopathic drugs in common use today were tested, or as homeopaths call it, "proved," in this way. It is important to note that Hahnemann based the selection of effective drugs on the beginnings of an experimental (and thus scientific) method that could be tested. This was a new idea for medicine, yet it was completely consistent with science as it was then understood. At the very least, it allowed for empirical verification or rejection of a particular rationale for therapy. This, in fact, had never been provided before. It took almost 150 years before the ideas that evolved from these tests began to be experimentally evaluated, however.

Hahnemann conducted these tests in a particular way. A modern approach to drug testing is to give a drug to a large number of people and then look for the frequency with which certain classes of symptoms (such as headache, depression, foot pain, fatigue, etc.) develop. Some of the people tested would be given an inert substance (a placebo) at random, and both the experimenters and the subjects given the medications would not be allowed to know which medication they had been given. Symptoms or patterns of symptoms in both the active and placebo groups would be compared and grouped, averaged, or counted in some manner. This is the statistical or mathematical approach and allows scientists to eliminate symptoms that develop spontaneously, by chance, or because of expectations, rather than from the drug. However, the statistical approach only allows for rather crude kinds of symptoms to be examined because they must be simplified, grouped together, and averaged. Unique and individual reactions, or unusual patterns of symptoms produced by the medications, cannot easily be counted and included in an analysis using this approach. The application of mathematics to human illness was not to come until after Hahnemann's death. Hahnemann was looking for certain unique and qualitative reactions to the drugs. Rather than study large numbers of people in a general way, Hahnemann studied a small number of people but studied each in great detail.

PROVINGS

Hahnemann painstakingly documented any and all symptoms, both mental and physical, that his "provers" had, before, during, and after the drugs were given to them. He was especially interested in those people who seemed sensitive to a particular medicine. He looked for the unusual, the unexpected, and the unique reactions that the provers had, and he would examine their symptom records and question them extensively, looking for these "strange, rare, and peculiar" symptoms as he later came to call them. Not being able or desiring to use mathematical averages as a guide for drug indications, he used uniqueness instead. This approach to experimentation gave homeopathy a radically different focus compared to the statistical approach to medicine that developed a hundred years later. With this type of testing as its basis, homeopathy became the medicine of the individual rather than the average, the unusual rather than the common, and later, the medicine of the personal rather than the impersonal. This approach also made it very difficult to study using the statistical methods of medical science that were to evolve later.

A second feature of these provings was also to produce an important difference between homeopathy and modern medicine. Hahnemann did not exclude any type or class of symptom from evaluation in the provings. Indeed, he made a deliberate attempt to include any and all symptoms experienced or observed by the prover that seemed to be a reaction to the remedy. Rather than give varying importance to parts of an illness based on how objective or subjective they were, or on how well they predicted a specific physical cause, Hahnemann included all symptoms in the belief that they expressed some unseen, unified, and intelligent "force" that organized all human health and illness. This was a premodern and medieval idea known as *vitalism*, and this "force" was considered the same as the spirit and the source of life. The vitalism concept fell out of favor in modern times as science and technology became better able to objectify, predict, and manipulate specific aspects of the physical world. What it did for homeopathy, however, was to maintain its holistic character in medicine, by approaching human illness as patients experienced it rather than from the perspective of disease or pathological classifications. Hahnemann came to feel that disease classifications were crude at best and completely artifactual and false at worst. He maintained that the only aspects of illness one could be sure about were the signs and symptoms the patient experienced and expressed. By following the total expression of these signs and symptoms, one could see how a patient was coping with and attempting to cure the problem. This was, remember, at a time before microscopes, stethoscopes, blood chemistry, and CAT scan machines, when the signs and symptoms *were* the only way to gain knowledge about the illness. Homeopathy became a system that focused intensely on individuals and took into consideration all of their symptoms, subjective and objective, physical, emotional, and mental—as an ecological whole.

These two aspects of homeopathic science, individualization and holism, are both the strength and weakness of homeopathy. Modern medical science was to go in a different direction, grouping patients into diagnostic categories and dividing their experiences into various parts for management by different specialties. The process of experiments that Hahnemann did on himself and other provers did not lend itself to this type of division. Patients, on the other hand, perceive their particular diagnosis as a single experience and often find that being grouped into a disease classification and treated in a uniform manner is unsatisfying and often ineffective. No two expressions of a disease are exactly the same, and a scientific method of accounting for this has yet to be developed. In this early and cumbersome way, Hahnemann attempted to explore the effects of drugs that took into account both the unique sensitivities of the individual patient and the unified way illness is experienced and progresses. Individualization and holism were inherent in homeopathic science from the beginning.

POTENCY

After proving a remedy in great detail on several people, Hahnemann began to test out the accuracy of these drug pictures for their usefulness in treating sick individuals. Because many of the drugs he used were toxic, he began to dilute them, giving them in smaller and smaller doses. Contrary to what was expected from such dose reduction, Hahnemann reported that if these drugs, or "remedies" as they came to be called, were given according to symptom pictures found in the provings, they worked better and for longer. He explained this by saying that when individuals were sick, they were often sensitive to very small amounts of drugs. Homeopathy, he reasoned, worked by inducing a mild but specific set of symptoms "similar" to the ones experienced by the patient, and so induced the patient's healing mechanisms to eliminate and "cure" the disease. Even very dilute preparations would induce this process if the patient was sufficiently sensitive to the drug.

Hahnemann then began to do something that today seems very peculiar but was not particularly strange for his time. He began to shake or "succuss" the dilutions as they were made in order to extract what he saw as the spiritlike or dynamic nature from the substance. We do not know why Hahnemann did this, but the idea was perfectly consistent with the mixed alchemical/chemical thinking of the age. Alchemists would frequently shake, stir, and perform various other manipulations on solutions in order to activate the vital or spiritlike forces believed to be inherent in all substances. Chemists did not realize that the vital substance of oxygen, for example, was a single element, nor did they know why it was needed for life. Although his original intent was to reduce the toxic effects from drugs, Hahnemann reported that the process of succussion between each dilution made the remedies more active and specific for those individuals who were sensitive to them. When prepared in this fashion, which Hahnemann called *potentizing*, the effectiveness of the drug depended even more on detailed matching of the total proving picture with the unique and complete symptom picture in the patient. When these pictures were matched carefully, according to Hahnemann, such potencies would stimulate a self-healing response precisely and patients would cure themselves of the disease.

This idea of potencies and "high dilutions" would prove to be one of the main areas of contention in the homeopathic system. Hahnemann and other early scientists understood that there must be a physical limit to how far you can dilute a substance before there is no longer any present. A problem arose because at the time of homeopathy's origin, science did not know what that actual limit of dilution was, and homeopathic practitioners were reporting remarkable effects at very low dilutions. It was realized later that if a substance was diluted at a ratio of one to one hundred for twelve times, the probability of having any original substance left in the preparation was practically zero. Yet dilutions much higher than this were used successfully for decades before this discovery was made. Not only is the dilution and potency issue one of the main contention points between homeopathic and allopathic medicine, it was and still is one of the main areas of conflict within homeopathy itself. The details of Hahnemann's (1982) approach were laid out in his book *Organon of Medicine,* which went through six editions and which he was constantly revising until his death.

COMPLEXITY

Nothing within us functions in isolation. No individual organ system or cell of our body is isolated. We continuously effect and are affected by our emotions, thoughts, and social and physical environment. For example, individuals exposed to cold viruses are much more likely to get infected and sick if they are under stress (Cohen, Tyrrell, & Smith, 1991) Every disease/healing process involves an interplay between the offending cause or agent of the disease and the person's self-healing response to that cause. In some cases, the agent is more dominant, as after trauma, overwhelming infections, epidemics, and other isolated acute illnesses. In many situations, however, a person's healing response is the dominant part of the illness, as in most chronic disease. In these situations, it is the self-healing, homeostatic mechanisms that must be assisted. It is this aspect of the disease/healing complex that homeopathy attempts to address.

Because of these multiple influences on disease and multiple pathways to healing, the treatment of disease/healing cannot be dogmatic. There are many ways to heal in most cases. No two individuals with the same diagnosis are exactly the same. Even in cases where we know the exact cause of the disease, as in measles, strep throat, or a herniated disc, for example, some individuals can be deathly ill with the problem and others not even notice it. Some people with a cold or allergies may have a dry, stuffy nose, others a wet, drippy one. Some have cough, others sore throat, some headache or swollen glands, others none of these symptoms. Except where a disease is specifically defined by a laboratory test or a pathology slide, most diagnoses are arrived at by convenience or social agreement (American Psychiatric Association, 1994; Rosenberg & Golden, 1992). Illness is variable and that variability is formed by our body's healing response to a greater degree than by the causes. Homeopathy attempts to address this variability of disease/healing by individualizing each drug selection in detail.

HOLISM

Any intervention, be it a drug, surgery, psychotherapy, or change in behavior, has effects on the entire body and mind—the entire ecological system of the person. The difference between therapies lies only in which part of this effect is assessed and used. Where a specific cause is the dominant factor in an illness, it makes sense to direct a therapy toward that factor and then attempt to minimize the side effects of therapy. If a person with a nasal infection, for example, develops bacterial meningitis (a serious infection in the brain), the healing action of the body has been overwhelmed by the cause, and the treatment is to eliminate the bacteria with high-dose antibiotics. The side effects of the antibiotics (such as hearing loss in some cases) are an unfortunate consequence of the treatment but are better than dying. If the nose infection becomes a chronic sinus problem, on the other hand, where the efforts of the body are the dominant factor in the disease/healing complex, a drug must act on the person so as to enhance those self-healing efforts. The side effects under these circumstances become the central effects of the therapy and are the very changes needed for a successful cure. Treatment efforts aimed at the bacteria in such a case will often have only a temporary effect. Homeopathy uses the total effects of a drug to enhance the body's healing efforts. It assumes that all aspects of a drug's effect can be useful when they are matched appropriately to what the total patient needs rather than just what the diagnosis calls for.

THE PRINCIPLES OF HOMEOPATHY

Homeopathy selects medications by matching detailed drug profiles with the complete picture of an ill person's symptoms. This matching process is called the law of similars, or like-cures-like, sometimes written in Latin as *Similia Similibus Curentur.* The homeopathic therapist first gets a detailed report of any symptoms, signs, pathologies, and other unique characteristics of the ill person. The practitioner then looks through descriptions of drug profiles or pictures detailed in homeopathic textbooks. These drug profiles are called, again in Latin, *Materia Medicas.* The homeopathic practitioner may use certain specific symptoms to guide the selection of the drug, but it is assumed that the most long-term and comprehensive effects will come from a remedy that produces symptoms similar to those a person has on all levels: physical, behavioral, and psychological. Such a remedy will induce and guide that person's healing response in the most complete and stable manner.

The goal of homeopathic therapy is to induce and guide the self-healing response of a person. Because the medications are not given to eliminate the cause of an illness or to overwhelm any particular disease agent, they are not administered in large or frequent doses. It is not the drug itself that helps the illness; rather, it is the person's reaction to the medication that leads to improvement. If a person is sensitive to the medication, the self-healing response can be induced with very small and infrequently repeated doses. This idea of giving the smallest amount of drug possible is called the "minimum dose." From the beginning of homeopathy's development, homeopathic physicians began to reduce the doses of medications to the minimum amount that would still elicit a healing response in the patient without producing direct toxic effects. It was soon noticed, however, that individuals who were ill were often unusually sensitive to certain drugs. Gradually drug dosages were further and further reduced and found to still have an effect. Later, it was discovered that in many of the dilutions used, there could no longer be any molecule of the original substance left in the remedy. The ill person was not responding to the preparation or administration process of the therapy. The nature and existence of this signal is one of the great unsolved mysteries in biological science and is the main obstacle to the acceptance of homeopathy by mainstream medicine.

The third principle involved in the application of homeopathy (after the principle of similars and the minimum dose to induce healing) is the ecological pattern of healing. Homeopathy has a set of clinical guides as to how a patient should respond after taking a correct homeopathic medication. These guides are about how symptoms should change and improve as the body improves in its capacity to heal. This principle states that when people are healing properly, they will get better first in areas that are crucial to their ability to function. For example, if an individual with nasal allergies also has confusion and fatigue, a proper response to a homeopathic remedy should result in improvement in the confusion and fatigue before or simultaneously with the improvement in the nasal allergies. Improvement of the nasal allergies but worsening of the fatigue or nasal function is not considered a good healing response. If the nasal allergy symptoms are so severe as to limit the person's function more than fatigue, then one would expect that the allergies would improve to a greater extent and before the fatigue. Judging what symptoms limit a person to the greatest extent is a variable and subjective process incorporating medical knowledge, patient preferences, and cultural values. Experience, clinical judgment, and the art of medicine still play a major role in decision making.

RESEARCH INTO HOMEOPATHY

If homeopathy is effective for the reasons that it purports, then it poses a serious challenge to both modern medicine and science, for it would edify not only the concept of diagnosis as important for therapeutic effectiveness but also the concept of molecular theory as the basis for biological and pharmacological action. To entertain this challenge requires demonstrating several phenomena. First, specific information would need to be stabilized and retained in solutions that contain no other molecules than hydrogen and oxygen. Second, this information must specifically signal extensive biological reactions from local areas of the body or diffuse or radiate through the body (also mostly made up of hydrogen and oxygen) to produce a comprehensive effect. Third, the effect must be a general biological phenomenon, effective in a variety of living systems, and fourth, the clinical effectiveness of homeopathic therapy as a system must be demonstrated.

Modern research into these four questions is still in its infancy, and so the answers must wait. Preliminary research is intriguing, much of it tending to support this system. Studies on the stability of information in water and changes in various structural patterns in potentized water have been reported (Berezin, 1990; del Giudice, 1990; Endler & Schulte, 1994; Resch & Gutmann, 1987). Information transfer from potency preparations to biological systems producing global effects has been reported in a number of models, both in vitro and in vivo (Bastide, 1994; Bellavite & Andrea, 1995; Doutremepuich, 1991; Linde et al., 1994). Finally, a number of clinical trials evaluating the effectiveness of the homeopathic system and its preparations have been done (Bellavite & Andrea, 1995; King, 1988; Kleijnen, Knipschild, & ter Riet, 1991; Majerus

1990; Righetti 1988). More research of this type will help shed light on these questions, but it is unlikely that our understanding of homeopathy will significantly advance until a mechanism is discovered.

Modern clinical investigation also provides a fundamental challenge to homeopathy. The clinical effects of homeopathy may be the consequence of the homeopathic assumptions and method. At any one time, 60 percent to 70 percent of people will report symptoms of some kind, even without extensive questioning, and more than 70 percent of patients who seek medical care will have symptoms that do not fit a specific diagnosis (Kroenke & Mangelsdorff, 1989). About 80 percent of these patients will improve on placebo or reassurance and probably any therapy that incorporates these aspects (Thomas, 1974, 1994). Because homeopathy extensively seeks out symptoms that may not be associated with a diagnosis, it runs the risk of eliciting symptoms that would by their very nature resolve with any therapy. By giving a treatment under those conditions, improvement may be falsely attributed to the therapy. If this is the mechanism of homeopathic effects, these effects would be their consequence rather than their cause.

IS HOMEOPATHY A CAUSE OR CONSEQUENCE?

Throughout its history, a number of attempts to combine homeopathic and modern biomedical concepts have been developed. These attempts to modernize homeopathic concepts occur in one of two ways. First, homeopathic drug pictures are linked with conventional diagnoses and "covered" with specific combinations of medicines. This results in loss of individualization and the holistic orientation, as symptoms of illness are lumped into generalized groups and lose their personal meaning. Diagnoses are largely created by professional organizations to simplify investigation and treatment (Lawrence, 1992). These diagnostic groups represent heterogeneous populations with variable prognoses and outcome preferences. Although in many cases these simplifications are useful, at other times, they create problems when applied too broadly. Attempts to modernize homeopathy by applying remedies to conventional diagnostic categories risk losing its appreciation of the complexity and holism inherent in illness and healing.

Second, attempts have been made to find and explain homeopathic effects based on some physical mechanism. These investigations assume that homeopathy must produce its effects following traditional assumptions of cause and effect (linearity), localized molecular action (physicality), and independence of the contextual influence of drug delivery (expectation and intention) from drug action. Although serially agitated dilutions may be found to have a physical nature and influence, it seems unlikely that current observations of global effects from homeopathic treatment can be explained using traditional pharmacological principles. Methods of investigation that look for correspondences rather than causes may be needed in order to detect subtle effects in complex systems that are not strictly casual. More descriptive and ecological approaches to the investigation of drug effects are needed in order to understand how these "drugs with eyes and ears" affect us.

If homeopathy works, it represents an important area for investigation as a method of stimulating self-healing that is sensitive to the body's complexity and ecology. If it does not work or if it appears to work because of the way homeopathic medicine is delivered, it represents an important area for investigating the mystery of placebo in ways as yet unfathomed. In either case, this system has a lot to teach us about healing and science and about the limitations and the frontiers of our current understanding.

REFERENCES

American Psychiatric Association. (1994). *Diagnostic and statistical manual of mental disorders (DSM-IV).* Washington, DC: Author.

Bastide, M. (1994). Immunological examples on UHD research. In *Ultra high dilution: Physiology and physics.* Dordrecht: Kluwer.

Bellavite, P., & Andrea, S. (1995). *Homeopathy: A frontier of medical science.* Berkeley, CA: North Atlantic Books.

Berezin, A. A. (1990). Isotopical positional correlations as a possible model for Benveniste experiments. *Medical Hypotheses, 31,* 43-45.

Cohen, S., Tyrell, D. A. J., & Smith, A. P. (1991). Psychological stress and susceptibility to the common cold. *New England Journal of Medicine, 325,* 606-612.

del Giudice, E. (1990). *Collective processes in living matter: A key for homeopathy.* Essen: Verlag fuer Ganzheitsmedizin.

Doutremepuich, C. (1991). *Ultra low doses.* London: Taylor & Francis.

Endler, P. C., & Schulte, J. (Eds.). (1994). *Ultra high dilution: Physiology and physics.* Dordrecht: Kluwer.

Haehl, R. (1992). *Samuel Hahnemann: His life and work.* London: Homeopathic Publishing.

Hahnemann, S. (1982). *Organon of medicine.* Los Angeles: Tarcher.

King, G. (1988). *Experimental investigations for the purpose of scientifical proving of the efficacy of homeopathic preparations.* Thesis, Tierarztliche Hochschule, Hanover.

Kleijnen, J., Knipschild, P., & ter Riet, G. (1991). Clinical trials of homeopathy. *British Medical Journal, 302,* 316-323.

Kroenke, K., & Mangelsdorff, A. D. (1989). Common symptoms in ambulatory care: Incidence, evaluation, therapy, and outcome. *American Journal of Medicine, 86,* 262-266.

Lawrence, C. (1992). "Definite and material": Coronary thrombosis and cardiologist in the 1920s. In *Framing disease: Studies in cultural history* (pp. 50-82). New Brunswick, NJ: Rutgers University Press.

Linde, K., Jonas, W. B., Melchart, D., Worku, F., Wagner, H., & Eitel, F. (1994). Critical review and meta-analysis of serial agitated dilutions in experimental toxicology. *Human and Experimental Toxicology, 13,* 481-492.

Majerus, M. (1990). *Kritische Begutachtung der wissenschaftlichen Beweisfuhrung in der homoopathischen Grundlagenforschung. Gesamtbetrachtung der Arbeiten aus dem frankophonen Sprachraum.* Thesis, Tierarztliche Hochschule, Hanover.

Resch, G., & Gutmann, V. (1987). *Scientific foundations of homeopathy.* Starnberger, Germany: Barthel & Barthel.

Righetti, M. (1988). *Forschung in der homeopathie.* Goettingen: Burgdorf Verlag.

Rosenberg, C. E., & Golden, J. (Eds.). (1992). *Framing disease: Studies in cultural history.* New Brunswick, NJ: Rutgers University Press.

Thomas, K. B. (1974). Temporarily dependent patients in general practice. *British Medical Journal,* 625-626.

Thomas, K. B. (1994). The placebo in general practice. *British Medical Journal, 344,* 1066-1067.

28 Eating in the Bioregion

DOROTHY BLAIR

Eating is not a solitary act. Eating is a profoundly social and ecological event that connects us in the most intimate and primary way to others, to our land, water, and soil, to the future, and to other species.

Poet Gary Snyder (1990, p. 184) describes eating as a "sacrament." Whatever place in the food chain we choose, our meals require the deaths of numerous and marvelous species of living things, no less wonderful in their complexity than ourselves. Our bodies will also one day be the food of other living creatures. Eating provides our most intimate association with the other, the sharing between life forms of organic chemicals carrying the energy necessary for life. To eat fully we need to be mindful of our debt.

Wendell Berry (1990) calls eating an "agricultural act." He writes, "How we eat determines how the earth is used" (p. 149). As eaters, we not only consume agricultural products, we also shape the relationship between agriculture and nature by our food choices. By ceding the responsibility for knowing how food is grown to the government, food manufacturers, and food retailers, we place ourselves "in exile from biological reality" (Berry, 1990, p. 148). Food choice becomes merely a matter of visual appeal and price.

The cost of turning our backs on the food system has been high. In the United States, one third of our national treasure of topsoil has been eroded in less than 200 years. Half of the topsoil in Iowa is gone (Pimentel, 1984). Municipal water supplies throughout the Midwest, California's central valley, and other intensively farmed areas are contaminated with pesticides and nitrates. Major aquifers are being depleted to irrigate subsidized crops, such as sugar beets and corn in Nebraska and rice in Texas, and excessive irrigation has resulted in serious salinization of soil in California, Hawaii, the Colorado River Basin, and along the Rio Grande (Worster, 1984).

Eating can be an act of "extensive pleasure" (Berry, 1990, p. 151), which is the intimate knowing of what and who is being eaten: the memory of the green pastures and sweet waters, the well-tended tomatoes picked at their peak of flavor, the proud squawk of the chicken as she laid the egg that now graces your plate and sauntered out into the barnyard. It is the joy of food uncontaminated by the off-flavor of inhumane factory farms, by worrisome chemicals or unjust working conditions. Knowing a good farmer, one can savor honest food grown with caring hands.

Sacraments based on the interconnectedness of human actions have little chance to thrive in American industrial society. Madison Avenue assumes that individuals are secular, self-seeking, and self-justifying (Douglas, 1984) and, thus, it promotes the individual uses of food at the expense of social considerations. Food is depicted as a matter of individual taste and of individual or, at most, family health. We eat our anonymous food quickly and often alone at fast-food restaurants or out of the microwave, mindlessly tossing away packaging more costly than the food itself. We eat in ways that we have been led to believe enhance our own personal health; "fresh" winter fruits arrive by air freight from Chile. In the land of Johnny Appleseed, bananas from Central America are our favorite fruit—bananas whose price has barely risen in decades due to cost-saving measures like using cheaper pesticides known to cause sterility in workers (Thrupp, 1989). In Honduras, banana plantations are so extensive that they have pushed landless peasant farmers to deforest steep and unstable rain forest slopes for their livelihood. Few notice or even care that half of our orange juice crop now comes from Brazil, where the poor often cannot afford food. There, exporters thrive, and the top fifth of the population earns twenty-six times more than the bottom fifth (Bello, 1994).

In our disconnected, postindustrial society, greed and goods substitute for solidarity. We expect our food in a seasonless stream, obtained with no more effort than pushing a cart down a supermarket aisle. We want those shelves well stocked with inexpensive food, because our rent and medical care are expensive, and we need to reassure ourselves that capitalism is really better than any other economic system.

Eating as Americans eat is an act of extreme ethnocentrism. We eat as if we were the only species and the only country that matters. We have colonized the world with our standards for consumption. While one fifth of the world's population lives without food security, grains are increasingly diverted from people to animal fodder. Meat consumption has risen in almost every country, and the rich monopolize scanty health care budgets with the medical sequelae of overconsumption.

We are eating out of place, we are living out of touch, and the system conspires to reinforce our ignorance and stimulate our appetite. We are not evil people. We are simply consuming in a vacuum.

THE BIOREGIONAL VISION OF FOOD

Bioregionalism is essentially a paradigm of coexistence "in place" as opposed to the industrial model of exploiting a world economy for our livelihood. In the case of eating, bioregionalism directs us to shape a diet from what our local environment can sustainably provide.

When I introduced this concept in a meeting of nutritionists, the shocked response was, "You mean, give up bananas and orange juice? What about our strides in public health?" The concept of eating a more locally produced diet is not only troubling from an economic perspective, it is antithetical to the prevailing concept of the public good. The global marketplace and free trade are eulogized as bringing the benefits of cheap food and goods for "all." Based on the economic axiom of comparative advantage, tomatoes should be produced where the factors of production—land, soil, water, chemicals, fuel, and labor (and environmental regulations)—are cheapest. Tomatoes should be imported by places that cannot match this "efficiency of production." Forgotten in the narrowness of this industrial vision of consumer welfare is the integrity and continuity of the life of those consumption units, the individuals who presumably live in the environment that is being despoiled for their own good. Cheap goods, food in particular, consume natural resources rather than sustain them. They are palliatives that divert our attention from the loss of our autonomy in an increasingly hierarchical and inequitable society, the loss of our local culture, and the loss of our sense of community.

In contrast, bioregionalism advocates a reorientation of the self to an identification with place. It is a means of grounding ourselves once again in nature and in community. To "live in place" is to be in and of the natural environment that surrounds us.

A bioregion is usually defined by a watershed, by plant and animal species, by cultural distinctiveness, and by a sense of place, and not by political boundaries or borders (Devall, 1988). Bioregions are a size that people can identify with. Identification with place evolves through knowing and celebrating the land, the waterways, and the life forms of each, and through learning traditional wisdom and lore. Living in place requires skilled use of what the local environment provides for food, shelter, energy, crafts, culture, and entertainment. Bioregional economics develops the potential of the region to increase its self-sufficiency by replacing imported goods with sustainably produced, local alternatives. The gift of bioregionalism is increased self-realization and self-reliance, "liberating the self" from the domination of impersonal market forces and hierarchical forms of corporate and bureaucratic control (Sale, 1985, pp. 44-47).

Arne Naess (1989, p. 99), the Norwegian philosopher and originator of deep ecology, has said that food should be "grown within the horizon." Trade and cash cropping should be reduced, ground collectivized, and preservation and storage localized. All ecosystems, except perhaps those desertified, highly eroded, or logged off, are capable of providing a wholesome and delicious diet to local people, within the constraints of carrying capacity. Food can be gathered, hunted, and grown in a manner that honors living species and the environment.

Orienting oneself to the bioregion involves learning how people historically lived off the land and fashioned sustainable diets. Indigenous peoples have an encyclopedic knowledge of local plants, animals, fish, and insects, choosing from among a wide variety of edible, local species to create a palatable and nutritious diet. They are also avid adopters of novel foods. Corn, beans, squash, and potatoes are examples of foods from as far away as Peru that were adapted by Native North Americans. On his arrival to the American colonies, William Penn observed peach orchards thriving throughout his new land grant. The seed was originally acquired from early Spanish settlements in Florida and traded by natives up the coast (Kimball & Anderson, 1988).

Colonists bent on maintaining their identification with their mother country have ignored most of the foods eaten by indigenous peoples. They have imported familiar grains, vegetables, fruits, and meats, along with their weed species, mixed with grains and animal fodder. Native Americans ate the dandelion greens introduced inadvertently by the colonists, as well as the purslane introduced purposefully by French Jesuits, but the English colonists of North America did not eat potatoes until they became popular in Europe. We have yet to become very familiar with the Jerusalem artichoke, which grows wild in much of the eastern United States, although many European groups have savored this crunchy root crop since it was introduced from America in the 1600s (Kimball & Anderson, 1988).

Bioregionalists are native to place. They explore the possibilities and fashion their diets from what pleases; what can be locally, sustainably, and humanely grown; and what does not draw them into the injustices of the marketplace. Bioregionalism is based on the tenet that we can care effectively only for our own backyards, the region we passionately and personally identify with. Food from outside our region comes with an invisible and incalculable price tag for the future of our species and others. A global food system guarantees that we will neither know enough nor care enough about these costs to eliminate them. The environmentally sensitive option is to draw our sustenance from the territory we can oversee, from farmers we know.

It is easy to dismiss a bioregional food system as impractical, but in fact the global food system is based on rather incredible impracticalities that we take for granted. Despite dwindling supplies of U.S. fossil fuels, we use four calories of fuel to produce one calorie of food and then transport that food an average of 1,300 miles (Bashin, 1987). The Food and Agriculture Organization of the United Nations and the World Bank continue to promote industrial farming and large dam projects despite the damages caused by these short-term, production-augmenting techniques. One third of the world's cropland is already experiencing moderate to severe erosion. Roughly 6 million hectares a year are completely desertified. About 20 percent of the world's irrigated land is either waterlogged or salinated (Goldsmith & Hildyard, 1991). In contrast, a bioregional food system asks consumers to make food choices based on where, how, and by whom that food was produced—not so impractical in comparison with a nearly complete disregard for the soil and its inhabitants in the name of profit.

BIOREGIONAL FOOD: WHERE WE ARE

The first steps toward a bioregional food system can be found in the existing traditions of many communities across the United States and elsewhere. Wherever people are growing their own food, are willing to go out of their way to buy from local farmers, or are maintaining local hunter/gatherer customs, the bioregional sentiment survives. Local hunters, although often despised by the animal rights community and criticized for their "male bonding" customs, are practicing bioregionalism.

Gatherers of berries, mushrooms, nuts, tubers, and succulent leaves are also keeping alive the local knowledge base required to live off the land. Avid naturalists such as Euell Gibbons (1962) and Lee and Roger Peterson (1977) make it easy to access some of that local wisdom and to reexplore the bounty of the bioregion.

Where states have preserved farmland around urban and suburban areas, there are ample opportunities to be close to our food sources. Among these are U-pick fruits and vegetables, farm stands, and small-scale butchering operations. Cows, lambs, pigs, and flocks of chickens may be sold directly to the public on butchering day. Local milk is still bottled and sold mostly in the area in which it is produced, although there are regional variations of glut and scarcity. Local varieties of dairy products such as ice cream, soft cheeses, and yogurt are staple bioregional products in the northeast United States. Local honey is also usually easy to come by.

Local farmers' markets would seem to be an obvious example of bioregionalism, but unfortunately for most existing markets, the designation of "local" reflects only the market site. Stall holders simply retail produce from other parts of the country. Luckily, municipalities are beginning to see the advantages of promoting local farmers, and a growing number of markets require that farmers bring only those goods they have produced themselves with local resources. This spurs creativity and greater self-reliance. In the context of a well-attended market, a mandate for locally produced goods alters the economics of local production. Face to face with farmers you know personally, price is less of a deciding factor. The pleasure of buying from a friend, sustaining local enterprise, and immersing oneself in a bustling, colorful market become overriding elements in the purchasing decision. It is one thing to support your neighbor's efforts to conserve soil and reduce pesticides in your own watershed, and quite another to buy anonymous supermarket produce, be it "organic" or not.

Community Supported Agriculture (CSA) is a major breakthrough in bioregionalism. The concept of a farmer/consumer partnership was brought to New England in 1985 by European Bio-Dynamic farmers (Groh & McFadden, 1990). In this revolutionary model of agriculture, farmers and consumers cooperate to provide security to farmers and wholesome, high-quality, local food to consumers. Families or individuals are shareholders in the farm's yearly production and pay a predetermined price for weekly supplies of organic vegetables, fruits, herbs, flowers, eggs, grains, legumes, meat, and milk products—whatever the farmer can produce of interest to shareholders. In some cases, farmers collaborate to offer more selection. The price of a share is determined by the farmer, preferably with the cooperation of active shareholders, to cover a salary, farming costs, labor, and equipment repair. The CSA movement is growing rapidly and predictably throughout the United States. There are roughly 480 CSAs at present in North America.[1]

The CSA model localizes food production while drawing former industrial eaters into a new kind of food web: one that connects the well-being of land and the local economy. Successful CSAs foster a long-term friendship and trust among farmers and their shareholders, a fondness for and identification with the farm, and a sense of purposeful community. The community of shareholders meet around farming issues and farm workdays. They are called upon to make decisions about the development of the farm and to decide what they would like to have produced there. Their resources may be tapped for farm improvements. The pleasures of eating farm produce become more extensive as the web of relationships increases.

CSA membership provides an education in eating local food. Shareholders are forced by the seasonal nature of local production to learn to use unfamiliar, season-extending vegetables. At Sycamore Cooperative Garden, a central Pennsylvania CSA of 30 shareholding families, we share recipes and news clippings to help subscribers deal with the variety and seasonal abundance of vegetables and herbs. We often include common nutritious "weeds," such as amaranth leaves and purslane, in the weekly vegetable delivery, along with appropriate recipes, to widen the shareholder's repertoire of edibles. Our shareholders are beginning to accept the unfamiliar, are more proficient in the use of herbs to enliven foods, and are much more knowledgeable about seasonality and the potential of the local food system to provide a wide range of crops. Our season lasts 20-22 weeks. To prolong local food availability, some CSAs have built winter storage areas for root crops.

BIOREGIONAL FOOD: GAPS, PROBLEMS, AND SOLUTIONS

Eating locally is a commonly proposed principle for those who would walk lightly on the Earth (Greenpeace, 1994). But bioregional eating is more often praised than achieved by the environmental community. Environmentally concerned people have changed their food habits in many ways to fit their perceived sense of social justice (Giesecke, 1992). A common response is to become vegetarian or to eat organic food grown 3,000 miles away so as to feel that one has done one's part to nudge the food system along. Why? Because eating bioregionally requires knowledge of place, and it takes time. Bioregionalism is a difficult mandate for time-stressed, out-of-place urban dwellers, especially for those who keep their distance from the kitchen. Extra time is needed to hunt out sources of bioregional food, to gather them together, and to deal with unprocessed foods in the kitchen. Most of us lack kitchen skills. The demographic profile of 1990s eaters includes many single restaurant grazers; frantic, working single moms; and two-worker families. Even pushed by a strong environmental ethic, few of these people would jump on the bioregional bandwagon unless it became a more convenient option.

Almost missing from the bioregional scene in the northeast United States, for example, are local grains, grain products, and legumes. The rise of large grain operations and steel roller mills in the American Midwest some 120 years ago nearly wiped out all small-scale, local grist mills. Only dedicated bioregionalists with their home stone grinders have experienced the heavenly flavor of freshly ground grains. Most cows still eat bioregionally, but even chickens in the northeast United States are eating feed from Midwest grain and soy farms.

The origin of grains and legumes seems to be of lesser importance than fruits, vegetables, and meats to most persons concerned with local eating, perhaps because freshness is not so critical, but also because grain growing shifted to the Midwest so long ago. Grains grown in the selenium-rich soils of the West do have a definite nutritional advantage over those grown in old Appalachian soils; however, selenium could be fortified in salt just as iodine has been since the 1920s. As major dietary staples, grains and legumes should be produced locally. Perhaps more than for any other crops, the relocalization of grain and legume production would create an amazing variety of opportunities for profitable local enterprise: the farming, milling, processing, and manufacturing of the multitude of products that are now produced by the largest transnational companies.

Bioregional eating must be part of a broader bioregional movement toward local self-reliance that allows less time spent earning wages and more time spent in ways that promote local exchange. Third-party bartering schemes give a jump start to a local economy, such as Ithaca, New York's "Ithaca Hour"—"money" worth an hour of time that may be exchanged only for locally produced goods and services (Glover, 1994). Local cooperative food stores are extremely important as vehicles for carrying local foods and food products and making their purchase more convenient. They can educate members about bioregionalism's importance, or even institute green taxes on nonregional foods and/or reward the purchasers of locally grown food with lower markups. As the movement to eat locally grows, so will the availability of local eating options, including prepared products and restaurant foods.

In the last 15 years, a few municipalities have made the revolutionary discovery that the food supply is a local concern. Individuals have formed food policy councils in places such as St. Paul, Minnesota; Onondaga County, New York; Philadelphia, Pennsylvania; and Toronto, Ontario, to examine the local area's current food system and potential to feed itself. They have worked on mechanisms for preserving local farmlands, facilitated CSAs that serve urban areas, and improved local farmers' markets (Dahlberg, 1992). The Philadelphia Food and Agriculture Task Force promoted the licensing of tailgate farmers' markets in inner-city areas. It was also a leader in promoting urban gardening (Dahlberg, 1994). More communities need to use the municipal food policy model to discover what shape the food system is in, what imported foods can be replaced with local food sources, and what regulatory actions can be taken to stimulate and link local food production, processing, and sales.

THE COSTS OF BIOREGIONALISM

We pay too little up front for our supermarket food. The real cost of growing food ecologically and on a small scale is a shock to consumers who are accustomed to the economies of large-scale, government-subsidized industrial production. Although their costs are much greater, local farmers are forced to keep prices in line with or lower than local supermarket prices. Even the most dedicated CSA shareholders balk at paying a share price that translates into a livable wage, although their farmer may work for them 80 hours a week. CSA earnings show an improvement over farmers' market earnings, but these efforts are still labors of love (Kelvin, 1994). The comparison with supermarket prices will likely become less meaningful to the bioregionalist who obtains most food from CSAs or other local outlets and rarely deals with mass-marketed food. Third-party bartering schemes may also help make locally produced food more affordable.

North America, with its rich soils and favorable, temperate climate, could easily foster many diverse, bioregional food systems. But the question remains whether our sacred tropical beverages—coffee, tea, and chocolate—must be eliminated. Should exceptions be made for caffeine addicts? And what about spices, citrus fruit, sugar, and so on? The sugar question could be easily fixed with a local supply of sugar beets, but the issue of how bioregional one's food consumption needs to be is surely moot at this point. We are far from growing the most basic things locally and further still from exploring the possibilities that our environment offers for free. The basic consideration that should inform our decision to import is whether import crops can be grown ethically at a distance and can be exchanged for our own surplus after our basic food needs are locally met. Perhaps the urge for caffeine would wane somewhat in a more self-reliant, less time-driven society. But people are unlikely to give up addictions voluntarily.

CONCLUSION

On the surface, bioregionalism may look like a hopeless anachronism. With the passage of the North American Free Trade Agreement and the General Agreement on Tariffs and Trade, the world is moving swiftly toward a globalized economy. The economic tenets of the postindustrial world are completely counter to bioregionalism, and, along with advertising, tend to colonize our minds with messages of passive consumerism and the ineffectualness of individual action. But empowerment is the heart of bioregionalism. Eating bioregionally is a profoundly political act. It is completely within the power of any individual through his or her own consumption choices to affect the local food system and reorient it toward local production and consumption. It is a matter of changing ourselves and our own backyard. Even the urban poor can choose to garden, or work to make gardening an option. Bioregionalism does not require economic power or political clout. It is accessible to anyone who chooses to make self-reliance and local potential a priority.

NOTE

1. The Bio-Dynamic Farm and Gardening Association, Kimberton Hills, PA, supplied this figure, but the number is constantly increasing as new CSAs develop. The Bio-Dynamic Farm and Gardening Association maintains a toll-free consumer hotline to provide potential subscribers with a brochure listing the CSAs in their state. It is 1-800-516-7797.

REFERENCES

Bashin, B. J. (1987). The freshness illusion. *Harrowsmith, 2*(7), 41-50.

Bello, W. (1994). *Dark victory*. London: Pluto Press, in cooperation with Food First, San Francisco, and Transnational Institute, Amsterdam.

Berry, W. (1990). *What are people for?* San Francisco: North Point Press.

Dahlberg, K. (1992). *Report and recommendations on the Saint Paul, Minnesota, food system* (Unpublished report). Kalamazoo: Department of Political Science, Western Michigan University.

Dahlberg, K. (1995). *Report and recommendations on the Philadelphia, Pennsylvania, food system* (Unpublished report). Kalamazoo: Department of Political Science, Western Michigan University.

Devall, B. (1988). *Simple in means, rich in ends*. Salt Lake City, UT: Peregrine Smith.

Douglas, M. (1984). Standard social uses of food: Introduction. In M. Douglas (Ed.), *Food in the social order: Studies of food and festivities in three American communities*. New York: Russell Sage Foundation.

Gibbons, E. (1962). *Stalking the wild asparagus*. New York: David McKay.

Giesecke, C. C. (1992). *Assessment of consumer behaviors promoting a sustainable food supply*. Doctorial thesis, Pennsylvania State University, State College, PA.

Glover, P. (1995). *Creating ecological economics with local currency*. Ithaca, NY: Unpublished E-mail article (ITHACAHOUR@ADL.COM).

Goldsmith, E., & Hildyard, N. (1991). World agriculture: Toward 2000 FAO's to feed thee world. *The Ecologist, 21*(2).

Greenpeace. (1994). *Stepping lightly on the Earth: A minimum impact guide to the home*. Washington, DC: Greenpeace Newsletter.

Groh, T., & McFadden, S. (1990). *Farms of tomorrow: Community-supported farms, farm-supported communities*. Kimberton, PA: Bio-Dynamic Farming and Gardening Association.

Kelvin, R. (1994). *Community-supported agriculture on the urban fringe: Case study and survey*. Emmaus, PA: Rodale Institute Research Center.

Kimball, Y., & Anderson, J. (1988). *The art of American Indian cooking*. New York: Lyons & Buford.

Naess, A. (1989). *Ecology, community, and lifestyle*. Cambridge: Cambridge University Press.

Peterson, L. A., & Peterson, R. T. (1977). *A field guide to edible wild plants*. Boston: Houghton Mifflin.

Pimentel, D. (1984). Energy inputs and U.S. food security. In L. Busch & W. B. Lacy (Eds.), *Food security in the United States* (pp. 99-114). Boulder, CO: Westview.

Sale, K. (1985). *Dwellers in the land: The bioregional vision*. San Francisco: Sierra Club Books.

Snyder, G. (1990). *The practice of the wild*. San Francisco: North Point Press.

Thrupp, L. A. (1989, May). Direct damage: DBCP poisoning in Costa Rica. *Dirty Dozen Compaigner, Pesticide Action Network*, pp. 1-2.

Worster, D. (1984). Thinking like a river. In W. Jackson, W. Berry, & B. Coleman (Eds.), *Meeting the expectations of the land*. San Francisco: North Point Press.

29 An Introduction to Permaculture

BILL MOLLISON

Permaculture is a design system for creating sustainable human environments. The word itself is a contraction not only of permanent agriculture but also of permanent culture, as cultures cannot survive for long without a sustainable agricultural base and land-use ethic. On one level, permaculture deals with plants, animals, buildings, and infrastructures (water, energy, communications). However, permaculture is not about these elements themselves but about the relationships we can create between them by the way we place them in the landscape.

The aim is to create systems that are ecologically sound and economically viable, which provide for their own needs, do not exploit or pollute, and are therefore sustainable in the long term. Permaculture uses the inherent qualities of plants and animals, combined with the natural characteristics of landscapes and structures, to produce a life-supporting system for city and country, using the smallest practical area.

Permaculture is based on the observation of natural systems, the wisdom contained in traditional farming systems, and modern scientific and technological knowledge. Although based on ecological modes, permaculture creates a *cultivated* ecology that is designed to produce more human and animal food than is generally found in nature.

Fukuoka (1978), in his book *The One Straw Revolution,* had perhaps best stated the basic philosophy of Permaculture. In brief, it is a philosophy of working with, rather than against nature; of protracted and thoughtful observation rather than protracted and thoughtless labor; and of looking at plants and animals in all their functions, rather than treating elements as a single-product system. I have spoken, on a more mundane level, of using aikido on the landscape, of rolling with the blows, turning adversity into strength, and using everything positively. The other approach is to karate the landscape, to try to make it yield by using strength and striking many hard blows. But if we attack nature, we attack (and ultimately destroy) ourselves.

Harmony with nature is possible only if we abandon the idea of superiority over the natural world. Levi-Strauss (1966) said that our profound error is that we have always looked upon ourselves as "masters of creation," in the sense of being above it. We are not superior to other life forms; all living things are an expression of life. If we could see that truth, we would see that everything we do to other life forms, we also do to ourselves. A culture that understands this does not, without absolute necessity, destroy any living thing.

We can exist on the Earth by using energy that is naturally in flux and relatively harmless and by using food and natural resources that are abundant in such a way that we don't continually destroy life on earth. Every technique for conserving and restoring the Earth is already known; what is not evident is that any nation or large group of people is prepared to make the change. However, millions of ordinary people are starting to do it themselves without help from political authorities.

THE PERMACULTURE INSTITUTE

The Permaculture Institute was established in 1981 to teach the practical design of sustainable land use and community development. In 1987, the institute acquired a five-acre property at Tyalgum, Australia, and it has since developed an extensive permaculture demonstration site. In addition to acting as a central information base for Permaculture groups and associations worldwide, it also provides hands-on experience for both Australian and overseas visitors who come to work and study in the research library.

Permaculture has had a profound influence on people worldwide, from ordinary farmers and suburban householders to government officials and teachers. There are currently projects in Zimbabwe, Botswana, South Africa, India, Nepal, Brazil, Ecuador, Mexico, and Micronesia. There are Permaculture groups and associations in many more countries. Permaculture has been at the vanguard of taking sustainable land-use training into the world's troubled regions and has been working for more than four years in Cuba, Palestine, and Cambodia. In

Vietnam, Permaculture trainers are working with the government farming organization to train 150,000 farmers in design techniques. We are currently holding discussions with the Rwandan government to organize courses for returning refugees.

BEGINNING WITH OURSELVES

Wherever we live, we should start to do something. We can start first by decreasing our energy consumption—you can actually live on 40 percent of the energy you are now using without sacrificing anything of value. We can refit our houses for energy efficiency. We can cut our vehicle use by using public transportation and sharing with friends. We can save water off our roofs into tanks, or recycle gray water to the toilet system or garden. We can also begin to take some part in food production. This doesn't mean that we all need to grow our own potatoes, but it may mean that we will buy them directly from a person who is already growing potatoes responsibly. In fact, one would probably do better to organize a farmer-purchasing group in the neighborhood than to grow potatoes.

In all permanent agricultures, or in sustainable human culture generally, the energy needs of the system are provide by that system. Modern crop agriculture is totally dependent on external energies. The shift from productive permanent systems (where the land is held in common) to annual commercial agricultures (where land is regarded as a commodity) involves a shift from a low- to a high-energy society, the use of land in an exploitive and destructive way, and a demand for external energy sources, mainly provided by the Third World as fuels, fertilizers, protein, labor, and skill.

Conventional farming does not recognize and pay its true costs: The land is mined of its fertility to produce annual grain and vegetable crops; nonrenewable resources are used to support yields; the land is eroded through overstocking of animals and extensive plowing; land and water are polluted with chemicals.

"Organic" agriculture is not enough on its own. You can farm organically, in the sense that you don't use persistent biocides or nitrates, and still erode your land and fail to serve your community. Organic agriculture does not necessarily relate components to each other; it takes no notice of the energy it uses. Organic farmers may build inappropriate houses, for example, that use up more energy than they produce in food. A fanatic organic farmer might have seaweed transported from thousands of miles away. Composting is the mainstay of most organic farming methods, yet composting wastes a lot of nutrients, time, and energy, as opposed to mulching, which wastes none of these. Organic agriculture looks at part of the system, and you can't look at only parts of the system and make the whole thing work.

What is most prized in modern agriculture is production, and it doesn't matter at what energy cost that production is achieved. It grows practically all of its soybeans to feed animals; fish are caught to be turned into powder and fed to pigs—to get one third of the protein of fresh fish. Beef agriculture has destroyed the world's drylands. Modern agriculture is now almost at the stage where it is so ridiculous, it should be a banned activity. And the world's largest agriculture is the European and American grass lawn. More resources are spent on maintaining these lawns than are spent on agriculture in the whole of Africa and India—more fossil fuels, fertilizer, even more manpower.

No more than 4 percent of the present agricultural landscape is needed to produce the food that people need. Once it was there to produce food for people; now it's there to produce money for large interests. With present-day agriculture, the Third World is made to feed the First World, the reverse of aid in its true sense.

When the needs of a system are not met from within the system, we pay the price in energy consumption and pollution. We can no longer afford the true cost of our agriculture. It is killing our world, and it will kill us.

All we need to live a good life lies about us, sitting at our doorsteps. Sun, wind, people, buildings, stones, sea, birds, and plants surround us. Cooperation with all these things brings harmony; opposition to them brings disaster and chaos.

REFERENCES

Fukuoka, M. (1978). *The one straw revolution: An introduction to natural farming.* Emmaus, PA: Rodale.

Levi-Strauss, C. (1966). *The savage mind* (2nd ed.). Chicago: University of Chicago Press.

30 Living the Good Life

HELEN NEARING

The majority of human beings, notably in industrial communities, dedicate their best hours and their best years to getting an income and exchanging it for the necessities and decencies of physical and social existence. Children, old people, the disabled, the sick, the voluntary parasitic are at least partially freed from livelihood preoccupations. Able-bodied adults have little choice. They must meet the demands of livelihood or pay a heavy penalty in social disapproval, insecurity, anxiety, and finally in physical hardship.

During the deepest part of the Great Depression, in 1932, my husband, Scot Nearing, and I moved from New York City to a farm in the Green Mountains of Vermont. At the outset we thought of the venture as a personal search for a simple, satisfying life on the land, to be devoted to mutual aid and harmlessness, with an ample margin of leisure in which to do personally constructive and creative work. With the passage of time and the accumulation of experience, we came to regard our valley in Vermont as a laboratory in which we were testing out certain principles and procedures of more general application and concern.

We left the city with three objectives in mind. The first was *economic*. We sought to make a depression-free living, as independent as possible of the commodity of labor markets, which could not be interfered with

---

AUTHOR'S NOTE: This chapter is excerpted from *Living the Good Life*, by Helen Nearing, copyright 1970 by Random House and reprinted by permission.

by employers, whether businesspeople, politicians, or educational administrators. Our second aim was *hygienic*. We wanted to maintain and improve our health. We knew that the pressures of city life were exacting, and we sought a simple basis of well-being where contact with the earth, and home-grown organic food, would play a large part. Our third objective was *social and ethical*. We desired to liberate and dissociate ourselves, as much as possible, from the cruder forms of exploitation: the plunder of the planet; the slavery of human and beast; the slaughter of men in war, and of animals for food.

We were against the accumulation of profit and unearned income by nonproducers, and we wanted to make our living with our own hands, yet with time and leisure for avocational pursuits. We wanted to replace regimentation and coercion with respect for life. Instead of exploitation, we wanted to use economy. Simplicity should take the place of multiplicity, complexity, and confusion. Instead of the hectic mad rush of busyness, we sought a quiet pace, with time to wonder, ponder, and observe. We hoped to replace worry, fear, and hate with serenity, purpose, and at-oneness.

Changing social conditions during the twenty years that began in 1910 cost us our professional status and deprived us of our means of livelihood. Whether we liked it or not, we were compelled to adjust to the new situation that war, revolution, and depression had forced upon the Western world. Our advancing age (we were approaching fifty) certainly played some part in shifting our viewpoint, but of far greater consequence were the world developments.

Beyond these social pressures, our choices were in our own hands, and their consequences would descend upon our own heads. We might have stayed on in the city, enduring and regretting what we regarded as essentially unsatisfactory living conditions, or we might strike out in some other direction, perhaps along a little-used path.

It would have been quite possible to live in the Vermont hills as one did in the suburbs of New York or Boston, by going frequently to market in nearby towns, buying to meet all one's needs in shops, using fruits and vegetables loaded with poisonous sprays and dusts and far removed from their production source, plus the processed and canned output of the food industry. Such a procedure was followed by several families in the valley, as long as they could afford it. Meanwhile, they paid the usual price in lowered vitality and ill health.

We were not at all pulled in this direction, partly because we believed in fresh, vital food, organically produced, and partly because our economy was planned on the assumption that we would produce and use everything possible, relying on cash spending for the smallest residue of goods and service procured outside the circle of our household establishment.

The basis of our consumer economy was the garden. By raising and using garden products, we were able to provide ourselves with around 80 percent of our food. Shelter, which ranks second to food in budget of the low-income household, we designed and constructed ourselves. For fuel we used wood, cut on the place. Some of our neighbors heated with oil, coal, gas, or electricity. We enjoyed work in the forest, which needed continual cleaning and weeding. And wood cut and used on the place necessitated no cash outlay but represented a direct return for our labor. Thoreau said of cutting one's own fuel: "It warms us twice, and the first warmth is the most wholesome and memorable, compared with which the other is mere coke. . . . The greatest value is received before the wood is teamed home."

Our Vermont economy provided food, shelter, and fuel, the big items among necessaries, mainly or entirely on a use basis. With rather wide limitations, we could have a supply of these things in direct proportion to the amount of labor time that we were willing to put into their production. Our purpose in going to Vermont, however, was not to multiply food, housing, fuel, and other necessaries, but to get only enough of these things to meet the requirements of a living standard that would maintain our physical efficiency and at the same time provide us with sufficient leisure to pursue our chosen avocations. Livelihood was no end in itself—rather, it was a vestibule into an abundant and rewarding life. Therefore, we produced the necessaries only to a point that would provide for efficiency. When we reached that point, we turned our attention and energies from bread labor to avocations or social pursuits.

Current practice in U.S. economy called upon those who had met their needs for necessaries to turn their attention forthwith to procuring comforts and conveniences, and after that to luxuries and superfluities. Only by such procedures could an economy based on profit accumulation hope to achieve the expansion needed to absorb additional profits and pay a return to those investing in the new industries.

Our practice was almost the exact opposite of the current one. Our consumer necessaries came mostly from the place, on a use basis. Comforts and conveniences came from outside the farm and had to be procured either by barter or through cash outlays. We bartered for some products—chiefly food that we could not raise in a New England climate. Cash outlay meant earning additional cash income. Consequently, we endeavored to do as Robert Louis Stevenson advised in his Christmas Sermon, "earn a little and spend a little less." Food from the garden and wood from the forest were the products of our own time and labor. We paid no rent. Taxes were reasonable. We bought no candy, pastries, meats, soft drinks, alcohol, tea, coffee, or tobacco. These seemingly minor items mount up and occupy a large place in the ordinary family's budget. We spent little on clothes and knickknacks. We lighted for fifteen years with kerosene and candles. We never had a television or radio. Most of our furniture was built-in and handmade. We did our trading in town no more than twice a month, and then our purchases were scanty.

"Civilization," said Mark Twain, "is a limitless multiplication of unnecessary necessaries." A market economy seeks by ballyhoo to bamboozle consumers into buying things they neither need nor want, thus compelling them to sell their labor power as a means of paying for their purchases. Because our aim was liberation from the exploitation accompanying the sale of labor power, we were as wary of market lures as a wise mouse is wary of other traps.

Readers may label such a policy as painfully austere, renunciatory, or bordering on deliberate self-punishment. We had no such feeling. Coming from New York City, with its extravagant displays of nonessentials and its extensive wastes of everything from food and capital goods to time and energy, we were surprised and delighted to find how much of the city clutter and waste we could toss overboard. We felt as free, in this respect, as a caged wild bird who finds himself once more on the wing. The demands and requirements that weigh upon city consumers no longer restricted us. To the extent that we were able to meet our consumer needs in our own way and in our own good time, we had freed ourselves from dependence upon the market economy.

Vermont life liberated us as consumers from the limitations, restrictions and compulsions of the city market. It had an even more profound effect on us as producers. A household economy based on a maximum of self-sufficiency gives the householder a maximum of responsibility.

Householders living under a use economy must provide their own goods and services, not only in sufficient amount, but at the proper time. Dwellers in a remote valley cannot send or phone to the corner grocery an hour before supper. They must plan and prepare during the previous season. If radishes are to be ready for the table on the first of June, they must be planted not later than the first week in May. If seeds are to yield the best results, the soil must be prepared before the planting day. Soil preparation with us necessitated compost. Compost piles, to be available in the spring, had to be set up by midsummer of the previous year. To enjoy fresh radishes on June 1, we began to get ready ten or twelve months in advance.

Similarly with the fuel supply. It is possible to burn green wood by putting it in the oven or under the stove and drying the outside fibers before the sticks go into the firebox. They will not burn really well, but neither will they put the fire out. Best results are obtained by splitting the wood in the open, leaving it in a heap until sun and wind have seared over the outside, then piling it in an open-sided woodshed for six months. This means, in practice, that the winter's wood supply should be under cover by the previous spring. If the wood can be cut one year in advance, put under cover, and burned the following year, so much the better.

Isolated self-contained households meet their needs for current repairs and upkeep as they meet the requirements for capital installation, by keeping on hand a modest supply of lumber, hardware, and simple tools and dealing with repairs and replacements at appropriate times. Such jobs, when completed, might not look professional, but they use the ingenuity and stretch the imagination of the householder and provide excellent training. After all is said and done, it is foolish and wasteful to let the professional building tradesman think out, plan, construct, and at the end of the job, thrill with the joy of work well done. "Shall we," asks Thoreau, "forever resign the pleasure of construction to the carpenter?"

Power age economy has substituted the specialized machine and the assembly line for the craftsman and has transformed many a skilled worker into a machine tender, with a resulting concentration, not upon excellence, but upon volume of product. The average city worker is asked to accept a wage or salary as a substitute for pride in workmanship and the satisfaction of mastery over tools and materials.

Our self-contained Vermont economy, with its dependence on our own productive efforts, reopened for us a great variety of competencies of which the average city dweller knows little. The most important group of these competencies was associated with the use of soil and the production and preparation of food. Building, equipping, and repairing dwelling units and making and repairing tools and implements presented us with a second sphere of productive functioning. Cutting logs and firewood and clearing woodland brought us into contact with forestry and its associated practices. In all of these fields we were compelled to think, plan, assemble materials and tools, and practice the techniques required to obtain the results we had in view.

City dwellers, accustomed to a wide variety of services, get to a point at which they believe that the essential questions of day-to-day living can be settled by arrangement, chiefly over a telephone. A customer with a ten-dollar bill can get wonderful results in a department store. But put the same person in the backwoods with a problem to be solved and an inadequate supply of materials and tools. There money is useless. Instead, ingenuity, skill, patience, and persistence are the coin current. The store customer who comes home with a package under his arm has learned nothing, except that a ten-dollar bill is a source of power in the marketplace. The man or woman who has converted materials into needed products via tools and skills has matured in the process. A telephone call and a charge account get results in a market center. Very different requirements are called into play in a household aiming at maximum self-sufficiency.

The school of hard knocks is merciless. One can argue with a storekeeper, a taxi driver, or even with a traffic officer. A square, a level, a bit of knotty pine, a badly mixed batch of concrete, a leaky pipe, or a short circuit are implacable. There they stand, pointing a finger of accusation at the careless or the ignorant or clumsy worker. If, under such conditions, one knows good work and wants it, there is only one thing to do—tear out the job and begin all over again.

Self-contained rural economies require a certain amount of cash with which to pay taxes, to buy hardware and tools, and in our case, to purchase clothing, which we never attempted to produce during our stay in Vermont. The city man who has learned to depend on a wage or salary feels a sense of uncertainty, bordering on terror, when he contemplates weeks, months, and years minus a paycheck. Where, he asks, is the money coming from? We felt a bit the same way when we plunged from the whirlpool of New York life into the tranquility of hills and forests. Money was the coin of the urban realm from which we came—the open sesame to the satisfaction of needs and wants. When we left the city, we felt we had left cash payment behind. When it reared its ugly head even in the Vermont wilderness, we kept it in its place and made it our business to see only that there was a surplus of receipts over expenditures. William Cooper, in his *Guide in the Wilderness,* said wisely, "It is not large funds that are wanted, but a constant supply, like a small stream that never dies. To have a great capital is not so necessary as to know how to manage a small one and never to be without a little."

Vermont life was "free" in the sense that it placed before the individual and the household a wide range of choices. There was no set pattern. The state of Vermont was scarcely in evidence. During the entire twenty years of our sojourn, we never saw a uniformed policeman pass along the dirt road in front of our house. Once a year, the town listers assessed the property, but their visits were brief and perfunctory. From day to day and year to year, we did as we pleased. Aside from our own thinking and direction, our lives need not have been planned or patterned.

There was a degree of neighborhood pressure toward social conformity. Otherwise we were our own masters as long as we paid our taxes and obeyed traffic laws on the state highways. The only management or discipline to which we were subject was self-imposed. In fact, the word *discipline* was in such disrepute among the families in the valley that its mention aroused sharp opposition.

With minor exceptions, every household group in the valley owned land, buildings, and tools in fee simple. Each household was, to that extent, economically self-contained. In a word, each household was a law unto itself and was based on a solid economic foundation—a piece of earth from which, in a pinch, it could dig its own livelihood. Only the tax collector, the truant officer, and the recruiting sergeant could break into the domestic castles. In extreme cases, the police, the sheriff, and the game warden could invade the premises, but only on complaint or suspicion of flagrant law violation. In such cases, law enforcement personnel went in groups and armed, as practically every rural Vermonter kept firearms and a stock of ammunition.

There is no positive force, in rural Vermont or in rural America, drawing communities together for well-defined social purposes. Churches, parent-teacher associations, farm unions, granges, farm bureaus, cooperatives, and improvement associations cover specified fields and perform particular functions. No one of these groups deals with general rural welfare, even to the extent that the service clubs in trading towns and small cities deal with general urban welfare.

Some may suggest that general welfare is the business of government, under the constitutions of Vermont and the United States. To a degree that is true, and the New England town meeting plays such a role in a restricted sense. Outside of New England and a few border states, however, the town meeting has not existed, and in New England, its functions have been sharply circumscribed by its infrequent, formal meetings and by the organization of rural life into sovereign households, each with its economic base in landownership and each with its arsenal prepared to defend its individualism to the death.

Atomism, separatism, and consequent isolation have increasingly played havoc with rural life in the United States, as the family has decreased in size while the household had shed some of its most essential functions. Meanwhile, rural mail routes, mail order houses, traveling markets, and salespeople have joined hands with rural telephone lines, rural electrification, school consolidation, radio and television, mass auto production, and roads to link the rural communities to urban markets and urban shopping and recreation centers. The resulting absence of group spirit and neighborhood discipline, the chaos and confusion of perpetual movement to and from work, to and from school, to and from the shows and the dances, has destroyed the remnants of rural solidarity and left a shattered, purposeless, functionless, ineffective, unworkable community.

Against this all-pervasive decline and dissolution of the fragile, tenuous structure of America's rural community life we attempted to make a stand in the Pikes Falls Valley in Vermont. Our chances of success were about equal to those of an alpine climber who throws himself against an avalanche.

Were we aware of this when we moved to Vermont in 1932? Certainly. We knew the social history of the United States; we had heard the issues discussed a hundred times. We did not know the details as we encountered them in our efforts to live among our neighbors and to build a local community in a disintegrating society. But had we known all and more, we would have persevered, because the value of doing something does not lie in the ease or difficulty, the probability or the improbability of its achievement, but in the vision, the plan, the determination, and the perseverance, the effort and the struggle that go into the project. Life is enriched by aspiration and effort, rather than by acquisition and accumulation. Knowing this and despite the odds against success, if we had to do it over again, we would—in all its social as well as economic aspects.

Index

About the Authors

Hunter "Patch" Adams is founder of the Gesundheit Institute in southern West Virginia and author of *Gesundheit* (1993).

Michael J. Balick is Director of the Institute of Economic Botany at The New York Botanical Garden in the Bronx, New York.

Philip Blackford is Executive Director of Canadian Outward Bound Wilderness Schools in Toronto, Ontario.

Dorothy Blair is Assistant Professor of Nutrition and of Science, Technology, and Society at Pennsylvania State University and copartner in Sycamore Gardens, an organic subscription farm.

Stephen Couchman is Director of Outward Bound's Centre for Change programs.

Jennifer Chesworth is a freelance writer and editor, organic gardener, and homeschooling mother residing in the Appalachian foothills of Ohio.

Mariana Chilton is a doctoral student in the Department of Folklore and Folklife at the University of Pennsylvania.

Robbie E. Davis-Floyd is a Research Fellow at the University of Texas at Austin and a cultural anthropologist specializing in medical and symbolic anthropology, gender studies, and futures research. She is author of *Birth as an American Rite of Passage* (1992) and coeditor of *Childbirth and Authoritative Knowledge: Cross-Cultural Perspectives* and *Cyberborg Babies: From Techno-Sex to Techno-Tots,* both forthcoming.

Strachan Donnelley is a philosopher and President of the Hastings Center in Briarcliff Manor, New York. He directs the Center's Ethics and Environmental Program.

James Duke is Executive Director of Herbal Vineyard, Inc., Fulton, Maryland, and Senior Scientific Adviser to Nature's Herbs, Spanish Forks, Utah. He served for thirty years as an economic botanist for the USDA and is the author of fifteen books on economic botany.

Michael W. Fox is Vice President of the farm animal protection and bioethics section of the Humane Society of the United States in Washington, D.C. He has written numerous articles about animal rights and the treatment of animals, including a weekly syndicated newspaper column. His book *Inhumane Society* was published in 1991.

Frank B. Golley is a Research Professor in the Institute of Ecology at the University of Georgia in Athens. His critically acclaimed *History of the Ecosystem Concept in Ecology* was published in 1993.

David J. Hufford is Professor of Humanities and Behavioral Science in the College of Medicine and Director of the Doctors' Kienle Center for Humanistic Medicine at Pennsylvania State University's Milton S. Hershey Medical Center in Hershey, Pennsylvania.

Ivan Illich is a historian and philosopher who currently holds positions at Pennsylvania State University and the University of Bremen (Germany). He is author of numerous books, including *Deschooling Society* (1971); *Tools for Conviviality* (1973); and *Medical Nemesis* (1976). *In the Vineyard of the Text* was published in 1993.

B. K. S. Iyengar developed the internationally practiced Iyengar Hatha Yoga method and is director of the Ramamani Iyengar Memorial Institute in Pune, India.

Jim Johnson is a certified personnel consultant with more than eighteen years of experience in providing technical services to both corporations and consumers. He has been a consultant to the computer industry since 1987 and is currently a columnist for three computer industry publications.

Judith H. Johnsrud is a specialist in the geography of nuclear energy. She was a legal representative of Citizens of Harrisburg in the original licensing of Three Mile Island. She is Director of the Environmental Coalition on Nuclear Power based in Pennsylvania and former chair of the National Solar Lobby and of the Sierra Club National Energy Committee.

Wayne B. Jonas is Director of the Office of Alternative Medicine at the U.S. National Institutes of Health and former director of the Medical Research Fellowship at the Walter Reed Army Institute of Research in Washington, D.C.

Dean Lerner is President of the B. K. S. Iyengar Yoga National Association of the United States. He is a senior Iyengar yoga instructor and a codirector of the Center for Well-Being in State College, Pennsylvania.

Marilyn Mardiros is Associate Professor of Nursing at the University of Ottawa. Her work focuses on primary health care, mental health, and health and anthropology.

Constance M. McCorkle helped pioneer the field of ethnoveterinary research and development as a member of the Department of Rural Sociology at the University of Missouri-Columbia. She is currently an independent consultant in agriculture, environmental management, and rural development, and is senior editor with World Bank and IIRR veterinary scientists of the 1996 volume *Ethnoveterinary Research & Development*.

Edna McHutchion is a registered nurse and chartered psychologist, as well as Associate Professor of Nursing at the University of Calgary and a director of the Canadian Palliative Care Association.

Carl Mitcham is Director of the Science, Technology, and Society Program at Pennsylvania State University. His *Philosophy and Technology* (1972, 1983) and *Bibliography of Philosophy and Technology* (1973, 1985) are standard works in the field. His most recent book is *Thinking Through Technology*.

Bill Mollison developed the philosophy and design concepts of permaculture, which focuses on positive ecological design for urban and rural properties. He is an honorary fellow of the Schumacher Society and, in 1993, was named an Outstanding Australian Achiever by the National Australian Day Council. In addition to his three-volume *Genealogies of Tasmanian Aborigines* (1968), he has written several definitive texts about permaculture philosophy and design. *Permaculture—A Designer's Manual* was published in 1988.

David Morris is cofounder of the Institute for Local Self-Reliance in Washington, D.C., and is now its vice-president. A specialist in community-based, environmentally benign economic development, he has been an adviser to business, government, and community organizations for more than 20 years and has written extensively on sustainability as it applies to communities.

Janice Morse is Professor of Nursing and Behvioral Science at Pennsylvania State University. She is also holds an honorary research associate at Massey University in New Zealand. In 1991, she was awarded the International Nursing Research Award from the American Nurses Association Council of Nurse Researchers. *The Illness Experience: Dimensions of Suffering* (with J. Johnson) was published in 1991.

Helen Nearing was the "grandmother" of the homesteading movement and director of the Good Life Institute in Harborside, Maine. She authored numerous books, including *Living the Good Life* (1970) with the late Scott Nearing, and *Simple Foods for the Good Life* (1994).

Phil Nuernberger is President of Mind Resource Technologies in Honesdale, Pennsylvania, and author of *The Quest for Personal Power* (1996), *Increasing Executive Productivity* (1992) and *Freedom From Stress* (1981), a best-selling standard work in psychology.

Robert N. Proctor is Professor of History at Pennsylvania State University. His books include *Racial Hygiene* (1988), *Value-Free Science?* (1991), and *Cancer Wars* (1995).

Janice Raymond is Professor of Women's Studies and Medical Ethics at the University of Massachusetts and author of *Women as Wombs: Reproductive Technologies and the Battle Over Women's Freedom* (1993).